Pocket Guide for Counseling the Nursing Mother

Debbie Shinskie, RN, IBCLC
Judith Lauwers, BA, IBCLC
Executive Director
Breastfeeding Support Consultants

JONES AND BARTLETT PUBLISHERS
Sudbury, Massachusetts
BOSTON   TORONTO   LONDON   SINGAPORE

World Headquarters	Jones and Bartlett Publishers Canada	Jones and Bartlett Publishers International
Jones and Bartlett Publishers 40 Tall Pine Drive Sudbury, MA 01776 978-443-5000 info@jbpub.com www.jbpub.com	2406 Nikanna Road Mississauga, ON L5C 2W6 CANADA	Barb House, Barb Mews London W6 7PA UK

Copyright © 2002 by Jones and Bartlett Publishers, Inc.

All rights reserved. No part of the material protected by this copyright notice may be reproduced or utilized in any form, electronic or mechanical, including photocopying, recording, or by any information storage and retrieval system, without written permission from the copyright owner.

Library of Congress Cataloging-in-Publication Data

Shinskie, Debbie.
  Pocket guide for counseling the nursing mother / Debbie Shinskie, Judi Lauwers.
    p. cm.
  Includes bibliographical references and index.
  ISBN 0-7637-1820-3 (alk. paper)
  1. Breast feeding--Handbooks, manuals, etc. 2. Lactation--Handbooks, manuals, etc. I. Title: Counseling the nursing mother. II. Lauwers, Judith, 1949- III. Shinskie, Debbie. Counseling the nursing mother. IV. Title.

RJ216.S463 2002
649'.33--dc21

2001038051

Production Credits
Acquisitions Editor: Penny M. Glynn
Associate Editor: Christine Tridente
Production Editor: Anne Spencer
Editorial Assistant: Thomas R. Prindle
Manufacturing Buyer: Amy Duddridge
Cover Design: Anne Spencer
Cover Image: Marcia Smith
Design and Composition: D&G Limited, LLC
Printing and Binding: Courier Stoughton

Printed in the United States of America.

05 04 03 02 01   10 9 8 7 6 5 4 3 2 1

Acknowledgments

The authors wish to express their gratitude to the following individuals for their roles in the preparation of this pocket guide:

Anne Spencer—Vice President of Design & Production (Production Editor)

Penny M. Glynn—Acquisitions Editor

Christine Tridente—Associate Editor

Amy Duddridge—Manufacturing Coordinator

Taryn Wahlquist—Associate Marketing Manager

Thomas Prindle—Editorial Assistant

Kelly D. Dobbs—Project Manager

Jan Lynn—Copy Editor

Claudia Bell—Designer and Layout Technician

Terrie Edwards and Donna Martin—Proofreaders

Chris Mulford, Kathy Romberger, Pat Houck, and Ruth Solomon—Reviewers

Sandra Breck—Research Consultant for *Counseling the Nursing Mother*, 3rd Edition

Jan Barger, Linda Kutner, and Carole Peterson—Contributing Authors for *Counseling the Nursing Mother*, 3rd Edition

Contents

1	Breastfeeding Promotion in the Modern World	1
2	The Lactation Consulting Profession	10
3	Empowering Women through Your Attitude and Approach	15
4	Counseling: Learning to Help Mothers	20
5	Client Consultations	27
6	The Science of Lactation	46
7	Maternal Health and Nutrition	72
8	Properties of Human Milk	93
9	Prenatal Considerations	126
10	Hospital Practices that Support Breastfeeding	139
11	Infant Assessment and Behavior	161
12	Getting Breastfeeding Started	196
13	Infant Attachment and Suckling	210
14	Breastfeeding Issues in the Early Weeks	230
15	Breastfeeding Beyond the First Month	259
16	Problems with Milk Production and Transfer	272
17	Changes in the Family	286
18	Special Counseling Circumstances	298
19	Breastfeeding Techniques and Devices	314
20	Temporary Breastfeeding Situations	345

21	High-Risk Infants	362
22	When Breastfeeding is Interrupted	373
23	Mothers and Babies with Long-Term Special Needs	383
24	Professional Considerations	411

Appendix A	417
Appendix B	426
Index	435

Special Subjects
Table of Contents

Periodically throughout this text, you will observe a tab at the top of a page, similar to the one above. This tab has been designed for easy referencing of content frequently used in clinical practice, as outlined below.

Anatomy	46
Weight Gain	183
Positioning	197
Latch-On	198
Sleepy Baby	206
Baby Resisting Breastfeeding	207
Sucking	211
Principles of a Good Latch	216
Frequency and Duration of Feeds	231
Nipple Soreness	235
Yeast	244
Engorgement	247
Mastitis	249
Plugged Duct	256
Slow Weight Gain and Poor Weight Gain	274
Failure to Thrive	276
Lactational Amenorrhea Method	292
Milk Expression	325
Alternate Feeding Methods	334
Jaundice	345
Relactation	354

Breastfeeding Promotion in the Modern World

Current Breastfeeding Recommendations

- Breastfeed exclusively for six months and continue breastfeeding with appropriate complementary food through twelve months and beyond
- Follow the Ten Steps to Successful Breastfeeding
- Exclusively breastfed infants
  - Receive no drinks or foods other than mothers' milk
  - May receive vitamin and mineral drops or medicines
  - Should not be given pacifiers or artificial nipples
  - Are fed in response to feeding cues, without limits on frequency or length of breastfeedings
  - Receive at least eight to twelve breastfeedings in 24 hours (including night feeds)

THE TEN STEPS TO SUCCESSFUL BREASTFEEDING

Every facility providing maternity services and care for newborn infants should

1. Have a written breastfeeding policy that is routinely communicated to all health care staff.
2. Train all health care staff in skills necessary to implement this policy.
3. Inform all pregnant women about benefits and management of breastfeeding.
4. Help mothers initiate breastfeeding within a half hour of birth.
5. Show mothers how to breastfeed and how to maintain lactation even if they should be separated from their infants.
6. Give newborn infants no food or drink other than breastmilk unless medically indicated.
7. Practice rooming in—allow mothers and infants to remain together—24 hours a day.
8. Encourage breastfeeding in response to feeding cues.
9. Give no artificial teats or pacifiers (also called dummies or soothers) to breastfeeding infants.
10. Foster the establishment of breastfeeding support groups and refer mothers to them on discharge from the hospital or clinic.

THE WORLD HEALTH ORGANIZATION'S INFANT FEEDING RECOMMENDATION

The scientific evidence: The optimal duration of *exclusive breastfeeding* and thus the optimal timing of when *complementary feeding* should begin—is an important public health issue that WHO keeps under continual review. Consistent with available scientific and epidemiological evidence, WHO's current recommendation is

> *Infants should be exclusively breastfed for the first 4 to 6 months of life. Thereafter, to meet their evolving nutritional requirements, infants should begin to receive nutritionally adequate and safe complementary foods while breastfeeding continues for up to 2 years of age or beyond.*[1]

In 1995, WHO published the report of the WHO Expert Committee on Physical Status;[2] this included a meticulous review of available scientific evidence, including the organization's own research, on the influence of exclusive and nonexclusive breastfeeding patterns on the growth of infants and children in a number of countries in disparate regions. The evidence showed that in predominantly breastfed infants, weight and growth velocity begin to fall at 3 months of age when judged against the current NCHS/WHO reference.[3] In contrast, weight and

---

[1] The World Health Organization's infant-feeding recommendation. *Weekly Epidemiological record.* 1995, 70:119–120; WHO's infant-feeding recommendation: http://www.who.int/nut/.

[2] *Expert Committee on Physical Status: The Use and Interpretation of Anthropometry.* World Health Organization. 1995, WHO Technical Report Series, No. 854.

[3] Ibid., p. 238. The current WHO/National Center for Health Statistics (Washington, D.C.) reference reflects the growth of children who were fed primarily with infant formula and who were of restricted genetic, geographic, and socioeconomic background. The Expert committee concluded that the combined effect of these limitations so seriously flaws the present international reference on both technical and biological grounds as to interfere with the sound health and nutritional management of individual infants and young children, and provides inaccurate community estimates of over and under nutrition.

growth velocity begin to fall at about 5 months of age when judged against a trial breastfed growth reference.[4] This suggested that whatever the underlying cause (e.g., inadequate nutrient supply, infection) nutrient intake in predominantly breastfed infants may become insufficient to meet their normal growth requirements from about 5 months of age (or even earlier, depending on the growth reference used). It was also clear that there was considerable variation in the age at which this insufficiency occurred.

On this basis the WHO Expert Committee and its Working Group on Infant Growth:

- Reconfirmed the suitability of WHO's current recommended timing of the introduction of complementary foods—that is, four to six months of age
- Urged that a new growth reference be developed based on breastfed infants who are living under conditions that favour achievement of genetic growth potential.

Given the worldwide variation in growth velocity and other health and development outcomes, an *age range* is an essential element of WHO's population-based infant feeding recommendation.

---

[4]Ibid., pp. 236–237. This conclusion was based on analysis of pooled data concerning infants predominantly breastfed for at least four months and partially breastfed for at least twelve months, from seven North American and European studies; deprived communities in India and Peru; seven centers in five countries (the WHO/HRP data set from Chile, Egypt, Hungary, Kenya and Thailand); and formula-fed infants in affluent populations. For additional detail in this regard, see *WHO Working Group on Infant Growth. An evaluation of infant growth* (document WHO/NUT/94.8). World Health Organization, Geneva: 1994.

INNOCENTI DECLARATION

Recognising that breastfeeding is a unique process that:

- Provides ideal nutrition for infants and contributes to their healthy growth and development
- Reduces incidence and severity of infectious diseases, thereby lowering infant morbidity and mortality
- Contributes to women's health by reducing the risk of breast and ovarian cancer, and by increasing the spacing between pregnancies
- Provides social and economic benefits to the family and the nation
- Provides most women with a sense of satisfaction when successfully carried out

and that recent research has found that:

- These benefits increase with increased exclusiveness of breastfeeding during the first six months of life, and thereafter with increased duration of breastfeeding with complementary foods, and
- programme intervention can result in positive changes in breastfeeding behavior.

We therefore declare that:

As a global goal for optimal maternal and child health and nutrition, all women should be enabled to practise exclusive breastfeeding and all infants should be fed exclusively on breastmilk from birth to four to six months of age. Thereafter, children should continue to be breastfed, while receiving appropriate and adequate complementary foods for up to two years of age or beyond. This child-feeding ideal is to be achieved by creating an appropriate environment of awareness and support so that women can breastfeed in this manner.

Attainment of this goal requires, in many countries, the reinforcement of a "breastfeeding culture" and its vigorous defence against incursions of a "bottle-feeding culture." This requires commitment and advocacy for social mobilization, utilizing to the full the prestige and authority of acknowledged leaders of society in all walks of life.

Efforts should be made to increase women's confidence in their ability to breastfeed. Such empowerment involves the removal of constraints and influences that manipulate perceptions and behaviour towards breastfeeding, often by subtle and indirect means. This requires sensitivity, continued vigilance, and a responsive and comprehensive communications strategy involving all media and addressed to all levels of society. Furthermore, obstacles to breastfeeding within the health system, the workplace, and the community must be eliminated.

Measures should be taken to ensure that women are adequately nourished for their optimal health and that of their families. Furthermore, ensuring that all women also have access to family planning information and services allows them to sustain breastfeeding and avoid shortened birth intervals that may compromise their health and nutritional status, and that of their children.

All governments should develop national breastfeeding policies and set appropriate national targets for the 1990s. They should establish a national system for monitoring the attainment of their targets, and they should develop indicators such as the prevalence of exclusively breastfed infants at discharge from maternity services, and the prevalence of exclusively breastfed infants at four months of age.

National authorities are further urged to integrate their breastfeeding policies into their overall health and development policies. In so doing they should reinforce all actions that protect, promote, and support breastfeeding within complementary programmes such as prenatal and perinatal care, nutrition, family planning services, and prevention and treatment of common maternal and childhood diseases. All health care staff should be trained in the skills necessary to implement these breastfeeding policies.

Operational Targets
All governments by the year 1995 should have:

- Appointed a national breastfeeding coordinator of appropriate authority, and established a multisectoral national breastfeeding committee composed of representatives from relevant government departments, non-governmental organizations, and health professional associations
- Ensured that every facility providing maternity services fully practises all ten of the *Ten Steps to Successful Breastfeeding* set out in the joint WHO/UNICEF statement "Protecting, promoting and supporting breastfeeding: the special role of maternity services"
- Taken action to give effect to the principles and aim of all the Articles of the International Code of Marketing of Breast-Milk Substitutes and subsequent relevant World Health Assembly resolutions in their entirety; and
- Enacted imaginative legislation protecting the breastfeeding rights of working women and established means for its enforcement

We also call upon international organizations to:

- Draw up action strategies for protecting, promoting, and supporting breastfeeding, including global monitoring and evaluation of their strategies
- Support national situation analyses and surveys and the development of national goals and targets for action; and
- Encourage and support national authorities in planning, implementing, monitoring, and evaluating their breastfeeding policies

The Innocenti Declaration was produced and adopted by participants at the WHO/UNICEF policymakers' meeting on "Breastfeeding in the 1990s: A Global Initiative, co-sponsored by the United States Agency for International Development (AID) and the Swedish International Development Authority (SIDA), held at the Spedale degli Innocenti, Florence, Italy, on 30 July - 1 August 1990. The Declaration reflects the content of the original background document for the meeting and the views expressed in group and plenary sessions.

A SUMMARY OF THE AMERICAN ACADEMY OF PEDIATRIC'S 1997 BREASTFEEDING RECOMMENDATIONS

1. Human milk is the recommended food for all infants with only rare exceptions. Optimally it is obtained by direct breastfeeding. If the infant is unable to breastfeed, expressed milk is the next choice and is fortified if necessary for the premature infant.
2. Breastfeeding should begin as soon as possible after birth, with the infant remaining with the mother throughout her recovery.
3. Newborns should be nursed when they exhibit early hunger cues, approximately eight to twelve times every 24 hours. If four hours have passed since the last feeding, infants should be aroused to nurse.
4. Rooming-in provides the optimal climate for a mother's attention to feeding cues and for offering frequent feedings.
5. Evaluation and documentation of breastfeedings should take place within the first 24 to 48 hours after delivery and again two to three days after hospital discharge.

6. Mothers are encouraged to keep a diary of feedings, voids, and stools in the early days.
7. Supplements for newborns are not recommended unless there is a medical indication.
8. Pacifiers are not encouraged.
9. If hospital discharge occurs before 48 hours after birth, all breastfeeding mothers and infants are to be seen between Day Two and Four after birth. All infants are to be seen by one month of age.
10. Exclusive breastfeeding is encouraged for the first six months of life. Breastfeeding is recommended to continue for at least 12 months and beyond as long as mother and infant desire to nurse.
11. Vitamin D, iron, and/or fluoride supplements may be necessary.
12. In the case of hospitalization of either the mother or the infant, breastfeeding is to be continued either directly or via milk expression.

2

The Lactation Consulting Profession

Functioning as a Lactation Consultant

Role in the Profession
- Become an International Board Certified Lactation Consultant (IBCLC)
- Must be an advocate first for the nursing dyad and secondly for the infant
- Have the knowledge, skills, and willingness to work at the baby's pace
- Suggest alternate care plans when what is prescribed by other members of a health care team could impact negatively on breastfeeding
- Keep knowledge current by reading relevant research and literature from all disciplines
- Share information and work collaboratively with physicians and other health care providers
  - Inform physicians of your services and help them understand your intentions
  - Provide evidence-based breastfeeding materials
  - Encourage mothers to share the positive aspects of breastfeeding with their physicians
  - Help physicians recognize a mother's need to be supported and validated
  - Encourage physician referral to support groups

Role with Mothers

- Promote health consumerism
- Provide options and advice
- Suggest ways in which they can interact with their physicians
- Coordinate their breastfeeding care
- Empower them to breastfeed with minimal intervention or complications
- Educate and gently guide them

Services to Mothers

- Prenatal and postpartum classes
- Daily rounds to all postpartum breastfeeding mothers
- Assistance with breastfeeding problems before and after their discharge
- Routine long-term follow-up
- Telephone warm line for counseling new mothers
- Periodic development or review of parent literature
- Referral to a peer support group
- Teaching of breastfeeding management
- Keeping up to date with new breastfeeding literature and practices
- Sharing of medical information

Practice Settings for International Board Certified Lactation Consultants (IBCLCs)

IBCLCs perform several duties in the following environments:

Hospital

- Observe a baby breastfeed before discharge
- Train staff in breastfeeding management
- Serve as a resource for hospital staff

- Develop breastfeeding policies, procedures, and documentation
- Develop handouts and reading materials for mothers
- Refer mothers to support groups and, when necessary, to another IBCLC or other health care professional
- Assist mothers in obtaining breastfeeding devices, and teach mothers how to use them
- Provide classes about infant feeding

Special Supplemental Food Program for Women, Infants, and Children (WIC) Clinic

- Breastfeeding women are favored in the WIC priority system
- Required to fund breastfeeding promotion and support
- Services of the IBCLC
  - Counsel mothers and work with other staff
  - Teach breastfeeding classes and facilitate support groups
  - Develop promotion and nutrition programs on breastfeeding
  - Participate in breastfeeding workshops, consortiums, and committees
  - Establish a system of networking for breastfeeding resources
  - Provide breastfeeding in-service programs
  - Supervise and train peer counselors
  - Develop and evaluate breastfeeding materials for clients

Physician Group

- Care for healthy normal babies and those experiencing difficulties
- Mostly a preventive practice rather than crisis management
- Services of the IBCLC
  - Teach breastfeeding classes

- Meet with pregnant women at least once
- Make rounds in the hospital to check on breastfeeding mothers
- Provide a series of follow-up telephone calls
- Provide a warm line for breastfeeding mothers
- Serve as the resource person to physicians and their staff
- Maintain supplies of breastfeeding products and literature
- Record breastfeeding statistics
- Facilitate a postpartum support group for mothers in the practice
- Make recommendations on treatments that impact breastfeeding

Home Health Care

- Provide follow-up to mothers and babies after their hospital discharge
- Receive referral from maternity discharge planners
- Average length of a lactation visit is 90 minutes
- First visit
  - Perform a breastfeeding assessment
  - Observe a breastfeed
  - Complete an assessment of the mother and infant if a qualified nurse
- Second visit (around Day Five or Six)
  - Assess the mother and baby
  - Perform a breast exam
  - Note that the baby should have at least six wet diapers and four stools per 24 hours
  - Baby's weight loss must be stabile and less than seven percent of birth weight

Private Practice

- Seasoned IBCLC with wide experience
- Customary to have, credentials beyond IBCLC (for instance, RN, MD, or RD)
- Small business that does its own marketing, billing, and fee collection

- Acquire referrals from past clients, physicians, hospitals, and telephone listings
- Be available to clients at established times, with coverage when unavailable
- Document consultations and complete reports to a client's physician
- Retain copies of all records for at least seven years
- Provide a client with insurance reimbursement forms
- Provide breast pumps and other devices for rental or sale

Relationship of Lactation Consultant and Peer Counselor

- Maintain a reciprocal referral system
- Train other counselors in counseling skills and breastfeeding information
- Serve as an advisor to a support group
- Co-sponsor and help organize outreach programs
- Speak at parent and counselor meetings
- Serve as a liaison between a support group and the medical community
- Review the written materials for educating counselors and parents

3

Empowering Women through Your Attitude and Approach

Health Consumerism

Role of the IBCLC
The IBCLC has an integral role in encouraging parents to become active health consumers for themselves and their baby.

- Encourage parents to take responsibility for their own actions
- Do not suggest parents change providers
- Educate mothers about breastfeeding through reading, conversations, classes, and meetings
- Emphasize that the mother knows her baby best
- Help her become attuned to her baby's behavior
- Help her understand her baby's needs
- Help mothers understand the difference between parenting issues and medical advice
- Present facts to help parents find options suiting their needs and goals

CONSUMER RIGHTS AND RESPONSIBILITIES

The mother has the right to

- Understand what she is giving consent to
- Receive information concerning a drug or treatment prior to its administration
- Know alternative methods
- Accept or refuse treatment or advice without pressure
- Know if a procedure is medically indicated or elective
- Have access to her complete medical records
- Seek another medical opinion
- Be kept informed of up-to-date information
- Be treated as an equal partner in her health care
- Have questions answered completely and courteously
- Be treated with respect
- Be provided with the best care possible, with a focus on prevention
- Make decisions regarding her own treatment and that of her infant
- Care for herself and her infant to the maximum extent of her ability

The mother has the responsibility to

- Find out what is available and to make informed choices
- Find caregivers who can help her reach her goals
- Listen to caregivers with an open mind
- Let her preferences be known in a courteous manner
- Carry through on a care plan
- Find out the approximate cost of a procedure in advance
- State why she changes caregivers, if applicable

Using an Adult Learning Approach

Approach Is One of Learning Rather Than Being Taught

The IBCLC's role in teaching adults includes
- Serving as a facilitator
- Developing a partnership with the mother and baby to form a problem-solving team
- Creating an effective learning climate
- Individualizing your approach to each dyad

The Learning Process

- Learning takes place at three levels
  - Tell me and I may remember
  - Show me and I may understand
  - Involve me and I may master
- Correspond to each mother's learning style

Humor as a Communication Tool

- Helps to develop relationships in which mothers will comply with the care plan
- The following are the health benefits of humor:
  - Causes a therapeutic biochemical change in the body
  - Speeds up heart rate, raises blood pressure, accelerates breathing, and increases oxygen consumption
  - Stimulates muscles and relaxes muscle tension, thereby reducing pain and anxiety
  - Stimulates the cardiovascular system, sympathetic nervous system, and production of catecholamines and endorphins, thus boosting the immune system

- Increases adrenaline in the brain, which stimulates alertness and memory, and enhances learning and creativity
- Returns respiration, heart rate, and muscle tension to below normal levels after an arousal state
- Humor enhances learning in the following ways:
  - Reduces tension and anxiety
  - Helps stimulate divergent thinking
  - Frees the flow of ideas
  - Stimulates both the right and left hemispheres of the brain
  - Increases the mother's ability to take risks
  - Enables the mother to feel more comfortable and more welcome to ask questions and offer input
  - Helps a mother to remember things better and longer

Components of Communication

The Spoken Word Is Seven Percent of the Message
- Avoid words and phrases that create doubt or undermine a mother's confidence
- Avoid sending mixed messages
- Supplement your verbal messages with demonstrations, visual aids, and written instructions

Voice Tone Is Thirty-Eight Percent of the Message
- Create a warm, friendly, and humorous atmosphere with voice tone
- Make sure your voice tone matches the message that you want to send
- Evaluate your voice's volume, rate, breathing, and pitch

Body Language Is Fifty-Five Percent of the Message

- Smiles add to a warm and inviting atmosphere
- Eye contact conveys a desire to communicate
- Posture conveys your interest or disinterest
- Body position conveys power or submission
- Touch can convey warmth, caring, and encouragement
- Cultural differences dictate appropriate body language
- Reading a mother's body language will help you to gather your impressions

4

Counseling: Learning to Help Mothers

Understanding the Counseling Process

Counseling Skills Enable You to Meet a Mother's Needs

Appropriate counseling skills will provide mothers with emotional support, physical comfort, and understanding; and enable them to take positive action.

- Emotional support
  - Validate her feelings, emotions, and concerns
  - Hear what she is saying as well as what she is not saying
  - Skills—attending, active listening, empathetic listening, reassuring, praising, and building hope
- Immediate physical comfort
  - First offer emotional support
  - Make suggestions to help her feel better physically
  - Define the problem and suggest actions
- Mother's understanding
  - Help her to understand herself and her feelings
  - Help her to define and understand a problem clearly
  - Help her to understand her options in resolving a problem

- Skills—listening, influencing, facilitating, informing, and problem solving
- Positive action
  - The goal of counseling is the mother's satisfaction and self-sufficiency
  - Initiate positive action through problem-solving, decision-making, and by developing plans together with the mother

Using Counseling Methods and Skills

Guiding Method

This counseling method is used to offer emotional support with limited direction through listening, questioning, and making supportive statements.

- Three forms of listening
  - Attending (passive listening)
    - Minimizes your tendency to intervene unnecessarily
    - Pausing and waiting for the mother to fill a silence enables her to take a more active role
  - Active listening (reflective listening)
    - Clarifies information, shows acceptance, and encourages a mother's response
    - Paraphrases what was said and reflects the message back to the mother
    - Mother's response lets you know if you understood correctly
  - Empathetic listening
    - Involves listening with your ears, eyes, and heart—tuning in to feelings, meanings, and behaviors being conveyed
    - Rephrases the content and feeling
- Facilitating
  - Directs the conversation to help pinpoint issues and feelings
  - Encourages a mother to provide more information and define the situation better

- Clarifying information
  - Admits your confusion and restates what you heard
  - Skills—active listening, asking open-ended questions, and interpreting information
- Open-ended questions
  - Begin with "who," "what," "when," "where," "why," "how," "how much," and "how often"
  - Balance your questions with other guiding skills
- Interpreting
  - Analysis containing your own thoughts and feelings
  - Draws together several statements
  - Adds your tentative conclusions to interpret what was said
  - Leaves the door open for the mother to process what you have said and to correct any misinterpreted message
  - Use when you have a clear impression of the stated information and when the mother needs help sorting out her feelings
- Focusing
  - Emphasizes a topic you think would be helpful to explore
  - Brings the mother back to important points
  - Pursues one aspect you feel could be useful
- Summarizing information
  - Go over highlights of the conversation to reinforce important aspects
  - Urge the mother to do the summarizing to demonstrate her understanding
- Influencing a mother
  - Gives reassurance to help the mother see a situation is normal
  - Be careful not to give the impression you are minimizing the importance of her feelings or concerns

- Builds hope to help in long-term conditions (for example, persistent sore nipples, fussy baby, unsupportive family, returning to work)
- Identifies strengths to help the mother focus on positive qualities
- See Table 4.1 for an example of guiding skills

Leading Method

This method places more responsibility for the direction of the discussion on you rather than the mother.

- Informing (educating)
  - Begins only after you have gathered enough information so your leads are not premature or incorrect
  - Communicates a problem or concern the mother is unable to solve
  - Corrects any misconception or mismanagement
  - Explains how something functions and the reasons behind it
  - Allows enough time to begin to explore concerns and to determine what a mother needs to know
  - Provides additional resources to lead the mother toward a solution
  - Suggests appropriate reading materials
  - Capitalizes on a teachable moment
  - Limits the amount of information at one time
- Problem solving
  - Facilitates the understanding of a problem and enables you and the mother to develop a plan of action
  - Leaves the decision to the mother in order to develop her self-sufficiency
  - See Chapter 5, "Client Consultations," for utilization of a problem-solving approach

TABLE 4.1 EXAMPLE OF EFFECTIVE USE OF GUIDING METHOD SKILLS

A pregnant woman says, "I'm afraid that breastfeeding might make my child too dependent."

Listening Responses	• Attending • Active listening • Empathetic listening	Hmmm, you do . . . . . You worry that breastfeeding will make your child too dependent on you. You want your baby to grow into an independent child and you are not sure whether breastfeeding will make that possible.
Facilitating Responses	• Clarifying • Interpreting • Asking open-ended questions • Focusing • Summarizing	Could you explain what you mean by 'too dependent'? You believe the close breastfeeding relationship will keep your child from exploring his world. In what ways do you think breastfeeding will make your child too dependent? Let's get back to your concerns about . . . (This would be used later if it becomes necessary to focus on the mother's primary concern.) We talked about . . . . (Repeat the main points of this topic.)
Influencing Responses	• Reassuring • Building hope • Identifying strengths	Being a parent can be confusing. Many bottle-feeding mothers also wonder how the attention they give their infant relates to the child's later independence. You know, research has actually shown otherwise. Babies given more attention and physical contact in the early years grow up to be more independent. It's great that you are concerned about your baby's independence. How do you feel you can encourage your baby to become independent?

Follow-Up Method
- Evaluate the session
- Research outside sources if necessary
- Arrange the next contact
  - Determine when the next contact needs to occur, if any
  - Contact through a telephone or an in-person visit
  - Make sure that the mother understands she may call you or another caregiver before the prearranged time
  - Establish who will initiate contact and what additional information or assistance you will provide

Questions for Evaluating a Counseling Contact
- What support did I give? In what other ways could I have supported the mother?
- Did the mother require immediate physical comfort? If so, what suggestions did I offer?
- Did I gather enough information so we both understood the problem? If not, what further information do I need?
- Did I provide appropriate information? Did the mother understand it? If not, what information do I need to provide to the mother during the next contact?
- Did the mother seem relaxed and talkative? If not, what skills can I use in a new approach during the next contact in order to encourage her to talk freely?
- What plan did the mother and I make? Is it workable? If not, what alternative actions could I suggest?
- Did the mother seem satisfied with the contact? If not, what areas should I explore in future contacts?
- What follow-up did the mother and I arrange? Is it adequate, or should I contact the mother sooner?

- Did I take usable notes during or after the contact? How were the notes from previous contacts with this mother helpful? How can I improve my documentation method?
- Did I form a partnership with this mother and empower her to be self-sufficient in her problem solving?
- Am I satisfied in my helping role with this mother? If not, what can I do to bring about greater satisfaction?

5

Client Consultations

Reaching Out through Anticipatory Guidance

- Provides an experienced support person
- Gives practical and timely information
- Supplies the mother with the self confidence to anticipate her own needs
- More effective than crisis intervention

Crisis Intervention

- Occurs after a problem has already been encountered
- Additional time spent problem solving negates time saved by not providing anticipatory guidance
- Ends in less positive results for the mother

Providing Anticipatory Guidance

- Requires more time in the early stages of breastfeeding
- Guides the mother one step at a time through breastfeeding
- Teaches the mother well in advance of critical periods
- The frequency of contact subsides after the first few weeks
- May be practical to use a hot line or warm line in some settings
- Be sensitive to the mother's cues that your contacts may be too frequent

Using a Problem-Solving Approach

Working Toward a Solution
- Step 1. Form your first hunch
  - Ask the mother what she thinks is the cause of the problem, and what she has tried to solve it
  - Form a hunch about the cause and possible solution to the problem
- Step 2. Look for hidden factors
  - Explore other factors that may contribute to the problem
  - Guiding skills are essential to this process
- Step 3. Test your hunch
  - Continually evaluate your hunch
  - Hidden factors and lack of information may obscure a problem
  - To test your hunch, use interpreting, focusing, and summarizing
  - If your hunch is correct, develop a plan of action with the mother
- Step 4. Explore alternative hunches
  - If your initial hunch is wrong, pursue other hunches
  - If your hunch is ill-defined throughout several contacts with the mother, develop a trial plan
  - Network with other IBCLCs
- Step 5. Develop a plan
  - You and the mother should come up with alternatives that fit the mother's situation and are specific to the problem
  - Set a time limit on the actions that are to be taken by the mother
  - The mother's reception of facts and hints will indicate whether she feels they will help her
  - Plan only two or three actions for a mother
  - Have the mother summarize the plan to show that she understands it
  - Follow up with the mother to learn if the plan worked

Situations When You Must See the Mother

- Sore nipples
- Severe engorgement
- Latch-on problems or incorrect positioning
- Poor weight gain of the baby
- Use of an electric breast pump by the mother
- Mother seems shy or nontalkative, or if you sense she has difficulty relating concerns to you in a telephone conversation
- Any time you feel uneasy about the situation or are unable to obtain sufficient information during telephone contact

Elements in a Consultation

Obtain Signed Consent

- To work with the mother and infant at this and all subsequent visits (see Chapter 24, "Professional Considerations")
  - To touch the mother's breasts or nipples for the purpose of assessment
  - To examine the infant, which includes a digital oral examination
  - To observe a breastfeed
  - To demonstrate or use any necessary equipment and techniques
- To release information to an insurance company
- To send reports to the primary physicians of the mother and infant, and to consult with them regarding their care
- To use the information obtained from a consult for educational purposes, which includes taking pictures
- To receive payment for your services and rental of equipment

Gather Information and Impressions through Guiding Skills and a History

- Mother's economic and employment status
- Mother's support network and its cultural beliefs and practices
- Mother's breastfeeding goals
- Health of the mother and infant, both past and present
- Mother's perception of the present problem and when it began
- Previous breastfeeding experience
- Medications taken by the mother and baby, both past and present
- Mother's diet, which includes the amount of fluids consumed daily
- Present situation and what the mother has tried in attempting to alleviate the problem
- Infant's feeding and growth patterns
  - Sleeping
  - Crying
  - Ability to socialize
  - Producing stools and voids (estimation of amounts in the last 24-hour period)
  - Any change in these patterns and, if so, when that change occurred

Perform a Physical Assessment of Mother and Infant

- Infant (see Chapter 11, "Infant Assessment and Behavior")
  - Daily weight status
  - Baby's intake and output
  - Signs of hydration
  - Caloric status
  - General health
- Mother's breasts and nipples

Assess a Feed
- Move at the baby's pace
- Help the mother into a comfortable position
  - Ask her to nurse and show what the baby does at the breast
  - Offer no suggestions or interventions until you have a clear picture of what is happening
  - If problems are perceived, suggest alternative methods or interventions
- Factors to consider when doing a feeding assessment:
  - Interactions between the mother and infant
  - Dynamics of the feeding process
  - Infant's oral and facial structure
  - Temperaments, behaviors, and emotional statuses of the mother and infant
  - Appearance and condition of the mother's breasts and nipples
  - Evidence of milk transfer

Develop a Plan with the Mother
- Determine what a mother needs to know
- Initially limit the plan to the essentials:
  - Feeding the baby
  - Pain relief
  - Maintaining or increasing milk production
- Help the mother understand what produced the situation and how she can avoid a recurrence
- Brainstorm options, and be mindful of the mother's reactions to your suggestions
- Encourage a mother to decide what will work for her
- State the care plan and ask the mother to repeat it
- Summarize with her if necessary to avoid any confusion
- If present, include the baby's father in developing a care plan
- Arrange for a follow-up visit

Document the Consultation
- Document all aspects of the consultation as appropriate for your setting
- Write a *physician report* if you are an IBCLC in private practice (see Figure 5.1)
  - Use professional letterhead
  - Address the report to the physicians for both the mother and baby unless only one is needed
  - Send the report within 24 hours of visiting with a client

Evaluate the Consultation

- Evaluate the mother frequently, as a change in situation may require a change in the care plan
- If a problem is not resolved ask the following:
  - Is there more to this problem than you first thought?
  - Do you need to do another complete assessment?
  - Is the mother compliant with the care plan?
  - Did you overwhelm the mother or suggest things she is unable to do?
  - Are there family members who are interfering?
  - Are you holding the mother to a plan that is not working because of your own expectations?
- Evaluate your counseling skills (see Figure 5.2)

Hospital Documentation

Use a Method That Will Not Seem Daunting to Staff
- Teach the mother to chart much of her own information
- Chart at least one time per hospital shift
- Avoid terms that give very little information (for example, good, fair, or poor)
- Find a form that works best for you (see Figures 5.3 through 5.6 and Table 5.1)

1. Date the patient was seen.
2. Names and addresses of the physicians for mother and baby.
3. Regarding: Name of the mother and baby and baby's date of birth.
4. Dear Dr. . . . ,
5. This patient was seen at your request, was self-referred, was referred by (include name if possible).
6. In addition, if you also called the physician's office to give a verbal report or faxed in a short report, you can mention this in your letter.
7. State the reason for referral.
8. Provide a brief description of the mother's history (general health, conception, pregnancy, and birth).
9. Provide an assessment of the mother's breasts and nipples.
10. Give a brief description of the baby's history (birth, Apgar scores, in-hospital feeding, current feeds, output, weights, behavior, and so forth).
11. Provide an assessment and the present status of the baby (muscle tone, activity, skin turgor, oral cavity, behavior, weight, and so forth).
12. Provide a feeding assessment, including feeding weights, if possible.
13. Provide your assessment of the situation.
14. List the suggestions that you made to the mother and the action plan that was developed.
15. List the arrangements for a follow-up with the mother.
16. If the patient was referred to you, thank the physician for allowing you to participate in the care of her/his patient. If the patient self-referred, you may comment about working with the physician with this couple ("It was a pleasure . . .").
17. Sincerely yours, . . . (Insert your name with all your credentials.)

Figure 5.1   Elements of a physician report

> 1. Understanding of the problem: Did I understand the mother and help her?
> 2. Breastfeeding information: Was the information correct and appropriate? Not too much or too little?
> 3. Clarity of instructions: Did the mother understand the information and advice?
> 4. Good counseling skills: Did I put her at ease and encourage her to share her feelings?
> 5. Partnership with mother: Was the mother drawn into the problem-solving process?
> 6. Encouraged mother's self-reliance: Did I foster greater self-assurance in the mother?
> 7. Balance: Did I achieve balance—no lecturing—between listening, educating, and problem solving?
> 8. Arrangements for follow-up: Did I make it clear when any further contact will take place and who will initiate it?
> 9. Overall impressions: Was the mother satisfied with the consultation?

Figure 5.2 Questions to evaluate counseling skills in a consultation

Develop a Plan of Care for Hospital Discharge

- Diary to record the baby's feeds, voids, and stools
- Instructions regarding what is normal and where to get help (see Chapter 11, "Infant Assessment and Behavior")
- Written care plan based on the assessment of the needs of the mother and infant (see Chapter 14, "Breastfeeding Issues in the Early Weeks," and Figure 14.9, "Engorgement care plan")

B-R-E-A-S-T Feed Observation

Mother's name: _____ Date: _____

Infant's age: _____ [Bracketed items refer only to the newborn infant, not to an older infant who sits up.]

SIGNS THAT BREASTFEEDING IS GOING WELL:	SIGNS OF POSSIBLE DIFFICULTY WITH BREASTFEEDING:

Body Position

___ Mother relaxed and comfortable.	___ Mother's shoulders tense, leans over baby.
___ Infant's body close to mother.	___ Infant's body away from mother's.
___ Infant's head and body straight.	___ Infant's neck twisted.
___ Infant's chin touching breast.	___ Infant's chin does not touch breast.
___ [Infant's bottom supported.]	___ [Only infant's shoulder or head supported.]

Responses

___ Infant reaches for breast if hungry.	___ No response to breast.
___ [Infant roots for breast.]	___ [No rooting observed.]
___ Infant explores breast with tongue.	___ Infant not interested in breast.
___ Infant calm and alert at breast.	___ Infant restless or fussy at breast.
___ Infant stays attached to breast.	___ Infant slips off breast.
___ Signs of milk ejection (leaking, after pains).	___ No sign of milk ejection.

Figure 5.3 Breastfeed observation form *(continues)*

Source: From Breastfeeding Management and Promotion in a Baby Friendly Hospital: An 18 Hour Course for Maternity Staff, UNICEF/WHO, 1993.

Emotional Bonding
- ___ Secure, confident hold.
- ___ Face-to-face attention from mother.
- ___ Much contact between mother and infant.

- ___ Nervous, shaking, or limp hold.
- ___ No mother/infant eye contact.
- ___ Little contact between mother and infant.

Anatomy
- ___ Breasts soft and full.
- ___ Nipples stick out—protractile.
- ___ Skin appears healthy.
- ___ Breast looks round during feeding.

- ___ Breasts engorged and hard.
- ___ Nipples flat or inverted.
- ___ Fissures or redness of skin present.
- ___ Breast looks stretched or pulled during feeding.

Suckling
- ___ Infant's mouth wide open.
- ___ Infant's lower lip turned outward.
- ___ Infant's tongue cupped around breast.
- ___ Infant's cheeks round.
- ___ Infant does slow deep sucks—bursts with pauses.
- ___ Can see or hear swallowing.

- ___ Infant's mouth closed and points forward.
- ___ Infant's lower lip turned inward.
- ___ Infant's tongue not visible.
- ___ Infant's cheeks tense or pulled in.
- ___ Infant does rapid sucks.
- ___ Can hear smacking or clicking.

Time Spent Suckling
- ___ Infant releases breast.
- ___ Infant suckled for ___ minutes.

- ___ Mother takes infant off breast.

Figure 5.3 Breastfeed observation form (*continued*)

Source: From Breastfeeding Management and Promotion in a Baby Friendly Hospital: An 18 Hour Course for Maternity Staff, UNICEF/WHO, 1993.

	0	1	2
L Latch	Too sleepy or reluctant. No sustained latch or suck achieved.	Repeated attempts for sustained latch or suck. Holds nipple in mouth. Stimulate to suck.	Baby grasps breast. Baby's tongue down. Baby's lips flanged. Rhythmical sucking.
A Audible swallowing	None.	Few with stimulation.	Spontaneous and intermittent—baby less than 24 hours old. Spontaneous and frequent—baby greater than 24 hours old.
T Type of nipple	Inverted.	Flat.	Everted (after stimulation).
C Comfort (breast/nipple)	Engorged. Cracked, bleeding, large blisters, or bruises. Severe discomfort.	Filling. Reddened/small blisters or bruises. Mild/moderate discomfort.	Soft. Nontender.
H Hold (positioning)	Full assist (staff holds infant at breast).	Minimal assistance (i.e., elevate head of bed; place pillows for support). Teach one side; mother does other. Staff holds and then mother takes over.	No assist from staff. Mother able to position and hold infant.

Figure 5.4 The LATCH method

Source: Jenson, D, Wallace, S, Kelsay, P (1994). "LATCH: A breastfeeding charting system and documentation tool." JOGNN, 23(1):29. Reprinted with permission of Lippincott-Raven Publishers and authors.

	Mother	Baby	Help
Signaling			
Positioning			
Fixing			
Milk Transfer			
Ending			

Total Score Possible—10

This is an assessment method for rating the progress of a mother and baby who are learning to breastfeed.
For every step, each person—both mother and baby—should receive an X before either one can be scored on the following steps. If the observer does not observe any of the designated indicators, a score of 0 is given for that person on that step. If help is needed at any step for either the mother or the baby, check Help for that step. This notation will not change the total score for mother and baby.

1. SIGNALING

- Mother watches and listens for the baby's cues. She may hold, stroke, rock, and talk to the baby. She stimulates the baby if he is sleepy, calms baby if he is fussy.
- The baby gives the following readiness cues—stirring, alertness, rooting, sucking, hand-to-mouth, vocal cues, and crying.

2. POSITIONING
- The mother holds baby in good alignment within latch-on range of her nipple. The baby's body is slightly flexed, and the entire ventral surface is facing the mother's body. The baby's head and shoulders are supported.
- The baby roots well at the mother's breast, opens his mouth wide with his tongue cupped and covering his lower gum.

3. FIXING
- The mother holds her breast to assist her baby as needed, and brings baby in close when his mouth is wide open. She may express drops of milk.
- The baby latches on, takes all of nipple and about 2 cm (1 inch) of areola into mouth, then sucks, demonstrating a recurrent burst-pause pattern.

4. MILK TRANSFER
- The mother reports feeling any of the following—thirst, uterine cramps, increased lochia, breast ache or tingling, relaxation, or sleepiness. Milk leaks from opposite breast.
- The baby swallows audibly; milk is observed in the baby's mouth; the baby may spit up milk when burping. Rapid "call up sucking" rate (two sucks/second) changes to "nutritive sucking" rate of about 1 suck/second.

5. ENDING
- The mother's breasts are comfortable; she lets her baby suck until he is finished. After nursing, her breasts feel softer; she has no lumps, engorgement, or nipple soreness.
- The baby releases his mother's breast spontaneously, and appears satiated. The baby does not root when stimulated. The baby's face, arms, and hands are relaxed, and the baby may fall asleep.

Figure 5.5 The mother-baby assessment method

Source: Mulford, C (1992). "The mother-baby assessment (MBA): An 'Apgar score' for breastfeeding." J Hum Lact, 8:79–82. Reprinted with permission of Human Sciences Press, Inc., and the author.

Check the answer that best describes the baby's feeding behaviors at this feed. Add the numbered responses and plot on graph.

1. When you picked baby up to feed was he/she

a. deeply asleep (eyes closed, no observable movement except breathing)	b. drowsy	c. quiet and alert	d. crying
3	2	1	0

2. In order to get the baby to begin this feed, did you or the nurse have to

a. just place the baby on the breast as no effort was needed	b. use mild stimulation such as unbundling, patting, or burping	c. unbundle baby; sit baby back and forward; rub baby's body or limbs vigorously at the beginning and during the feeding	d. baby could not be aroused
3	2	1	0

3. Rooting (definition: at touch of nipple to cheeck, baby's head turns toward the nipple, the mouth opens, and baby attempts to fix mouth on the nipple). When the baby was placed beside the breast, he/she

a. rooted effectively at once	b. needed some coaxing, prompting, or encouragement to root	c. rooted poorly even with coaxing	d. did not try to root
3	2	1	0

4. How long from placing baby at the breast does it take for the baby to latch on and start to suck?
   a. starts to feed at once (0–3 minutes)
   b. 3–10 minutes
   c. more than 10 minutes
   d. did not feed

   3 _____ 2 _____ 1 _____ 0 _____

5. Which of the following phrases best describes the baby's feeding pattern at this feed?
   a. baby did not suck
   b. sucked poorly; weak suckling; some sucking efforts for short periods
   c. sucked fairly well; sucked off and on, but needed encouragement
   d. sucked well throughout on one or both breasts

   0 _____ 1 _____ 2 _____ 3 _____

6. How do you feel about the way the baby fed at this feeding?
   a. very pleased
   b. pleased
   c. fairly pleased
   d. not pleased

   _____ _____ _____ _____

Figure 5.6 The infant breastfeeding assessment tool (*continues*)

Source: Matthews, MK (1988). Developing an instrument to assess infant breastfeeding behavior in the early neonatal period. Midwifery, 4(4), 154–165. Reprinted with permission of Churchill Livingstone and the author.

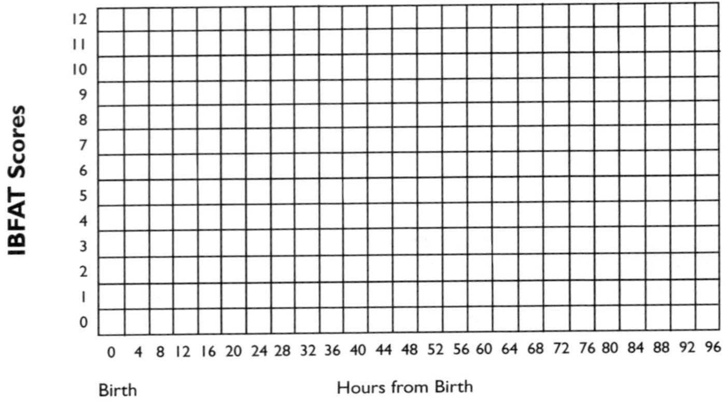

Date of Birth ____________
Infant No. ____________
Time of Birth ____________
Sex ____________
Time of First Breastfeed ____________
Birth W. ____________
Discharge W. ____________

Time ____________
Date ____________

Figure 5.6 The infant breastfeeding assessment tool (*continued*)
Source: Matthes, MK (1993). Assessments and suggested interventions to assist newborn breastfeeding behavior. *J Hum Lact*, 9:243–48. Reprinted with permission of Human Sciences Press, Inc., and author.

TABLE 5.1 CHARTING WITH BREASTFEEDING DESCRIPTORS FOR DOCUMENTATION OF FEEDS

You may chart two types of feeds in one session. For example, a mother and her baby may need considerable assistance with attachment. After the latch is achieved, the baby demonstrates nutritive sucking with audible swallows. This would be charted as FBF/GBF. Another example: You observe a baby that has some difficulty latching and the mother is poorly positioned. After offering assistance, the mother and her baby overcome the obstacles and have an excellent feed with lots of swallows. This would be charted as "Initial PBF/ after assistance EBF. Any rating below *Excellent Breastfeed* or *Good Breastfeed* will require further documentation that describes the problem and any help that is given.

DESCRIPTOR	MEANING	ELEMENTS OBSERVED
EBF	Excellent breastfeed	• Baby can latch on without difficulty. • Baby's sucks are nice and deep with a nice steady rhythm. • Pauses are brief, and baby quickly resumes sucking again. • Can hear baby swallowing frequently, sometimes with each suck. • Mother does not need assistance positioning baby or latching him on. • No nipple discomfort.

(*continues*)

TABLE 5.1 CHARTING WITH BREASTFEEDING DESCRIPTORS FOR DOCUMENTATION OF FEEDS (continued)

DESCRIPTOR	MEANING	ELEMENTS OBSERVED
GBF	Good breastfeed	• Baby can latch on without any difficulty. • Baby's sucks are nice and deep with a nice steady rhythm. • Pauses are brief, and baby resumes sucking again without being moved or prodded. • Some swallowing is heard. • Mother requires a little help with positioning or latch-on. • No nipple discomfort.
FBF	Fair breastfeed	• Baby is able to latch on to the breast and stay on. • Baby's sucks are short and quick with an occasional nice deep suck; no steady rhythm. • Mother has to stroke or prod baby to resume sucking. • An occasional swallow may be heard, but no swallowing is usually heard. • Mother requires a lot of assistance with positioning and latch-on. • Mother possibly experiencing nipple discomfort.

PBF	Poor breastfeed	- Baby roots for the breast and licks the nipple.
- Baby latches on, but has difficulty doing it.
- Once latched-on, baby does not stay on the breast or if he does he does not suck.
- No swallowing is heard.
- Mother requires a lot of assistance with positioning and latch-on.
ABF	Attempted breastfeed	- Mother could have nipple discomfort or pain.
- Baby roots and licks at the nipple.
- Baby unable to latch on to the nipple.
- Mother requires a great deal of assistance.
OBF	No breastfeed	- No effort from baby at the breast (too sleepy, lethargic, no interest).
- Baby pushes away from the breast, fights or cries, or both.
- Despite lots of assistance, mother unable to accomplish a feed.

Printed by permission of Breastfeeding Support Consultants (Barger, Kutner, 1996).

ANATOMY

The Science of Lactation

Anatomy of the Breast

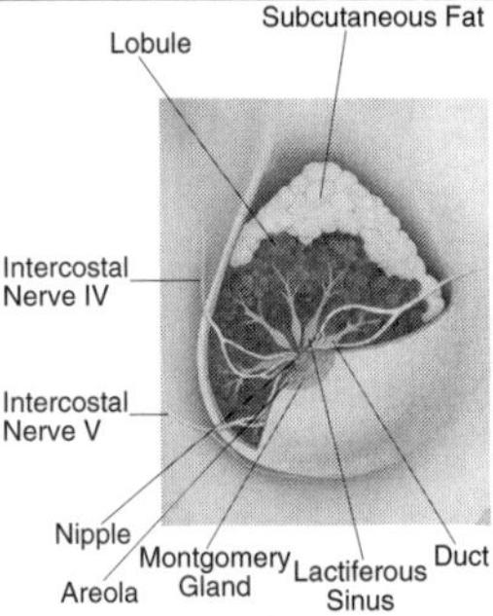

Figure 6.1 Frontal view of lactating breast

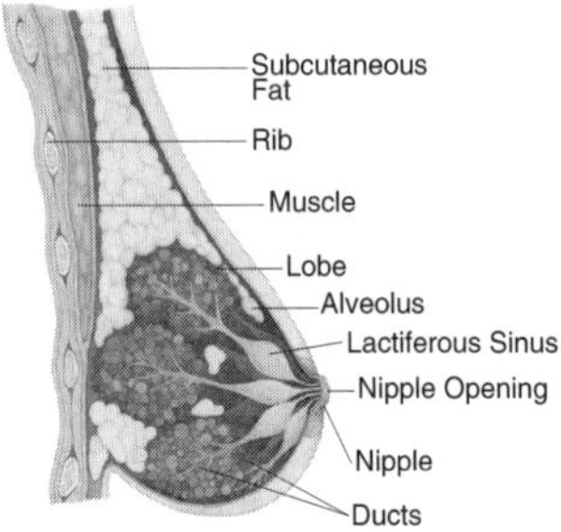

Figure 6.2 Side view of lactating breast

Nipple
- Is flexible and able to be molded to conform to the baby's mouth during a feed
- Nerve endings trigger the production and release of milk
- Composed of smooth muscle fibers that function as a closing mechanism for the lactiferous sinuses
- Contains 15 to 25 ductule openings (nipple pores) at its end
- Only six or seven nipple pores function during any particular feed—these alternate from one feed to the next

Montgomery Glands
- Have a pimply appearance
- Located on the areola
- Secrete an oily substance that protects the skin and allows the skin to breathe and remain pliable
- Taste and smell of the secretion may enable the baby to find the nipple
- Washing the nipples possibly removes these secretions, dries out the breast skin, and reduces the scent

Supportive and Sustaining Tissue
- Nerves
  - Fourth, fifth, and sixth intercostal nerves
  - Innervate smooth muscles in the nipples and blood vessels
- Innervation
  - The epidermis is supplied with few nerves
  - In the deeper part, the dermis is amply supplied, insensitive to light touch, and highly responsive to suckling stimulation
- When the baby grasps the breast well and suckles vigorously, he
  - Stimulates the deeper nerves
  - Activates milk production and release mechanisms
  - Activates Montgomery glands and milk duct openings

- If the baby is weak or tired, or sucks on the nipple alone, he
  - Does not adequately stimulate the deeper nerves
  - May lower milk production and decrease let-downs
- If the baby cannot nurse, the mother
  - Must express milk from her breasts
  - Will often notice a gradual decline in her milk production

Fatty Tissue

- The amount of fatty tissue in the breast primarily determines breast size
- Fatty tissue does not contribute to milk synthesis or its transport

Connective Tissue

- Fibrous bands (Cooper's ligaments)
- Attaches the breast to overlying skin and underlying fibrous tissue that encloses the muscles
- Keeps the breasts from sagging
- Grows during pregnancy
- Has a pattern of cyclic growth and deterioration throughout a menstrual cycle
- Retracts after lactation has ceased

Blood and Lymph Systems

- Needs of the breast increase during menstruation and pregnancy
- Blood flow increases to support tissue building
- Frequent suckling signals the need to increase milk production
  - More blood becomes available
  - Provides nutrients needed to produce milk
- Lymph in the breast does the following:
  - Flows mostly into nodes in the axilla
  - Traps bacteria that travels up the ducts from the nipple and from the bloodstream

- Breast engorgement causes the following:
  - Halts the flow of blood and lymph due to increased pressure from milk in the ducts
  - Causes tissues to become edematous
  - Slows the lymphatic system
  - Increases the risk of local infection
  - Causes inadequate removal of bacteria and cell particles from the breast
  - Leads to poor drainage of the duct and alveolus

Glandular Tissue
- The breast is a gland composed of many smaller individual glands, or lobuli
- Lobuli are
  - Made up of many milk-producing alveoli
  - Connected to a system of ducts from which milk flows out of the breast to the infant

Milk-Producing Tissue
- Milk is produced in alveoli, which have the following characteristics:
  - Are tiny individual glands
  - Consist of epithelial cells that are encased in a smooth muscle layer (myoepithelial cells)
  - Are surrounded by numerous capillaries that supply nutrient-rich blood
  - Select the ingredients for milk production
  - Receive oxytocin and prolactin, which signals them to release and produce more milk
  - During pregnancy, alveoli enlarge and cells undergo rapid multiplication
  - Are clustered in groups
    - Takes 10 to 100 alveoli to form a lobule (see Figures 6.1 and 6.2)
    - Takes 15 to 20 smaller lobuli to make up one lobe

- When lactation begins, the following actions occur:
  - Cells in the center of the lobule undergo fatty degeneration and are eliminated in the first milk as colostrum
  - Outer alveoli remain to produce milk, which is ejected into the cavity in the center of the lobule
- Majority of the lobuli are in the lower half of the breast
  - Located toward the axilla against the chest wall
  - Concentrated mainly in the bottom portion of the breast and toward the underarm
- Myoepithelial cells (smooth muscle layers) do the following:
  - Enclose the alveoli and ductules in overlapping bands
  - Multiply and greatly increase in size during pregnancy and lactation
  - Decrease in size and number when breast-feeding ends
  - Contract when exposed to oxytocin, which is released during suckling
  - Cause the contraction that squeezes the lobule, which forces milk down the ducts

Milk-Transporting Tissue

- Milk flows through a system of lactiferous ductules, secondary ducts, ducts, lactiferous sinuses, and nipple pores
  - In the first half of pregnancy, the sprouting and growth of ducts and alveolar development intensify
  - In the second half of pregnancy, duct and alveolar tissues become more specialized in preparation for their milk-related functions
- A mature lactating breast contains 15 to 25 duct systems
- Each duct widens beneath the areola to form a *lactiferous sinus*
  - Lactiferous sinuses narrow considerably in the nipple
  - Feeding each duct are 20 to 40 smaller ducts (secondary ducts) that have a lobule on each one

- Lobuli are supplied with milk through the ductules by 10 to 100 alveoli
- The total number of alveoli varies from 3,000 to 100,000

Question of Insufficient Mammary Tissue

- In rare cases, a woman lacks functional breast tissue to produce sufficient milk
- Symptoms include the following:
  - No noticeable change in breast size during pregnancy or lactation
  - One breast is appreciably smaller than the other
  - Previous or family history of lactation failure
  - Inadequate milk production despite appropriate feeding management
- Woman with ductal atresia
  - A milk duct opening is absent
  - Milk is prevented from being ejected from that particular duct
- Woman has had breast surgery
  - Augmentation usually does not destroy functional breast tissue or sever ducts, nerves, or blood vessels
  - Reduction is more intrusive and can interfere with lactation
    - Resection with transplantation of the nipple severs all ducts, rendering lactation impossible
    - Removal of portions of the breast with transposition of the nipple, areola, and ducts is compatible with breastfeeding, as long as nerve supply to the breast is left intact
  - Check with the surgeon to learn if any functional breast tissue was affected
  - Surgery for early-stage breast cancer
    - Lactation can be encouraged after surgery
    - Breastfeeding is possible from both the untreated and treated breast after conservative surgery and radiation
- Woman has had chest or cardiac surgery that involved the duct

- Consider a possibility of insufficient ductwork if:
  - Mother has great difficulty producing enough milk
  - Breastfeeding management issues have been ruled out
- Supplements may be needed if:
  - Mother has tried all means of increasing production
  - Mother is unable to keep up with the infant's requirements

Mammary Growth and Development

Baby's Breast Congestion at Birth

- Baby may secrete colostrum-like fluid (witch's milk)
- Fluid consists primarily of epithelial cells which have been shed
- Thought to be caused by an influx of hormones from the mother through the placenta

Mammary Growth between Puberty and Pregnancy

- Structural growth of the breast is very apparent during puberty
- Only a small amount of alveolar development occurs
- During ovulatory cycles, there is a slight development of functional breast tissue
- Onset of menstruation
  - Hormonal balance is altered by an increased production of estrogen
  - Produces the growth of ducts and connective tissue
- Major changes are complete about 12 to 18 months after the first menstrual period
- Breast fullness occurs as follows before menstruation:
  - Blood supply increases
  - Fluid retention increases in tissues

Mammary Growth during Pregnancy

- During the first trimester (conception to three months), the following occurs:
  - Estrogen and progesterone levels cause the duct system to multiply
  - Nipple and areola increase in circumference and pigmentation
  - Montgomery glands enlarge or elongate and begin to secrete an oily substance protecting the nipple and areolar skin
- During the second trimester (four to six months), the duct system continues to develop
- During the last trimester (seven to nine months), the following occurs:
  - Breast weight increases by as much as 1 to $1^1/_2$ pounds through the following:
    - Blood supply and body fluids (lymph) supporting alveolar growth
    - Multiplying number of alveoli
  - Colostrum is present
  - General breast development continues
  - If a premature delivery occurs, lactation is possible for the mother
- From the time alveoli begin to develop, the following occurs:
  - Alveolar cells wear out and are constantly being replaced
  - Ductwork proliferates, which explains why adolescent mothers can lactate despite recent pubescent changes

Lactogenesis

- Is the establishment phase of milk synthesis and secretion
- Stage I lactogenesis has the following characteristics:
  - Starts at the beginning of the third trimester
  - Increases occur in lactose, total proteins, and immunoglobulin
  - There is a decrease in sodium and chloride

- Stage II lactogenesis has the following characteristics:
  - Starts on the second or third day postpartum
  - Colostral phase ends and transitional milk is produced
  - Blood flow within the breast increases
  - Copious milk secretion begins
- Stage III lactogenesis, also called *galactopoiesis*, has the following characteristics:
  - Begins about 10 days after Stage II
  - Marks the establishment and maintenance of mature milk
- The period of involution following lactogenesis has the following characteristics:
  - Normal process marked by the decreasing size of an organ
  - Breast slowly returns to its prepregnant state
  - Takes about three months with slow, gradual weaning
  - Abrupt weaning causes marked involution in a matter of days or weeks

Hormonal Impact on Lactation

- Estrogen
  - Is produced in the ovaries and placenta
  - Causes growth of duct work and connective tissue between ducts in the breast
- Progesterone
  - Is produced in the ovaries and placenta
  - Aids in development of milk-secreting cells in the breast
  - Inhibits prolactin's effects during pregnancy
- Placenta retained following delivery
  - Is accompanied by progesterone
  - Could impair milk synthesis
- Prolactin
  - Is produced in the anterior pituitary
  - Stimulates alveolar growth in the breast during pregnancy

- Increases in the mother's blood soon after initiation of sucking stimulus
- Tells the breast to speed up milk synthesis
- Prolactin levels are higher when:
  - Baby is attached effectively at the breast
  - Baby is not given artificial nipples or pacifiers
  - Baby has unlimited access to the breast as frequently and as long as he wants—usually every one to three hours
  - Baby breastfeeds during the night when prolactin release is greatest
- Oxytocin
  - Is produced in the hypothalamus and is transported via nerve fibers to the posterior pituitary for storage
  - Suckling stimulates nerve endings in the nipple
  - Impulses are carried through the hypothalamic region to the posterior pituitary
  - Released by the posterior pituitary and is taken by blood to the breasts
  - Muscle layer around each milk-producing cell contracts during letdown—called the milk ejection reflex
  - In response, hindmilk (high-fat milk which adhered to the alveolar lining at the end of the previous feed) is pushed down the ducts and out through the nipple pores
  - When milk ejects, the rhythm of suckling changes from rapid to regular deep, slow sucks, about one per second

Hormonal Imbalances that Affect Lactation

- Incidence of hormone imbalances causing breastfeeding problems is extremely low
- Women at risk for hormone imbalance and milk insufficiency are as follows:
  - Women who had difficulty conceiving
  - Women who have become pregnant by reproductive technology

- Signs of hormone imbalance are as follows:
  - Breastfeeding problems
  - Vague feeling of physical discomfort
  - History of previous thyroid problems
  - Menstrual irregularities
- Placental retention
  - Can inhibit lactation by causing hormones to remain at pregnancy levels
  - Signs that placental fragments may have been retained are as follows:
    - Absence of breast fullness
    - Absence of changes in breast secretions
- Sheehan's syndrome causes the following to occur:
  - Mother's blood pressure drops so low that blood fails to circulate to the pituitary gland
  - Some or all cells in the pituitary gland stop working permanently
  - Breasts remain soft after delivery
  - Mother may not be able to produce any milk
  - This is an irreversible condition and may rule out the prospect of breastfeeding a future baby
- Prolactinoma
  - Is a pituitary tumor that secretes prolactin
  - Can cause secondary amenorrhea or galactorrhea
  - Is not a reason for a mother not to breastfeed
- Hypothyroidism
  - Is caused by a deficiency of thyroid secretion
  - Receiving replacement therapy with natural or synthetic hormone preparations can totally eliminate symptoms
  - Properly managing a mother who is receiving thyroid supplementation enables her to breastfeed without compromising her baby's health
  - If a mother is severely hypothyroid and is receiving an unusually high dosage of thyroid supplement, the following occurs:
    - Additional thyroid supplement passes to the baby through her milk

- May mask latent hypothyroidism in the baby while he is being breastfed
- Many hospitals routinely screen for hypothyroidism in newborns in conjunction with screening for phenylketonuria

Colostrum Production
- Contains water, minerals, fat droplets, lymphocytes, and similar cells
- Contains cast-off alveolar cells which form a unique combination of nutrients
- Designed to meet the nutritional and immunologic needs of a newborn
- Acts as a natural lubricant
- Is bactericidal—substance that destroys bacteria—because of lysozyme content
- Estrogen and progesterone act directly on the alveolar epithelium to suppress secretion of colostrum

Milk Synthesis
- When the placenta is delivered, the following actions occur:
  - Estrogen and progesterone levels drop sharply
  - Prolactin production in the anterior pituitary rises
  - Alveoli are signaled to start producing and secreting milk
- When an infant is allowed free access to the breast, the following occurs:
  - Colostrum is replaced with transitional milk
  - Milk production and breast fullness increase between the second and fifth day postpartum
- With initial milk production, many women experience normal breast fullness
  - Is a normal physiologic response
  - Can be mistaken for engorgement if the mother or care provider is unfamiliar with the process

- Estrogen and progesterone of pregnancy act locally on alveoli causing the following to occur:
  - Milk production and secretion are inhibited
  - Estrogen and progesterone levels drop after delivery
- Prolactin promotes milk synthesis as follows:
  - Prolactin levels increase gradually during pregnancy
  - Levels reach a peak of 20 times the normal value near term
  - Levels increase again tenfold in response to suckling
  - Prolactin levels range three to five times above the level of a menstruating female after three months' postpartum
  - Further stimulation doubles the level above the baseline through the second year of lactation
- Milk production is dependent on frequency of drainage and degree of drainage of each breast
- Feedback inhibitor of lactation (FIL)
  - Is an apparent human whey protein
  - Causes autocrine inhibition of milk synthesis
- Autocrine control
  - Is defined as local control within the gland
  - In the breast, the control agent is a secretory product from one type of cell that influences the activity of this same type of cell
  - Suggests that milk left in the breast inhibits the production of more milk
    - Mother produces only what her baby needs
    - Protects the mother's energy expenditure during lactation
  - The level of prolactin released is affected significantly by feeding frequency and nipple stimulation
  - During times when the baby is not nursing, prolactin is prevented from being released by the **prolactin inhibitory factor (PIF)**
  - Suckling inhibits the PIF, thereby allowing the release of prolactin

- In the absence of effective and frequent suckling to remove milk, prolactin production decreases and autocrine inhibition begins
- In the beginning, frequent and necessary feeds are necessary to ensure an increase in the number and sensitivity of prolactin receptors for when prolactin levels fall to normal

Milk Ejection Reflex (Letdown)

- When the baby suckles, contact between his tongue and the mother's nipple stimulates the nerve endings
- It sends a message to the hypothalamus, which relays a message to the anterior pituitary and the following actions occur:
  - Prolactin inhibitory factor is lowered
  - Prolactin is able to be released
- As suckling continues, the following occurs:
  - Posterior pituitary gland secretes oxytocin
  - Smooth muscles around the alveoli and uterus contract due to oxytocin
  - Milk is forced down through the duct system to the lactiferous sinuses underneath the areola
- Although milk ejection is bilateral, milk is prevented from flowing freely from the nonsuckled breast by sphincters at the ends of the ducts
- Letdown brings milk into the ducts, making milk accessible to the baby through suckling as follows:
  - Initially causes an active expulsion of milk through pressure within the lactiferous sinuses and ducts; lasts for a relatively short time, and then the flow subsides
  - Positive pressure is maintained within the breast
  - Milk flow continues with further suckling
- A letdown provides for free flow of milk and has the following characteristics:
  - Is essential to move fat globules down through the ducts
  - Are several within a single feed

- Initial letdown is usually only noticeable with a large quantity of milk moved at this time
- In the absence of letdown, the infant receives only a third of the milk available
- Enables the infant to receive the majority of the milk's fat content, which tends to stick to the duct lining
- Forces hindmilk down into the lactiferous sinuses
- Mixes hindmilk with foremilk, (high-protein milk at the beginning of a feed), which has collected in the sinuses since the previous feed
- Infant receives more fatty milk after letdown as the feed progresses
- Limiting nursing time on one breast in order for the mother to switch to the other breast can cause the following to occur:
  - Baby receives a large volume of foremilk that contains fewer calories
  - Baby may experience gastric upset and low weight gain
- To assist letdown, a mother needs the following:
  - Quiet location
  - Comfortable position
  - Routine to begin each feed
- For a mother who reports no symptoms of letdown, study the following:
  - Observe a baby's swallowing during a feed, which will be more pronounced than at the beginning of the feed
  - Monitor the number of wet diapers and stools a baby has during a 24-hour period
  - From the end of the first week through the first month, the baby should have six or more wet diapers and four or more stools each 24 hours

Signs of a Functioning Letdown Reflex

- Tingling sensation or feeling of fullness or tightening in the breasts
- Leaking from the other breast while nursing

- Leaking when thinking about the baby or hearing a baby cry
- Uterine contractions (afterpains)—especially noticeable in multipara
- Feelings of relaxation or well-being
- An increased thirst
- Filling of the lactiferous sinuses that can be felt with the fingers
- Areola is drawn toward the baby's lips
- Changes in sucking pattern during a feed—sucking slows or the baby begins to gulp
- Baby's swallowing is heard
- Baby is satisfied and gaining weight
- Baby has at least six wet diapers and four stools each 24 hours after Day Five without water or formula supplements
- Baby's stools change from dark meconium to yellow, soft, and seedy by Day Five postpartum

Inhibited Letdown
- Times of stress, pain or fatigue may result in the following:
  - Secretion of oxytocin can be inhibited
  - Adrenaline is released; believed to negate the effects of oxytocin on the myoepithelial cells
- Occurs when nipple stimulation is weak because the baby is not attached effectively
- See Table 6.1 for its signs, causes, and treatment
- See Figure 6.3 for examples of relaxation techniques

Variations in Breast Structure and Function

Examining the Mother's Breasts
- Is not necessary to examine every woman's breasts and nipples
- May be necessary when a difficulty arises due to the nipples or breasts

(continues on page 65)

TABLE 6.1 SIGNS, CAUSES, AND TREATMENT OF AN INHIBITED LETDOWN

Signs of an Inhibited Letdown

- The baby is frustrated after a short time at the breast.
- The baby pulls away from the breast repeatedly.
- The baby is not gaining weight.
- The baby has fewer than six wet diapers per 24 hours, or has dark, concentrated urine.
- The baby has fewer than four stools per 24 hours, or meconium is still present on the fifth day of life or beyond.
- The mother has engorged breasts.
- The mother has sore nipples.

Causes of an Inhibited Letdown

- Letdown is not well established.
- Mother is extremely tired or overextended.
- Mother is tense or pressured.
- Mother is caught in the cycle of little milk, worry, less milk.
- The baby is not latched onto the breast effectively.

Actions for the Mother

- Allow the baby ample time at the breast until he unlatches himself or falls asleep. For a baby who falls asleep and remains latched, try breast compression to encourage further suckling to enable letdown and good milk flow.
- Nurse in a quiet spot away from distractions.
- Avoid embarrassing or stressful situations for feedings.

- Ask someone to massage your upper back, especially along the sides of the backbone.
- Massage your breasts before feeds. See Chapter 19, "Breastfeeding Techniques and Devices," for a description of breast massage.
- Use warm compresses before feeds.
- Express a little milk, and gently stimulate the nipple.
- Drink juice, water, or noncaffeinated tea before and during feeds.
- Condition a letdown by setting up a routine for beginning a feed.
- Use relaxation and breathing techniques.
- Use breast compression while the baby is nursing.
- Stimulate the nipples manually before nursing.
- Concentrate your thoughts on the baby and on milk flow. Turn on a water faucet so that the sound of running water can help to stimulate letdown.
- Nap or rest when the baby rests.
- Lie down to nurse.
- Nurse the baby in bed at night.
- Increase skin-to-skin contact with the baby at feeding times. Remove your bra and shirt, and have the baby in a diaper only.
- Simplify daily chores and establish priorities.
- Get help with household, car pooling, and other responsibilities.
- Discuss causes of tension, and eliminate or minimize them.
- Take a break from the daily routine with an evening out, shopping, a walk, lunch with friends, and so on.
- Develop confidence in your mothering skills.

- Spend a few minutes before going to sleep to analyze your own relaxation techniques (e.g., movements, positions, and room darkness). Repeat these techniques at other times for relaxation.
- Remove distractions—for example, find a quiet spot, and take the phone off the hook.
- Get comfortable—for example, empty your bladder; find a cozy chair or bed; get pillows for support; remove eyeglasses, shoes, or tight clothing; adjust room temperature.
- Listen to relaxing music.
- Take a deep breath and let it out slowly. Repeat this several times.
- Breathe steadily and rhythmically, noting the faint movement of your body and breathing slowly to relax further.
- Tense your entire body and relax slowly. Concentrate on one muscle at a time, starting from your toes and progressing up to your facial muscles, until your limbs, eyelids, and all body parts feel heavy.
- Use massage or warm compresses on any tense parts of your body.
- Take a warm shower or bath.
- Close your eyes and move them back and forth or up and down. Then rest your eyes and feel the release of tension. Relax your eyes by thinking about a ship sailing away from you and disappearing over the horizon.
- Allow your mind to drift into a sleepy state and think pleasant thoughts—for instance, enjoyable moments, pleasures, and dreams.
- Think about your baby, of your milk flowing, or of water rushing.
- Think about and write down or talk with someone about your fears, stresses, tensions, and what you feel causes them to occur. Then let your mind drift or think of pleasant thoughts and feel the release of tension.
- Visualize some strenuous or precarious activity, such as walking across thin ice, and then pretend it has ended and you are at ease.

Figure 6.3 Relaxation techniques for the mother

(continued from page 61)

- Before touching a mother's breasts, ask for permission and explain the purpose
  - Most women associate breast examination with illness or cancer prevention
  - Make sure the mother knows you are examining her breasts in preparation for breastfeeding
  - Ensure the mother's privacy to help her feel comfortable
  - Be sensitive to modesty that can make examination uncomfortable for the mother
  - Reassure the mother that small and large breasts alike will produce milk
- Ask the mother if both of her breasts became larger and the areola became darker during pregnancy
- Examine both breasts at the same time for the following:
  - Observe their symmetry
  - Note the skin's elasticity as well as any engorgement, lumps, swelling, or redness
  - Look for evidence of past breast surgery, which may have severed some ducts
  - Note the size and shape of the nipples and the size of areola
  - Learn how the nipples respond to stimulation, in response to either cold or touching

Differences in Nipples

- Nipples that protrude upon stimulation
  - Aid an infant in finding and centering on the breast
  - Provide tissue for the infant to grasp in order to draw the breast into his mouth
- Nipple inversion—nipple retracts inward— has the following characteristics:
  - Is found in 28 to 35 percent of all women during early pregnancy
  - Skin gains elasticity by the third trimester of pregnancy and only a small percentage still have inversion at delivery

- Little relationship exists between the degree of protrusion and the ability of the infant to nurse well
- With a good latch, the baby takes a large portion of the breast into his mouth and forms a cone-shaped teat
- Milk transfer depends more on breast pliability than on configuration of the nipple
- Nipples are classified into five types
  - See Table 6.2 for the basic types of nipples
  - Stimulation through touch, cold, or gentle compression reveals whether inversion is present
  - Pinch test will demonstrate the ability of the nipple to protract (see Chapter 19, "Breastfeeding Techniques and Devices")

Working with Nipple Inversion

- For a baby to receive milk, the breast tissue must reach back to the hard palate
  - When the breast will not stretch to accommodate this pattern, the baby has difficulty maintaining suction
  - Only a very small percentage of women with truly inverted nipples have difficulty getting a baby to latch on
- Inverted nipples may begin to respond to correction techniques during the last trimester of pregnancy
  - Premature labor can be increased by nipple stimulation in some women
  - Always check with a physician before beginning any techniques that involve nipple stimulation
  - Neither breast shells nor the Hoffman technique cause nipple elongation
- See Chapter 19 for instructions on the following methods that decrease nipple inversion—most information about these methods is anecdotal
  - Form the nipple by hand or with the aid of ice just before a feed
  - Wear breast shells prenatally

- Wear breast shells between feeds to gently place pressure on the skin and stretch and push the nipple forward
- Use an inverted syringe to help elongate the nipple
- Use suction from a breast pump

Lumps in the Breast

- The normal state of a lactating breast is lumpy
- Enlarged milk-filled alveoli are distributed throughout the tissues
- Other lumps can occur due to a plugged duct or breast infection (see Chapter 14, "Breastfeeding Issues in the Early Weeks")
- If a lump does not move downward and begin to break up within three days
  - It may be caused by a condition unrelated to breastfeeding
  - It must be examined by a physician to identify the cause of the lump
- Lumps associated with fibrocystic breasts
  - Change with the menstrual cycle
  - Shrink and become less noticeable after menstruation
- Galactocele
  - Is a cyst caused by closing or blockage of a milk duct
  - Contains a thick, creamy milk-like substance
  - May be discharged from the nipple when a cyst is compressed
  - Can be aspirated
  - Some are removed surgically to prevent refilling
  - Presence of a galactocele is compatible with breastfeeding
- Intraductal papilloma
  - Is a nontender breast lump
  - Is a benign tumor within a duct
  - Is usually associated with a spontaneous bloody discharge from one breast

TABLE 6.2 FIVE BASIC TYPES OF NIPPLES

Type of Nipple	Before Stimulation	After Stimulation

Common Nipple
The majority of mothers have what is referred to as a *common nipple*. It protrudes slightly when at rest and becomes erect and more graspable when stimulated. A baby has no trouble finding and grasping this nipple and can pull in a large amount of breast tissue and stretch it to the roof of his mouth.

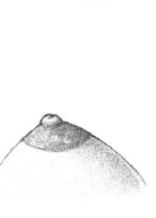

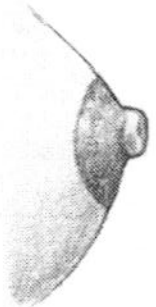

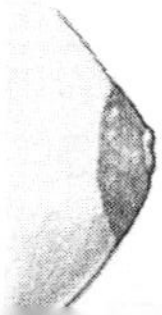

Flat Nipple
The flat nipple has a very short shank that makes it less easy for the baby to find and grasp. In response to stimulation, this nipple remains essentially unchanged. Slight movement inward or outward can be present, but there is not enough movement to aid the baby in finding and initially grasping the breast on center. This type of nipple may benefit from the use of a syringe to increase protractility.

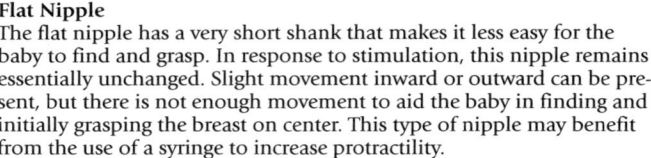

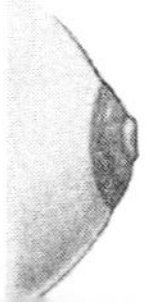

Inverted-Appearing Nipple
An inverted-appearing nipple may appear inverted but becomes erect after stimulation. This type of nipple needs no correction and presents no problems with the ability to grasp.

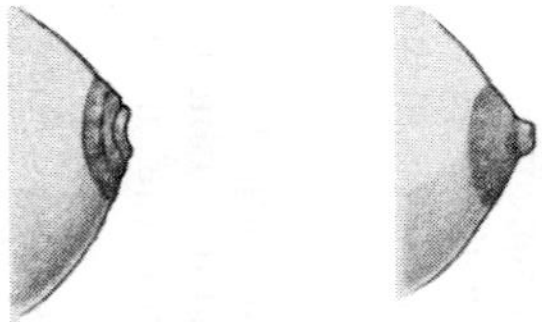

Retracted Nipple
The *retracted nipple* is the most common type of inverted nipple. Initially, this nipple appears to be graspable. However, upon stimulation, it retracts, which makes attachment difficult. This type of nipple responds well to techniques to increase nipple protrusion.

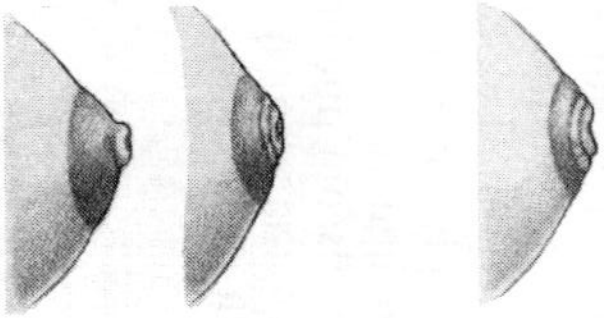

Inverted Nipple
The truly *inverted nipple* is retracted both at rest and when stimulated. Such a nipple is very uncommon and more difficult for a baby to grasp. All the techniques used to enhance protractility of breast tissue can be used to improve a baby's attachment to an inverted nipple. Even if the nipple remains retracted, the baby should be able to latch on if the mother helps form her breast into his mouth.

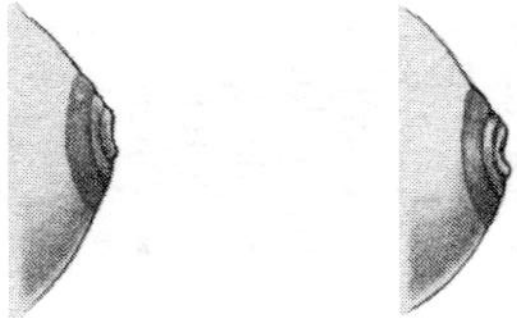

- Bloody discharge
  - Caused by trauma (most frequent)
  - Intraductal papilloma (secondary)
  - Fibrocystic breast (slightly less frequent)
  - Breastfeeding may continue after a serious disease is ruled out, the discharge stops, or the duct is surgically removed
- Lump due to malignancy
  - May need to discontinue breastfeeding; not compatible with treatments for breast cancer
  - Often, infant refuses to nurse from the cancerous breast
  - Explore breast rejection whenever a lump is found
  - Be careful not to confuse long-term breast rejection with temporary refusal to nurse for several feeds
  - If the physician locates a lump, a biopsy may be performed under local anesthesia to rule out cancer, usually without interruption in breastfeeding
    - Small risk that a milk fistula may develop as a result of the biopsy
    - May result in milk leaking from the biopsy incision site
    - Occasionally healing of the site may require temporary interruption of breastfeeding in that breast

Regular Breast Self-Examination

- Best time for a lactating woman is immediately after a feed, when the breasts are least full
- If menstruating, examine them on the seventh to tenth day after menses has begun
- Examine your breasts at the same time each cycle to increase familiarity with them in relation to hormonal influences
- See Figure 6.4 for examination method

Pick a regular time of the month to examine your breasts. When you are not pregnant, the best time is right after your menstrual period. Your breasts will feel lumpy and irregular during pregnancy and lactation. The idea is to get to know the particular contours of your breasts. After examining them, ask your physician to do a breast exam during your next visit, so he can confirm that what you feel is normal.

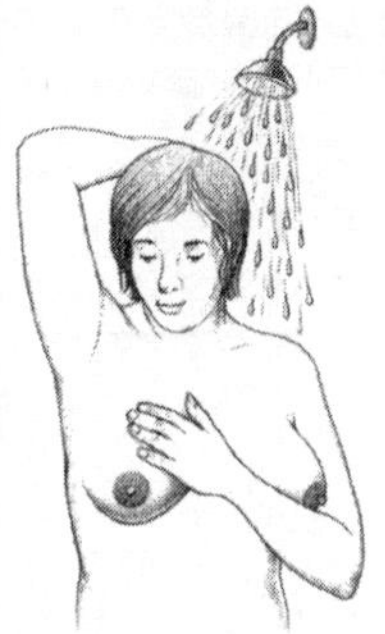

Examine your breasts during your bath or shower. Your fingers will glide easily over wet skin. Keeping your fingers flat, press gently in a circular motion over the entire breast area. Use your right hand to examine the left breast; your left hand for the right breast. Check for any lumps, hard knots, or thickenings.

Now look at your breasts in a mirror, first with your arms at your sides, then with your arms extended over your head. Look for any changes in the appearance of your breasts, a swelling, a dimpling of skin, or any changes in the nipple.

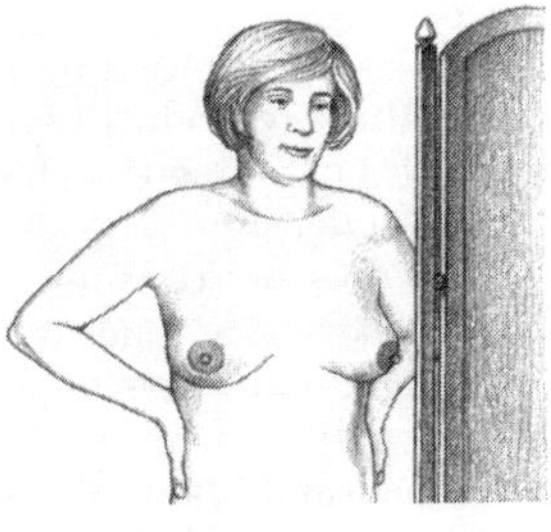

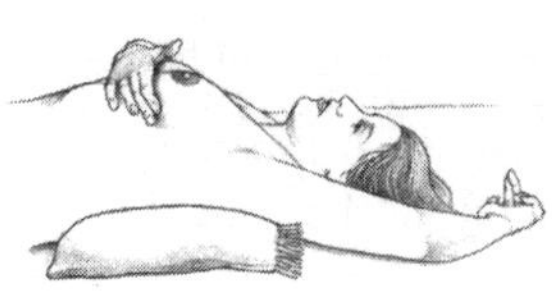

Finally, lie down and repeat the examination in a circular motion. Place your arm above your head and a pillow under your chest on the side you are examining. Using the opposite hand, be sure to check the entire area around the breast.

Figure 6.4 Breast self examination

Maternal Health and Nutrition

Nutritional Issues in Pregnancy and Lactation

Calcium
- Women who lactate are not more prone to osteoporosis
- Calcium mobilizes from a mother's bones during lactation
- Mothers recover their bone mass after weaning
- A mother's reproductive history, including lactation, is not a long-term indicator of her bone mineral density
- If one does not consume enough calcium, the body takes what it needs from its bones
- Women do not have to drink milk in order to make milk
- Women can obtain calcium through the sources presented in Table 7.1
- Women who do not eat enough calcium-rich foods are advised to take calcium supplements—there are no significant side effects from taking a supplement of between 500 and 1000 mg/day
- Pregnant or lactating women need to consume 1200 to 1500 mg of calcium daily

TABLE 7.1 GOOD SOURCES OF CALCIUM

Food	Calcium (mgs per serving)
Yogurt, plain (8 oz)	415
Cheddar cheese (2 oz)	408
Sardines, drained (3 oz)	372
Milk, skim or low-fat protein-fortified (8 oz)	352
American cheese (2 oz)	348
Yogurt, fruit-flavored (8 oz)	345
Milk, whole, low-fat or skim (8 oz)	297
Watercress (1 cup chopped)	189
Chocolate pudding, instant (1/2 cup)	187
Collards (1/2 cup cooked)	179
Buttermilk pancakes (3–4)	174
Pink salmon, canned (3 oz)	167
Tofu (4 oz)	145
Turnip greens (1/2 cup cooked)	134
Kale (1/2 cup cooked)	103
Shrimp, canned (3 oz)	99
Ice cream (1/2 cup)	88
Okra (1/2 cup cooked)	74
Rutabaga, mashed (1/2 cup cooked)	71
Broccoli (1/2 cup cooked)	68
Soybeans (1/2 cup cooked)	66
Cottage cheese (1/2 cup)	63
Bread, white or whole wheat (2 slices)	48

Water
- Lactating women need to drink water to satisfy their thirst
- It is easy for lactating mothers to remember to drink water if they drink something every time they nurse
- No data supports the concept of increasing a mother's fluid intake to increase her milk volume

- Women who consume excessive amounts of fluid actually produce less milk
- Restricting fluids has not been proven to decrease milk volume
- With fluid restriction, a mother will experience a decrease in urine output, but not in her milk output

Offering Nutrition Advice to Breastfeeding Women

Substances to Limit or Avoid

- Medications
  - Always consult a physician before taking any over-the-counter and prescription medication
  - Physicians may not be aware of a mother's medication use while she is breastfeeding
  - The International Board Certified Lactation Consultant (IBCLC) is an important source for information
  - Women need a clear understanding of substances they can and cannot consume during lactation
  - See Chapter 8, "Properties of Human Milk," for more discussion about drugs and social toxicants
- Nicotine and tobacco
  - The effects of passive smoke inhalation on a breastfed baby are of great concern
  - A baby ingests much more nicotine from smoke in the air than from nicotine in milk
  - Nicotine levels in milk are dependent on the number of cigarettes a mother has smoked and the amount of time between cigarettes
  - Mothers who smoke should be advised to quit
  - If a mother is unable to quit, she should cut back as much as possible, smoke away from the baby, and smoke after feedings to limit her baby's exposure

- Alcohol
  - A safe level of consumption while breastfeeding has not been determined
  - It enters the bloodstream and quickly migrates to a mother's milk
  - It is metabolized from human milk at about the same rate as from the body—1½ to 2 hours per ounce of absolute alcohol
  - Its occasional use timed around breastfeeds is not reported to have any harmful effects on a breastfed infant
- Caffeine
  - The American Academy of Pediatrics states that it is acceptable for lactating women to drink up to five cups of coffee per day
  - Caffeine is transmitted to the infant through a mother's milk
  - Caffeine is not easily eliminated from the body by very young infants
  - Susceptible infants may experience fussiness or excessive wakefulness
  - Regular coffee drinkers have lower hemoglobin and hematocrit with lowered human milk iron
- Allergens
  - Some evidence supports that a fetus and a young, breastfed infant can be sensitized to allergens while in utero and through breastfeeding
  - Babies born to parents with allergic manifestations have a greater possibility of developing the same allergies
  - Avoidance of allergen foods such as cow's milk, eggs, and fish in late pregnancy and lactation can lower the incidence of allergies
  - Most foods are acceptable in a mother's diet unless they are known to cause allergic reactions in the mother or father or are consumed in excessive amounts
  - See Chapter 8 for discussion of the substances found in human milk

Pregnancy and Lactation Diets

- A study of breastfeeding mothers during the first six months postpartum found the following:
  - Larger reductions in hip circumference than in mothers who did not breastfeed
  - Greater weight loss at one month postpartum than in mothers who did not breastfeed
  - Changes were similar regardless of the infant feeding method used at six months
- A study of breastfeeding duration up to 24 months found the following:
  - During the first three months, breastfeeding mothers do not lose weight more rapidly than mothers who do not breastfeed
  - Between three to six months, there is a significantly better weight reduction when mothers continue breastfeeding
  - Between one to twelve months, there is an average weight loss of 2 kg more in breastfeeding mothers than in those who do not breastfeed
  - Between nine and twelve months, a reduction in fat over the triceps area occurs in breastfeeding mothers that is not seen in those who do not breastfeed
- Encourage healthful eating habits (see Figure 7.1, Table 7.2, and Table 7.3)
- Provide specific food suggestions to accompany teaching of the basic principles of nutrition
- Translate the required number of servings from a food pyramid into meals with the proper number of calories
- Provide sample meal plans (see Table 7.4)
- A mother who is nursing twins:
  - Needs extra calories (approximately 500) to produce enough milk for the second baby
  - Can add foods at meal or snack times
  - Can increase the serving sizes

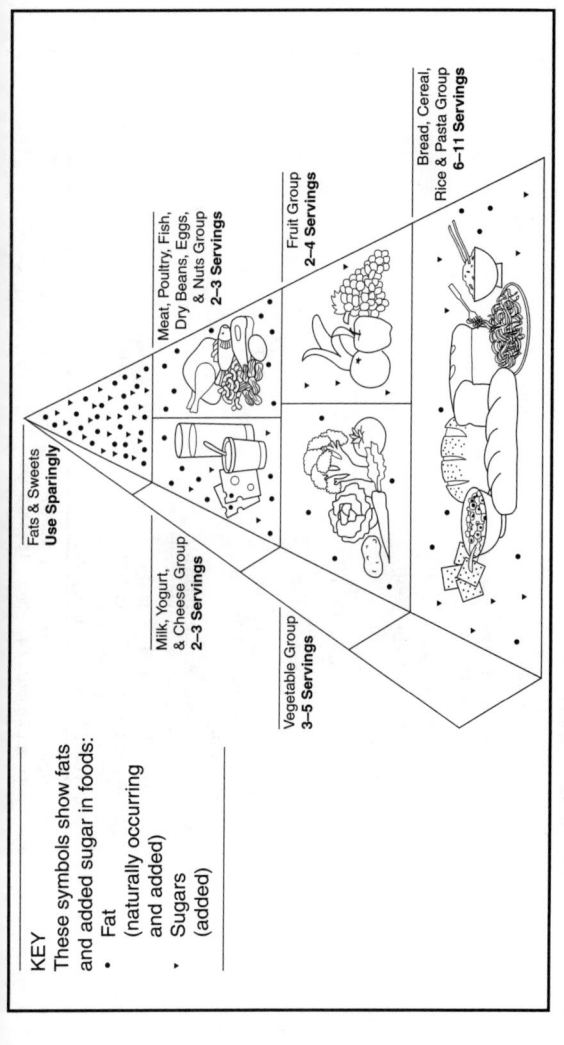

Figure 7.1 The food pyramid

TABLE 7.2 MENU SUGGESTIONS BASED ON THE FOOD PYRAMID

Food Group	Minimum Recommended Number of Servings Daily (with Sample Food Servings)	Nonpregnant (1900 Calories)	Pregnant or Lactating (2200 Calories)
Milk or milk products	1 cup low fat milk or yogurt; 1 1/2 oz. cheddar cheese; 1 cup pudding; 1 1/4 cups low fat ice cream; 2 cups cottage cheese; 1 cup tofu (soybean curd)	2	3
Meats and meat substitutes	Cooked lean meat, fish, or poultry; cheddar cheese; 1/2 cup cottage cheese; 1 cup dried beans or peas; 4 tbsp. peanut butter	5–7 ounces	7 ounces
Eggs		1	1–2
Fruits	(Include Vitamin C-rich choice): 1/2 cup cooked or juice; 1 cup raw; 1 medium-sized fruit	2–4	3–4
Vegetables	(Choose from dark leafy and starch vegetables. Variety is recommended.): 1/2 cup cooked; 1 cup raw	3–5	4–5
Grains	(Whole grain, fortified, or enriched): 1 slice breat; 1 cup ready-to-eat cereal; 1/2 cup cooked cereal, pasta, or grits	6–11	9–11

Data from The Food Pyramid: How to make it work for you. *Consumer Reports on Health*, September, 1996; Charbonneau, K. "Nutrition Continuum." *International Journal of Childbirth Education* 8:16–18, 1993.

TABLE 7.3 SUGGESTIONS FOR DIET IMPROVEMENT

PRACTICES	SUGGESTIONS FOR MOTHERS
Meal Planning	• Plan meals in advance, preferably on a weekly or monthly basis. • Include all food pyramid groups daily.
Shopping	• Prepare shopping lists according to meal plans. • Read labels carefully. • Select fresh, high quality foods. • Limit purchases of convenience foods.
Cooking Practices	• Use preparation methods which preserve nutritive quality—steaming, stir frying, boiling for short periods in a small amount of liquid. • Remove the fatty portion from meats before cooking or by broiling, boiling, or draining off fat.
Eating Practices	• Plan regular family meals and nutritious snacks. • Select foods which provide a well-balanced diet when eating away from home. • When psychological factors cause a desire to eat, substitute another activity or choose nutritious low calorie foods.

TABLE 7.4 SAMPLE MEAL PLAN

Sample Menu One

Breakfast	Cereal, honey nut cornflakes + skim milk 4 oz	156 calories
	Fruit juice (100%), apple 6 oz	84 calories
	1 medium banana	138 calories
Snack	Sliced turkey (low fat)	47 calories
Lunch	Whole wheat bread, 2 slices	140 calories
	Low-fat mayonnaise, 1 tablespoon	68 calories
	Lettuce	4 calories
	Tomato slice	20 calories
	Vegetable juice 6 oz	35 calories
Snack	Low-fat or nonfact yogurt 1 cup	210 calories
Dinner	Hamburger (extra lean ground beef or ground turkey)	213 calories
	Whole grain bun	113 calories
	Tomato slice, lettuce, onion	34 calories
	Spinach and tomato salad	26 calories
	w/ low-fat dressing	20 calories
	Skim milk 8 oz	86 calories
Snack	3 low-fat graham crackers	165 calories
	Skim milk 8 oz	86 calories
TOTAL		1,645 calories

Sample Menu Two

Breakfast	1 English muffin	134 calories
	Peanut butter, 2 tablespoons	188 calories
	Jelly	54 calories
	Skim milk 8 oz	86 calories
Snack	4 rye crackers	90 calories
	Low-fat swiss cheese 1 oz	50 calories
	Orange juice (100%) 6 oz	78 calories
Lunch	Bowl chicken vegetable soup	166 calories
	4 saltine crackers	50 calories
	Apple	65 calories
	Skim milk 8 oz	86 calories
Snack	1/4 cup raisins	129 calories
Dinner	Broiled chicken 3 oz	175 calories
	Broccoli 1/2 cup	22 calories
	Rice, brown 1/2 cup	109 calories
	Dinner roll	75 calories
	Spinach and tomato salad	26 calories
	w/ low-fat dressing	20 calories
	Skim milk 8 oz	86 calories
Snack	1/2 cup nonfat ice cream	110 calories
TOTAL		2,093 calories

Source: Medela, Inc., Rental Roundup, Vol. 10, Number 1, Winter 1993. *http://www.nutribase.com*

Vegetarian Diets

- Vegetarian diets are classified as follows:
  - Vegan—foods from plant sources only
  - Lacto-vegetarian—dairy products, in addition to plant foods
  - Ovo-vegetarian—plant foods plus eggs
  - Lacto-ovo-vegetarian—plant foods, dairy products, and eggs
  - Fruitarian—fruits, nuts, olive oil, and honey
- A well-balanced, vegetarian diet supplies a pregnant or lactating woman with the nutrients necessary to support her body functions and the healthy growth of her baby (see Table 7.5)
- During lactation, a mother can define the appropriate extra sources of calories, protein, and calcium, and can plan food combinations that will provide the eight essential amino acids (see Table 7.6)
- A poorly managed, vegetarian diet severely restricts the types of foods a mother is permitted to eat and can have the following results:
  - A serious deficiency in protein
  - Inadequate growth of a fetus or breastfed infant
  - An inadequately nourished mother
- Always watch for any of the following severe vegetarian regimens that can be harmful to a mother's pregnancy or her lactation by emphasizing one specific food group while neglecting others:
  - Zen macrobiotic diet
  - Fruitarianism
  - Restricted diets
  - Arbitrarily adopted patterns

TABLE 7.5 A NUTRIENT AND VITAMIN CHART

Key Nutrient	RDI for Ages 23–50	Important Sources	Important Functions
Water and liquids	N 4 C P 6–8 C L 8+ C	Water, juice, milk.	Carries nutrients to and waste products away from cells. Provides fluid for increased blood and amniotic fluid volume. Helps regulate body temperature and aids digestion. Comments: Often neglected. Is an important nutrient.
Protein amino acids	N 50 g P 60 g L 64 g	Animal: Meat, fish, eggs, milk, cheese, yogurt. Plant: Dried beans and peas, peanut butter, nuts, whole grains and cereals, soy milk, meat substitutes.	Constitutes part of the structure of every tissue cell, such as muscle, blood, and bone. Supports growth and maintains healthy body cells. Constitutes part of enzymes, some hormones and body fluids. Helps form antibodies that increase resistance to infection. Builds and repairs tissues, helps build blood and amniotic fluid. Supplies energy. Comments: Fetal requirements increase by about 1/3 in late pregnancy as the baby grows.

(continues)

TABLE 7.5 A NUTRIENT AND VITAMIN CHART (continued)

Key Nutrient	RDI for Ages 23–50	Important Sources	Important Functions
Minerals			
Calcium	N 800–1200 mg P 1200 mg L 1200 mg	Animal: Milk, cheese, yogurt, egg yolk, whole canned fish, ice cream. Plant: Whole grains, almonds, filberts, green leafy vegetables.	Combines with other minerals within a protein framework to give structure and strength to bones and teeth. Assists in blood clotting. Functions in normal muscle contraction and relaxation, and normal nerve transmission. Helps regulate the use of other minerals in the body. Comments: Fetal requirements increase by about 2/3 in late pregnancy.
Phosphorus	N 1000 mg P 1200 mg L 1200 mg	Animal: Milk, cheese, lean meats.	Helps build bones and teeth. Comments: Calcium and phosphorus exist in a constant ratio in the blood. An excess of either limits utilization of calcium.
Iron	N 18 mg P 30–60 mg L 18+ mg	Animal: Liver, red meats, egg yolk. Plant: Whole grains, leafy vegetables, nuts, legumes, dried	Aids in utilization of energy. Combines with protein to form hemoglobin, the red substance in blood that carries oxygen to and carbon dioxide from the cells. Prevents nutritional anemia and its accompanying fatigue. Increases resistance to

		fruits, prune and apple juice.	infection. Functions as part of enzymes involved in tissue respiration. Provides iron for fetal storage. Comments: Fetal requirements increase tenfold in final 6 weeks of pregnancy. Supplement of 30–60 mg of iron daily recommended by National Research Council. Continued supplementation for 2–3 months post-partum is recommended to replenish iron.
Zinc	N 15 mg P 20 mg L 25 mg	Animal: Meat, liver, eggs, and seafood, especially oysters.	A component of insulin. Important in growth of skeleton and nervous system. Comments: Deficiency can cause fetal malformation of skeleton and nervous system.
Iodine	N 150 μcg P 175 μcg L 200 μcg	Animal: Seafood. Plant: Iodized salt.	Helps control the rate of body's energy use, important in Thyroxine production. Comments: Deficiency may produce goiter in infant.

(continues)

TABLE 7.5   A NUTRIENT AND VITAMIN CHART (continued)

KEY NUTRIENT	RDI FOR AGES 23–50	IMPORTANT SOURCES	IMPORTANT FUNCTIONS
Magnesium	N 400 mg P 450 mg L 450 mg	Plant: Nuts, cocoa, green vegetables, whole grains, dried beans, peas.	Co-enzyme in energy and protein metabolism, enzyme activator, tissue growth, cell metabolism, muscle action. Comments: Most is stored in bones. Deficiency may produce neuromuscular dysfunctions.
Fat-Soluble Vitamins			
Vitamin A	N 800 RE P 1000 RE L 1200 RE	Animal: Butter, whole milk, cheese, fortified lowfat milk, liver. Plant: Fortified margarine, green and leafy vegetables, orange vegetables, fruits.	Assists formation and maintenance of skin and mucous membranes that line body cavities and tracts, such as nasal passages and intestinal tract, thus increasing resistance to infection. Essential in development of enamel-forming cells in gum tissue. Helps bone and tissue growth and cell development. Functions in visual processes, thus promoting healthy eye tissues and eye adaptation in dim light. Comments: Is toxic to the fetus in very large amounts. Can be lost with exposure to light.

Vitamin D	N 5 μcg P 10 μcg L 10 μcg	Animal: Fortified milk, fish liver oils. Plant: Fortified margarine, sun on skin.	Promotes the absorption of calcium from the digestive tract and the deposition of calcium in the structure of bones and teeth. Comments: Toxic to fetus in excessive amounts. Is a stable vitamin.
Vitamin E	N 8 mg P 10 mg L 13 mg	Vegetable oils, leafy vegetables, cereals, meat, eggs, milk.	Tissue growth, cell wall integrity, red blood cell integrity. Comments: Enhances absorption of Vitamin A.
Water-Soluble Vitamins			
B; Vitamins and folic acid	N 400 μcg P 800 μcg L 600 μcg	Liver, green leafy vegetables, yeast.	Hemoglobin synthesis, involved in DNA and RNA synthesis, co-enzyme in synthesis of amino acids. Comments: Water-soluble vitamins are interdependent on each other. Deficiency leads to anemia. Can be destroyed in cooking and storage. Supplement of 200–400 μcg/day is recommended by the National Research Council. Oral contraception use many reduce serum level of folic acid.

(continues)

TABLE 7.5 A NUTRIENT AND VITAMIN CHART (continued)

Key Nutrient	RDI for Ages 23–50	Important Sources	Important Functions
Niacin	N 13 mg P 15 mg L 18 mg	Pork, organ meats, peanuts, beans, peas, enriched grains.	Coenzyme in energy and protein metabolism. Comments: Stable; only small amounts lost in food preparation.
Riboflavin	N 1.2 mg P 1.5 mg L 1.7–1.9 mg	Animal: Milk products, liver, red meat. Plant: Enriched grains.	Aids in utilization of energy. Functions as part of a co-enzyme in the production of energy within body cells. Promotes healthy skin, eyes, and clear vision. Protein metabolism. Comments: Severe deficiencies lead to reduced growth and congenital malformations. Oral contraceptive use may reduce serum concentrations.
B1-Thiamin	N 1.0 mg P 1.4 mg L 1.5 mg	Pork, beef, liver, whole grains, legumes.	Co-enzyme in energy and protein metabolism. Comments: Its availability limits the rate at which energy from glucose is produced.
B6 Pyrodoxine	N 1.6 mg P 2.2 mg L 2.1 mg	Unprocessed cereals, grains, wheat germ, bran, nuts, seeds, legumes, corn.	Important in amino acid metabolism and protein synthesis. Fetus requires more for growth. Comments: Excessive amounts may reduce milk production in lactating women.

B12	N 2.0 μcg P 2.2 μcg L 2.6 μcg	Animal: Milk, cheese, eggs, meat, liver, fish. Plant: Fortified soy milk, cereals, meat substitutes.	Assists in the maintenance of nerve tissue. Coenzyme in protein metabolism, important in the formation of red blood cells. Comments: Deficiency leads to anemia and central nervous system damage. Is manufactured by microorganisms in intestinal tract. Oral contraceptive use may reduce serum concentrations.
Vitamin C	N 60 mg P 80 mg L 100 mg	Citrus fruits, berries, melons, tomatoes, chili peppers, green vegetables, potatoes.	Tissue formation and integrity, "cement" substance in connective and vascular substances, increases iron absorption. Comments: Large doses in pregnancy may create a larger than normal need in infant. Benefits of large doses in preventing colds have not been confirmed.

L, lactating; N, nonpregnant; P, pregnant; RDI, reference daily intake.

From Worthington-Roberts B and Williams SR. *Nutrition in Pregnancy and Lactation*, St. Louis, MO, Times Mirror/Mosby College Publishing: 1989 and *www.nal.usda.gov*.

TABLE 7.6 COMPLETE PROTEIN CASSEROLES

Directions: Choose one ingredient from each of the five columns in the table. Mix together ingredients from the first four columns. Pour into a greased 2-quart casserole dish and bake 30 minutes at 375°F. Top with one choice from column five and bake 15 minutes longer at 325°F. Salt to taste. Serve with bread and a salad.

GRAIN: 2 CUPS COOKED	BEANS: 1 CUP COOKED	SAUCE: 1 CAN SOUP AND 3/4 CUP WATER	VEGETABLES: TO MAKE 1 1/2 CUPS	TOPPINGS: TO MAKE 3 TO 5 TABLESPOONS
Brown rice	Soybeans	Cream of tomato soup	Browned celery and green onions	Wheat germ
Macaroni, enriched or whole wheat	Dried lima beans	Cream of potato soup	Mushrooms and bamboo shoots	Slivered almonds
Corn	Dried whole or split peas	Cream of mushroom soup	Browned green pepper and garlic	Fresh whole wheat bread crumbs
Spaghetti, enriched or whole wheat	Kidney beans	Cream of celery soup	Cooked green beans	Sesame seeds
White rice, converted	Lentils	Cheddar cheese soup	Cooked carrots	Chopped peanuts
Noodles, enriched, or whole wheat	Garbanzos (chickpeas)	Cream of pea soup	Browned onion and pimento	Sunflower seeds

Reprinted by permission of Nutrition Services, Allegheny County Health Department.

- Vitamin B12 is available only from animal sources
  - Vegetarian diets, particularly strict vegan diets, can be deficient in this vitamin
  - Even mothers with a low consumption of animal foods can be at risk for this deficiency
  - Low intake of Vitamin B12 by a mother leads to low levels of it in her milk
  - Be alert for the following signs in four- to eight-month-old infants that suggest a Vitamin B12 deficiency:
    - Anemia
    - Growth failure
    - Neurologic delay
    - Tremors
    - Excess skin pigmentation
  - Supplementation of Vitamin B12 during pregnancy and lactation is essential when a mother's diet limits or excludes sources of this vitamin

Weight Loss and Exercise

- A gradual loss of the excess weight accumulated during pregnancy is best
- It is suggested that a mother reduce calories by 300 per day to gradually lose weight, but to add more foods if any of the following occurs:
  - The mother begins losing weight too rapidly
  - The mother becomes easily fatigued
  - The baby does not seem satisfied at the mother's breast
- In well-nourished women, a modest reduction in calories enables gradual weight reduction and the continued and appropriate infant growth
- Well-nourished, healthy women can safely lose up to one pound (0.45 kg) per week as long as milk production continues to increase appropriately
- The loss of one pound per week is appropriate after lactation is established

- A mother's caloric intake should not go below 1800 kcal/day
- Caution mothers against liquid diets and diet medications
- Exercising is safe for most women as many as four to six times per week, and can begin six to eight weeks postpartum when a mother is breastfeeding
- An infant's acceptance of a mother's postexercise milk is not a problem in most cases
- Any mother considering a change in diet or exercise should discuss her plans with her caregiver

Properties of Human Milk

Colostrum: The Early Milk

Secretion of Colostrum
- Is thick, sticky, rich-looking, and clear to golden yellow in color
- May be secreted prenatally and for up to ten days postpartum
- In the first 24 hours, the infant takes approximately seven to fourteen ml per feeding
- Increased production over the next 36 hours until intake is approximately 500 ml in a 24-hour period by day five or six

Properties of Colostrum
- Residual mixture of materials present in the mammary glands and ducts
- Concentrated with protein suited to early and rapid newborn growth
- Contains approximately 57 kcal/100 ml (17 kcal/oz)
- Richer in sodium, potassium, chloride, protein, fat-soluble vitamins, and minerals
- Contains less fat and lactose than mature milk
- Contains many living cells that engulf and digest disease organisms

- Contains many antibodies such as the following:
  - Immune globulin A (IgA)—occurs in the highest concentration
  - Secretory IgA—obtained only through mother's milk until approximately six months of age and is not present in artificial baby milks
  - Immune globulin G (IgG)
  - Immune globulin M (IgM)

Function of Colostrum

- Aids in rapid gut closure
- Facilitates the establishment of bifidus flora that promotes the growth of beneficial bacteria
- Provides protection against pathogens such as polio, Coxsackie B virus, several types of staphylococci, and Escherichia coli
- Produces a laxative effect to aid the elimination of meconium from an infant's bowels
- Is needed in the first few days of life—a baby's kidneys are not meant to handle large fluid volumes and are put under stress by the additional water in an artificial feed that dilutes the colostrum's effects

Transition to Mature Milk

Secretion of Mature Milk

- The color and consistency of human milk varies according to the milk type and the specific additives in the mother's diet
- Transitional milk is produced approximately from seven to ten days to two weeks postpartum and it then gives way to mature milk production
- Mature human milk is secreted as approximately
  - One-third foremilk
    - Is low in fat
    - Has a thin appearance

- Collects in the lactiferous sinuses
  - Is readily available to an infant at the beginning of each feed
- Two-thirds hindmilk
  - Is much higher in fat
  - Is richer looking than foremilk
  - Contains fat that washes from the walls of the ducts and ductules as milk is let down

Appearance of Mature Milk

- Its typical bluish cast is caused by the presence of casein, which is a component of the proteins in milk
- Its greenish color is caused by additives in vitamin or iron supplements that are taken by the mother, or in rare cases, it is caused by stagnant milk from a plugged duct
- Its yellow color is caused by the presence of an excessive amount of Vitamin A—from either foods or a supplement
- Its black color can result from the use of the drug minocycline

Milk Volume

- Its volume depends on the regular removal of milk from the breast through nursing, manual expression, or pumping
- The removal of milk from the breast by a baby is the most efficient type of milk removal
- Babies can self-regulate their feeds to meet their individual needs for optimal growth
- A mother's milk supply is determined on a feed-to-feed basis through the amount of milk the baby removes each time
- The removal of milk at one feed signals the amount needed for the next feed
- Milk removal, in addition to a baby's feeds, does not decrease milk volume—in fact, it can and

probably will increase the volume due to more frequent removals
- Minor variations occur in the amount produced by each breast, the amount produced on different days, and the amount produced in response to an infant's suckling pattern
- Lactation only ceases totally in cases of extremely malnourished mothers
- The actual point in which milk volume decreases or ceases to be produced has not been determined

Composition of Human Milk

Composition Continually Changes

- Milk changes throughout lactation as a child grows
  - It varies in its sensory qualities and provides richly changing experiences in taste and odor
  - It is high in immunoglobulins and protein during the first several weeks postpartum
  - Its fat content decreases during the later months of lactation
  - It meets three-quarters or more of an infant's major nutrient needs during months six through twelve
  - Its output during the second year is equivalent to at least one 8-oz glass of milk daily and is still valuable to a toddler's diet in both quantity and composition
- Milk also changes during a feed
  - During the first four minutes, as much as 80 to 90 percent of the milk volume can be consumed, but a major portion of the high-fat milk is obtained later in that feed
  - Between the 11th and 16th minute, nearly one-sixth of the milk's calories are consumed
  - At the end of a feed, four to five times as much fat and one and a half times as much

protein are consumed than at the beginning of the feed
- No limits should be placed on the amount of time a baby is at each breast—the mother should continue to nurse until the baby decides his needs are met and ends the feed

Calories

- Colostrum contains 17 kcal/oz
- By two weeks, the average caloric content of mature human milk is 20 kcal/oz
- Around four months, the caloric content is approximately 26 kcal/oz
- Variations in the caloric content of mature milk are the result of variations in fat
- If a feed is not long enough for the infant to receive fatty hindmilk, the baby may receive only half of the available calories

Fat

- Fat provides 50 to 55 percent of an infant's energy needs
- It is the most variable of all the constituents present in human milk
  - The amount of available fat depends on a mother's body fat stores
  - Fat that is stored during pregnancy is easier to mobilize for lactation than other fat that is stored in a mother's body
  - The level of fat stored in a mother's body is lower in a severely malnourished mother, which is usually not an issue in developed countries
  - A lower fat level exists when the letdown reflex is inhibited
  - The fat content decreases after five or six months

- The following fat content changes occur within a feed as it progresses:
  - The longer the baby nurses, the higher the milk's fat content will be during that feed
  - If the fat content is low, a baby will stay at the breast longer to gain a higher fat yield
- Fatty acids
  - Linoleic and linolenic acids have significance in the quality of myelin laid down
  - Arachidonic acid (AA) from linoleic acid and docosahexaenoic acid (DHA) from linolenic acid are essential for the development of visual acuity
- If a baby is not gaining sufficient weight, the following may be occurring:
  - The baby may not be nursing long enough at each feed
  - The baby may not be nursing frequently enough throughout the day and night
- If the baby is removed from one breast too early, the following may occur:
  - The baby does not receive fatty hindmilk
  - The baby fills up on foremilk from both breasts
  - Colicky behavior and poor nourishment

Carbohydrates—Lactose

- Present in human milk in high levels (seven percent)
- Represents almost all of the carbohydrates in milk
- Provides 40 to 45 percent of energy
- Increases in concentration by approximately ten percent during the first six months of lactation
- Is slowly digested for the steady release of glucose into the bloodstream
- Is specific to newborn growth in the following ways:
  - Enhances calcium absorption, thereby helping prevent rickets
  - Helps supply energy to an infant's brain

- Helps keep in check the growth of harmful organisms in an infant's intestine
- Is essential to the development of an infant's central nervous system

Protein

- Colostrum contains about three times more protein than mature milk
- Out of all the milk produced by mammals, human milk contains the least amount of protein, which results in the slowest growth rate
- A distribution of specific proteins is ideally suited to infant growth
- Infants have the ability to use proteins with an extremely high efficiency
- The content of protein in milk seems to remain relatively constant, regardless of a mother's nutritional status or dietary practices
- Proteins are easily digested and well absorbed
- The whey (clear fluid when milk stands) to casein ratio changes throughout lactation—90:10 in early milk, 60:40 in mature milk, and 50:50 in late lactation
- **Lactoferrin**—the iron-binding protein in whey—has the following characteristics:
  - Inhibits the growth of iron-dependent bacteria (E.coli) in the gastrointestinal (GI) tract
  - Protects babies against GI infections
  - Renders intestinal iron unavailable to the pathogens in a baby's gut
  - Protects infants from infections such as salmonella, E.coli, and Candida albicans
  - May be saturated if a newborn is given an iron supplement, which enables the proliferation of E.coli
  - Does not provide its protection to a baby if he receives any other type of feeding
- **Lysozyme**—another whey protein—has the following characteristics:
  - Is one of over 20 active enzymes present in human milk

- Provides an antimicrobial factor against enterobacteriaceae and gram-positive bacteria
- Human milk contains eight essential amino acids

Vitamins

- Generally, all vitamins are available in human milk in sufficient quantities
  - Excessive maternal doses of Vitamin B6 (300 to 600 mg/day) can reduce milk production
  - Strict lacto-ovo-vegetarians may be deficient in Vitamin B12, which results in megoblastic anemia and neurologic malfunctions in infants (see Chapter 7, "Maternal Health and Nutrition," on vegetarian diets)
- **Vitamin E**
  - Colostrum is particularly rich in Vitamin E
  - Vitamin E is also highly concentrated in mature milk
  - A deficiency in infancy can result in anemia; therefore, breastfeeding is a preventive measure against anemia in infancy
- **Vitamin D**
  - Much debate occurs over an infant's need for Vitamin D supplementation
  - Circumstances that increase the risk of Vitamin D deficiency are as follows:
    - Darkly pigmented skin
    - Living in a cold climate
    - Residing in the inner city
    - A maternal vegetarian diet
    - A restricted maternal diet
  - At risk babies may require supplements and must receive sufficient sunlight—30 minutes per week wearing only a diaper or two hours per week fully clothed without a hat
- **Vitamin K**
  - Is present in small amounts, which provides an infant with that essential vitamin
  - Is routinely given to newborns by either an intramuscular injection or an oral dose to promote blood clotting

- The infant is protected through his fetal stores and the prophylactic dose given at birth until
  - He receives sufficient milk from his mother
  - His intestine matures enough to manufacture its own
- Vitamin K does not promote a greater risk for bleeding for babies who are fed human milk than those who are fed infant formula
- Increasing a mother's dietary intake is not shown to increase the amount present in her milk
- There is no current screening method that identifies babies at risk for hemorrhagic disease if not given a newborn injection of Vitamin K, therefore a source other than human milk is currently recommended
- Giving a prophylactic dose of Vitamin K appears to be the best way to offer a generalized protection to newborns

Minerals

- There is a lower percentage of minerals in human milk, as compared to cow's milk, which minimizes the fluid load on a baby's immature kidneys
- Calcium is absorbed much more efficiently from human milk
- Cow's milk has a higher mineral content and does the following:
  - Is a significant contributor to dehydration due to stressful situations such as hot weather or diarrhea
  - May require additional water intake by the infant to expel solutes
  - May cause higher weight gains because thirst is often misinterpreted as hunger and more formula is given to the baby instead of the water he needs
  - The baby experiences a sudden weight gain after switching from breastfeeding to bottle feeding due to water retention associated with increased body sodium

- Regardless of the climate where they live, babies who are exclusively breastfed do not require water supplements
- Increased feeds will satisfy the baby's need for more fluids when the climate is hot
- **Iron**
  - In the final six to eight weeks of pregnancy, a healthy nonanemic mother lays down iron stores that will provide her baby with enough iron through her milk for the first few months postpartum
  - Blood from the umbilical cord also contributes iron that an infant stores in his liver
  - Small quantities of iron in a mother's milk will meet the requirements of an exclusively breastfed, full-term infant for six months
  - Premature infants may need iron supplementation because they may not have received a sufficient quantity of iron while in utero
  - Iron is absorbed more efficiently from human milk than from cow's milk, partially due to the high Vitamin C level in human milk
  - Sixty percent of the iron in human milk is absorbed by a baby while only four percent of the iron in artificial baby milk is absorbed
  - Routine supplementation of iron is questionable because lactoferrin loses its ability to inhibit the growth of bacteria when it is saturated with iron
- **Fluoride**
  - Breastfed infants have fewer dental caries and better dental health
  - Fluoride supplements reduce the occurrence of cavities by 50 to 60 percent during the development of primary and secondary teeth
  - In communities with fluoridated drinking water, breastfed babies receive fluoride through their mother's milk
  - If the water supply contains less than 0.3 ppm (parts per million) of fluoride, fluoride supplementation is recommended after the age of six months

Other Constituents
- There are over 200 known components
  - Their complete significance has not been determined
  - Further investigation is needed
- Among the constituents are:
  - Trace elements such as copper, zinc, manganese, silicon, aluminum, and titanium
  - More than 20 human milk enzymes
  - Nitrogen compounds
  - Prostaglandins, bile salts, and epidermal growth factors
- Every mother's milk differs slightly due to individual genetic codes; thus every breastfed infant receives a totally unique product

Health Benefits of Human Milk

Immunologic Properties
- Anti-infective agents maintain a very low bacterial level within milk for many hours
  - Protect the infant and the mother's breast
  - Can destroy the bacteria in an infant's GI tract before they affect the infant
  - Components coat the infant's GI tract to prevent other offending organisms and molecules from entering
  - Protects against the following diseases—some chronic childhood diseases, Crohn's disease, juvenile diabetes, childhood lymphoma, multiple sclerosis, and heart disease
- At birth, an infant is suddenly exposed to microorganisms to which the mother is already immune
  - A mother's immunity is passed to her baby across the placenta before birth and through her colostrum and milk after birth
  - If a new microorganism is introduced, a mother will most likely produce the appropriate

antibodies and pass them to the baby through her milk
- A breast locally produces antibodies due to the organisms passed into it by a suckling infant

Anti-Infective Agents

- **IgA**
  - Protects an infant's GI tract against penetration by organisms and antigens
  - Is probably the most important antiviral defense factor
  - Is at its highest level in human milk immediately after birth
  - Remains at a continuous and significant level for at least six or seven months
- **Lymphocytes and macrophages**
  - Are living white cells
  - Engulf and digest bacteria
  - Synthesize IgA and other protective substances
- **Growth factors**
  - Enhance an infant's development
  - Enhance the maturation of the immune system, the central nervous system, and organs such as skin
- **Lactase and lipase**
  - Are digestive enzymes
  - Protect babies born with immature or defective enzyme systems
- **Lysozyme**—Breaks up bacteria in the bowel
- **Bifidus factor**
  - Works with the low pH of stools
  - Helps special bacteria grow in an infant's intestine
  - Prevents other harmful bacteria from growing
- **Mucins**
  - Protect against bacterial infections, including neonatal sepsis and meningitis
  - Protect against rotavirus

- **Oligosaccharides**—Protect against urinary tract infections in both the child and mother
- **Thyroid hormones**
  - Contains three essential thyroid hormones which are not present in cow's milk and conventional infant formulas
  - May prevent hypothyroidism, mask diagnosis, and protect a baby until weaning
- See Tables 8.1, 8.2 and 8.3

Protection for the Infant

- **Otitis Media**
  - Exclusive breastfeeding for at least four months appears to be the best protection against otitis media
  - After weaning, the protection is still at work—even four months after breastfeeding stops, the risk of otitis media is lower
- **Necrotizing Enterocolitis (NEC) and Sepsis**
  - NEC is six to ten times more likely to occur in artificially fed babies
  - NEC is 20 times higher for babies fed artificial baby milk (ABM) who are born after 30 weeks' gestation
  - NEC is three times more likely to occur in babies who receive mixed feeds than in those who are exclusively breastfed
  - The incidence of nosocomial sepsis is decreased in hospitalized breastfed babies
- **Maternal antigens**
  - When a mother contracts an infection, her body responds by producing antibodies in her milk that help protect her breastfed baby
  - Some viruses may be transmitted through human milk
  - The presence of antibodies counteracts the virus, offsetting the potential harm to the baby

TABLE 8.1 ANTIBACTERIAL FACTORS FOUND IN HUMAN MILK

Factor	Shown In Vitro to Be Active Against
Secretory IgA	E. coli (also pili, capsular antigens, CFA1), C. tetani, C. diphtheriae, K. Pneumoniae, S. mutans, S. sanguins, S. mitis, S. agalactiae, S. salvarius, S. pneumoniae, C. burnetti, H. influenza. H. pylori, S. flexneri, S. boydii, S. sonnei, C. jejuni, N. meningitidis, B. pertussis, S. dysenteriae, C. trachomatis, Salmonella (six groups), Campylobacter flagelin, S. flexneri virulence plasmid antigen, C. diphtheriae toxin, E. coli enterotoxin, V. cholerae enterotoxin, C. difficile toxins, H. influenza capsule, S. aureus enterotoxin F, Candida albicans
IgG	E. coli, B. pertussis, H. influenza type b, S. pneumoniae, S. agalactiae, N. meningitidis, 14 pneumococcal capsular polysaccharides, V. cholerae lipopolysaccharide, S. flexneri invasion plasmid–coded antigens, major opsonin for S. aureus
IgM	V. cholerae lipopolysaccharide
IgD	E. coli
Free secretory component*	E. coli colonization factor antigen I (CFA1)
Bifidobacterium bifidum	Enteric bacteria
Growth factors (oligosaccharides, glycopeptides)	
Other Bifidobacteria growth factors (alpha-lactoglobulin, lactoferrin, sialyllactose)	
Factor-finding proteins (zinc, vitamin B12, folate)	Dependent E. coli

Complement C1-C9 (mainly C3 and C4)	Killing of S. aureus in macrophages
Lactoferrin*	E. coli, E. coli/CFA1, Candida albicans
Lactoperoxidase	Streptococcus, Pseudomonas, E. coli, S. typhimurium
Lysozyme fumigatus	E. coli, Salmonella, M. lysodeikticus, growing Candida albicans and Aspergillus fumigatus
Unidentified factors	S. aureus, B. pertussis, C. jejuni, E. coli, S. typhimurium, S. flexneri, S. sonnei, V. cholerae, L. pomona, L. hyos, L. icterohaemorrhagiae, C. difficile toxin B, H. pylori
Nonimmunoglobulin (milk fat, proteins)	C. trachomatis, Y. enterocolitica
Carbohydrate	E. coli enterotoxin, E. coli, C. difficile toxin A
Lipid	S. aureus, E. coli, S. epidermis, H. influenzae, S. agalactiae
Ganglioside GM_1	E. coli enterotoxin, V. cholerae toxin, C. jejuni enterotoxin, E. coli
Ganglioside GM_3	E. coli
Phosphatidylethanolamine	H. pylori
Sialyllactose	V. cholerae toxin, H. pylori
Mucin (milk fat adhesion globulin membrane)	E. coli (S-fimbrinated) sialyloligosaccharides on sIgA(Fc) E. coli (S-fimbrinated)
Glycoproteins (receptor-like) + oligosaccharides	V. cholerae
Glycoproteins (mannosylated)	E. coli
kappa-Casein*	H. pylori, S. pneumoniae

(continues)

TABLE 8.1 ANTIBACTERIAL FACTORS FOUND IN HUMAN MILK (continued)

Casein	H. influenza
Glycolipid Gb$_3$	S. dysenterae toxin, shigatoxin of shigella and E. coli
Fucosylated oligosaccharides	E. coli heat-stable enterotoxin, C. jejuni, E. coli
Analogues of epithelial cell receptors (oligosaccharides)	S. pneumoniae, H. influenza
Milk cells (macrophages, neutrophils, B and T lymphocytes)	By phagocytosis and killing: *E. coli, S. aureus, S. enteritidis* By sensitized lymphocytes: *E. coli* By phagocytosis: *Candida albicans***,***, *E. coli* Lymphocyte stimulation: *E. coli*, K antigen, tuberculin Spontaneous monokines: Simulated by lipopolysaccaride Induced cytokines: PHA, PMA + ionomycin Fibronectin helps in uptake by phagocytic cells

*Factors found at low level in human milk can be antibacterial at higher levels, for example, secretory leukocyte protease inhibitor (antileukocyte protease) has antibacterial (E. coli, S. aureus) and antifungal (growing C. albicans and A. fumigatus) activity.

**Fungi.

***Contain fucosylated oligosaccharides.

TABLE 8.2 ANTIVIRAL FACTORS FOUND IN HUMAN MILK

Factor	Shown In Vitro to Be Active Against
Secretory IgA	Polio types, 1, 2, 3. Coxsackie types A9, B3, B5, echo types 6, 9, Semliki Forest virus, Ross River virus, rotavirus, cytomegalovirus, reovirus type 3, rubella varicella-zoster virus, herpes simplex virus, mumps virus, influenza, respiratory syncytial virus, human immunodeficiency virus, hepatitis C virus, hepatitis B virus, measles
IgG	Rubella, cytomegalovirus, respiratory syncytial virus, rotavirus, human immunodeficiency virus, Epstein-Barr virus
IgM	Rubella, cytomegalovirus, respiratory syncytial virus, human immunodeficiency virus
Lipid (unsaturated fatty acids and monoglycerides)	Herpes simplex virus, Semliki Forest virus, influenza, dengue, Ross River virus, Japanese B encephalitis virus, sindbis, West Nile, human immunodeficiency virus, respiratory syncytial virus, vesicular stomatitis virus
Non-immunoglobulin macromolecules	Herpes simplex virus, vesicular stomatitis virus, Coxsackie B4, Semliki Forest virus, reovirus 3, poliotype 2, cytomegalovirus, respiratory syncytial virus, rotavirus

(continues)

TABLE 8.2 ANTIVIRAL FACTORS FOUND IN HUMAN MILK (continued)

Alpha2-macroglobulin (like)	Influenza haemagglutinin, parainfluenza haemagglutinin
Ribonuclease	Murine leukaemia
Haemagglutinin inhibitors	Influenza, mumps
Mucin (glycoprotein/lactadherin)	Rotavirus
Chondroitin sulphate (-like)	Human immunodeficiency virus
Secretory leukocyte protease inhibitor (colostrum levels)	Human immunodeficiency virus, Bifidobacterium bifidum, Rotavirus
sIgA + trypsin inhibitor	Rotavirus
Lactoferrin	Cytomegalovirus, human immunodeficiency virus, respiratory syncytial virus, herpes simplex virus type 1, hepatitis C
	Induced interferon: Virus, PHA, or PMA and ionomycin
	Induced cytokine: Herpes simplex virus, respiratory syncytial virus
Milk cells	Lymphocyte stimulation: Rubella, cytomegalovirus, herpes, measles, mumps, respiratory syncytial virus

Factors found at low levels in human milk, known to be antiviral at higher levels:
Prostaglandins E2, F2 alpha (parainfluenza 3, measles)
Gangliosides GM1-3 (rotavirus, respiratory syncytial virus)
Heparin (cytomegalovirus, respiratory syncytial virus)
Glycolipid Gb4 (human B19 parvovirus)

TABLE 8.3 ANTIPARASITIC FACTORS FOUND IN HUMAN MILK

Factor	Shown In Vitro to Be Active Against
Secretory IgA	Giardia lamblia
	Entamoeba histolytica
	Schistosoma mansoni (blood fluke)
	Cryptosporidium
	Toxoplasma gondii
	Plasmodium falciparum (malaria)
IgG	Plasmodium falciparum
Lipid (free fatty acids and monoglycerides)	Giardia lamblia
	Entamoeba histolytica
	Trichomonas vaginalis
	Giardia intestinalis
	Eimeria tenella (animal coccidiosis)
Unidentified	Trypanosoma brucei rhodesiense

Tables 8.1, 8.2, and 8.3 from Proceedings of Breast Milk and Special Care Nurseries: Problems and Opportunities Conference. Melbourne, August 1995. Copyright J. T. May and Australian Lactation Consultants Association Victorian Branch, 1995. Updated August, 1998. Reprinted by permission of the Department of Microbiology, La Trobe University, Australia.

- **Immunizations**
  - The research responses of breastfed babies somewhat vary
  - Breastfed and artificially fed infants have similar levels of protection after immunization
  - Infants who are fed human milk have better immune response to immunizations

Allergy Protection

- When an infant is fed human milk, the GI tract develops more quickly and prevents foreign proteins from entering the infant's system
- Even giving babies a single feeding of ABM in their first days of life can increase the rates of allergic disease
- All formulas, including soy formulas, carry the risk of being an allergen
- Cow's milk is the most common food allergen in infants
- Three-fourths of cow's milk allergies begin in the first two months of life
- Allergy symptoms are more prevalent in infants who are fed a cow's milk-based formula than in breastfed infants
- Almost no antibodies exist in the immature intestines of a newborn
  - Human milk contains high levels of antibodies, especially IgA
  - Human milk is thought to provide anti-absorptive protection on the lining of the infant's intestines
- Breastfeeding does not totally eliminate food allergies, but it greatly reduces their incidence and delays their onset
- Infants may show the following symptoms in response to foods that are ingested by their mothers:
  - Spitting
  - Vomiting
  - Gas
  - Diarrhea
  - Colic-like behavior
  - Skin rash

Human Milk for the Premature Infant

- The milk of women who deliver prematurely contains a higher concentration of sodium, chloride, nitrogen, and immunoprotective factors

- Giving human milk to premature infants can help prevent NEC and improve their neurodevelopment
- The consumption of human milk is associated with higher IQ scores during childhood
- There is much debate about the special needs of premature babies
  - One issue is whether it is necessary to supplement a mother's milk
  - Much emphasis has been placed on keeping up with the missed intrauterine growth by increasing protein and energy in a preterm diet
  - Optimal brain growth is often not considered
  - The composition of human milk and how it relates to preterm diet needs is not yet well understood
- Human milk has ideal protein balance for babies who weigh 1500 g or more (about 3 lbs, 5 oz)
- Mother's milk is not considered to be adequate as a sole source of nutrition for babies who weigh less than 1500 g
  - Supplements of protein, calcium, and potassium phosphate may be needed in these cases
  - If an infant's diet is not supplemented, they may experience fractures of the long bones during rapid growth phases
  - Supplements should be used with caution—some additives have an adverse effect on the anti-infective properties of human milk

Impurities in Human Milk

Secretion of Substances into Milk

- In most cases, substances are secreted in low concentrations
- Secreted substances usually pose no danger to an infant
- The infant may experience adverse effects if the contaminants are not altered or eliminated by his GI system

Effects of Contaminants on the Breastfeeding Infant
- Almost any substance present in the mother's blood is present in some amount in her milk
- Medication that is considered safe to take during pregnancy is not necessarily safe to take during lactation
  - During pregnancy, the mother's liver and kidneys detoxify and excrete substances for a fetus via the placenta
  - During lactation an infant must handle a drug totally on his own after it has reached his circulation
- See Figure 8.1

Giving Advice about Medications
- Few drugs are contraindicated in breastfeeding
- Only one to two percent of a dose of medication will cross into a mother's milk
- Although a drug can be safe for a fetus and breastfeeding infant, it could affect the mother in the following ways:
  - Letdown reflex
  - Milk production
  - Milk secretion
- The effects of medications can be minimized in the following ways:
  - Selecting a less offensive drug
  - Scheduling to take a drug so that the least possible amount of it gets into the milk
  - Taking the drug immediately after nursing or three to four hours before the next feed
  - Avoiding breastfeeding when the drug is at its peak level in the milk
  - Avoiding medications with a long plasma half-life
- If a medication is untested for safety during lactation, weigh the options with the baby's physician
- See Table 8.4

> Factors to consider in the infant's exposure
> - Size of the molecules in the substance
> - Solubility of the substance in water or fat (diffuses more easily into milk)
> - Binding capacity of the substance with protein
> - pH of the substance
> - The milk/plasma ratio
> - Route of administration (oral, **intramuscular**, **intravenous**)
> - Short or long-acting version of the drug
> - Activity or inactivity of components of the substance
> - Rate of detoxification in the mother's system
> - Whether the substance accumulates in the mother's system
> - Duration of use
> - Time the substance is ingested relative to the feed
> - Number of days postpartum when the substance is consumed
> - Age and size of the infant (premature, fullterm, older baby)
> - Amount of milk the infant consumes (exclusively breastfed or supplemented)
> - Absorption of the substance in the infant's gut
> - Safety in giving the substance to the infant directly

Figure 8.1 An infant's exposure to substances secreted in human milk

- The IBCLC's role regarding medications
  - Encourage mothers to take responsibility for their decisions and actions
  - Help mothers pose questions
  - Present drug information objectively and cite references for such information to avoid placing yourself in a vulnerable legal position
  - Do not deviate from facts or attempt to interpret information

- Ask the following questions to obtain information from mothers to clarify situations:
  - Does she feel she needs the drug, or can she choose an alternative course
  - Can other safer drugs or procedures be substituted
  - Do the benefits of the drug outweigh the possible risk to her baby
  - Does exposure to the drug pose less of a risk to the baby than use of ABM
  - Would another medical opinion be helpful
- Not share personal experiences or opinions that conflict with research
- Use recommended sources such as *Medications and Mother's Milk* by Hale (1999) and *Drugs in Pregnancy and Lactation* by Briggs, Freeman, and Yaffe (1998)

Social Toxicants

- **Nicotine and tobacco**
  - Children of parents who smoke in the home are more susceptible to respiratory ailments
  - Second-hand exposure has been linked to an increased incidence of otitis media
  - If the mother smokes immediately before feeding her baby and she smokes 20 cigarettes daily, the following can possibly occur:
    - Nausea and vomiting in her baby
    - Diminished milk secretion
    - Lower fat concentration in her milk
    - An inhibited letdown reflex
    - Slower weight gain in her baby
  - See Chapter 7 for further discussion
- **Caffeine**
  - Infants react to their mothers' consuming six to eight servings of caffeinated beverages daily, and these symptoms will disappear within one week after caffeine is discontinued
  - Caution mothers against a high intake of herbal teas as a substitute for caffeinated

drinks—they may contain active ingredients that can be secreted into human milk and cause toxic effects in infants
- Cathartics such as buckhorn bark and senna may cause cramps and diarrhea in infants
- Camomile tea may sensitize an infant to ragweed pollen and cause an allergic reaction
- See Chapter 7 for further discussion
- **Alcohol**
  - An infant can have psychomotor scores one standard deviation below the mean when mothers consume at least four drinks daily
  - Babies will consume less milk after their mothers ingest alcohol
  - Excessive amounts of alcohol completely block the release of oxytocin and prevent letdown from occurring
  - One or two drinks socially is not a contraindication for breastfeeding; the mother can breastfeed when she feels normal again
  - See Chapter 7 for further discussion
- **Drugs of abuse**
  - Breastfeeding mothers should be advised to avoid all drugs of abuse
  - The AAP Committee on Drugs considers the following drugs of abuse to be contraindicated during breastfeeding: Amphetamines, cocaine, heroin, marijuana, and phencyclidine hydrochloride (angel dust)
  - There is concern about a mother's ability to care for her infant when she is abusing drugs
  - Mothers intending to breastfeed are more likely to decrease or stop their substance abuse
  - **Marijuana**
    - Can have a direct effect on a mother's ability to produce sufficient quantities of milk
    - There are no untoward effects on breastfed babies

TABLE 8.4 MEDICATIONS FOR THE BREASTFEEDING MOTHER

Breastfeeding is contraindicated	Anticancer drugs (antimetabolites)
	Radioactive substances (stop breastfeeding temporarily)
Continue breastfeeding: Side effects are possible; monitor the baby for drowsiness	Psychiatric drugs and anticonvulsants
Continue breastfeeding: Use an alternative drug, if possible	Chloramphenicol, tetracyclines, metronidazole
	Quinolone antibiotics (e.g., ciprofloxacin)
Continue breastfeeding: Monitor the baby for jaundice	Sulphonamides, dapsone
	Sulfamethoxazole + trimethoprim (co-trimoxazole)
Continue breastfeeding: Use an alternative drug (may inhibit lactation)	Estrogens (including estrogen-containing contraceptives)
	Thiazide diuretics
	Ergometrine

Continue breastfeeding: Safe in the usual dosage; monitor the baby	Most commonly used drugs Analgesics and antipyretics: Short courses of paracetamol, acetylsalicylic acid, ibuprofen; occasional doses of morphine and pethidine Antibiotics: Ampicillin, amoxacillin, cloxacillin and other penicillins; Erythromycin Antituberculars, antileporotics (see dapsone earlier) Antimalarials (except mefloquine, anthelminthics, antifungals) Bronchodilators (e.g., salbutamol), corticosteroids, antihistamines, antacids, drugs for diabetes, most antihypertensives, digoxin Nutritional supplements of iron, iodine, and vitamins

Source: *Breastfeeding and Maternal Medication, Recommendations for Drugs in the Eight WHO Model List of Essential Drugs, Division of Diarrheal and Acute Respiratory Disease Control*, UNICEF/WHO, 1995. Printed with permission.

- **Heroin**
  - Passes to an infant through a mother's milk
  - May lead to increased sleepiness, a poor appetite, an undernourished baby, uncoordinated and ineffective suckling reflexes, tremors, restlessness, and vomiting
- **Cocaine**
  - Is a powerful central nervous stimulant with a plasma half-life of about 30 minutes
  - Is metabolized and excreted slowly over a prolonged period of time
  - Causes irritability, jitteriness, tremors, and increased heart and respiratory rate in infants
  - After the effects of cocaine have subsided, a mother's milk is likely to contain significant quantities of benzoecgonine—an inactive metabolite of cocaine
  - Mothers can be advised to pump and dump their milk for 24 hours after ingestion of cocaine

Breast Implants

- The compound used in breast implants—polydimethylsiloxane (PDMS)—was not found in a few samples of milk from mothers with implants
- Mylicon drops, which contain PDMS, are frequently recommended for infant colic
- Greater amounts of silicone are found in other substances, such as cow's milk formulas

Environmental Contaminants

- Studies continue on environmental pollutants found in human milk and lead to the conclusion that there is no firm scientific basis for advising against breastfeeding
- The benefits of breastfeeding far outweigh the possible danger of contaminants

- Women returning to work are increasingly exposed to chemical pollutants
- The following guidelines will help reduce exposure:
  - Limit the use of domestic sprays such as pesticides and household cleaners
  - Limit the consumption of freshwater fish due to chemical wastes washed into and concentrated in lakes and streams
  - Avoid fatty meats and remove excess fat
  - Thoroughly wash or peel fresh fruits and vegetables
  - Avoid crash diets that release accumulated toxic substances that are stored in body fat
  - Avoid occupations involving possible chemical exposure
  - Avoid permanently moth-proofed garments that may contain dieldrin—a chemical absorbed through skin

Artificial Feeding

Risks of Artificial Baby Milk

- Artificial feeding is referred to as one of "the largest uncontrolled in vivo experiments in human history"
- The United States is not immune to the dangers of artificial milks
- Incorrect and inadequate use of infant formula accounts for about one million deaths every year worldwide
- See Table 8.5

Deficiencies and Contaminants in Infant Formula

- Can contain micronutrients or macronutrients in either excessive or deficient amounts
- May completely lack essential elements
- May contain contaminants
- Are deficient in the essential fatty acids necessary for proper brain development and visual acuity

TABLE 8.5   HEALTH RISKS ASSOCIATED WITH ARTIFICIAL FEEDING

HEALTH RISK AS IDENTIFIED IN STUDIES	RATIOS REPORTED IN STUDIES NOT BREASTFED : BREASTFED
Infants are hospitalized more often.	15:1 and 10:1 (two studies)
Infants get sick more often and when sick they are more sick.	21:8
Infants are more likely to get certain childhood cancers	6:1 and 8:1 (two studies)
Gastroenteritis is more common in infants.	6:1
Infants are more likely to suffer from ulcerative colitis and Crohn's Disease.	3:1
Infants have more bronchitis and pneumonia.	5:1 and 2:1 (two studies)
Infants are more likely to die from SIDS.	3:1 and 5:1 (two studies)
Premature infants are more likely to develop necrotizing enterocolitis (NEC).	20:1
Infants are more likely to develop juvenile diabetes that requires insulin each day.	2:1 and 7:1 (two studies)
Women are at a greater risk for breast cancer.	2:1
Women are at a greater risk for ovarian cancer.	1.6:1

- Cannot currently replicate human milk's complex fatty acid pattern—even after adding fats derived from a variety of sources such as fish heads, egg yolks, and genetically engineered marine algae
- May contain excessive concentrations of Vitamin D, which is toxic in high doses
- May be deficient in chloride
- May be contaminated with aluminum
- May contain bacteria, which can cause sepsis and meningitis; frequently occurs in powdered formula

Infant and Maternal Health Risks

- IQ levels may be eight points lower in formula-fed babies than in breastfed babies
- One bottle of formula can change a baby's gut flora for three weeks
- Digestion of cow's milk sensitizes a baby to the proteins found in cow's milk
- Feeding an infant cow's milk can provoke an allergy later during re-exposure
- Feeding soy formulas to female infants can change their menstrual patterns later in life
- Women who do not breastfeed have an increased risk of osteoporosis

Dangers in Preparation of Formula

- Mothers may attempt to stretch a supply by diluting it, which can lead to water intoxication and seizures
- Mothers may not have access to refrigeration, clean water, or adequate waste facilities
- Infants are at a greater risk for lead intoxication from a water source
- Infants are susceptible to methemoglobinemia from water that contains nitrate
- Mothers may not mix formula correctly—they may be undereducated and may not understand directions well enough to mix formula properly
- Even when formula is mixed according to its directions, it may have wide variations in its final composition

- The formula's composition in the can may not be totally uniform when its milk source varies from season to season
- Formula powders can pack down in the can, resulting with one scoop of powder containing a greater or lesser quantity of powder by weight
- The mother may fail to wash the formula can and can opener, thus leaving behind residue from pesticides and animal droppings

Impact of Formula Use on the Family
- The following are examples of the economic burden of purchasing formula and feeding equipment:
  - In the United States, formula use can cost over $1400 annually
  - Women and family members will often go hungry because their food money is spent on artificial formulas and medications to deal with increased sickness resulting from formula use
- The mother experiences an earlier return of fertility, shorter birth intervals, maternal depletion, a higher number of pregnancies, and earlier maternal death
- Mothers are at increased risk for developing premenopausal breast cancer, ovarian cancer, and osteoporosis
- There is a loss of time and convenience

Impact of Formula Use on the Community
- Its production consumes valuable land and resources
- Production errors create a burden on society as a whole
- It uses fuel distribution and disposal, thus using additional resources
- It contributes to environmental pollution
- Researchers are burdened by an ever-increasing need to improve infant formulas
- The use of formulas monopolizes time and resources that could be used productively for

unavoidable health concerns, to help women breastfeed, and to make safe human milk available for those infants whose mothers cannot provide it
- Using formula is an expenditure of health care workers' time for the education of parents in the proper use of infant formula
- Using formula also is an expenditure of the parents' time in caring for children who are acutely and chronically ill due to the lack of human milk intake
- The increase in health care dollars is passed along to the consumer

Choosing and Preparing an Artificial Baby Milk
- Investigate the allergy history of the entire family
- Make the choice of a human milk substitute with the baby's physician
- Consider a family's circumstances when deciding the choice between using ready-to-feed, concentrated, or powdered formulas (i.e., finances, storage, and water)
- Pay careful attention to the expiration dates and label instructions of formulas
- Record the lot number of each can in the event of a recall or class action lawsuit
- Use only clean or sterile utensils because the baby is not receiving infection protection from human milk
- Wash the formula cans thoroughly to remove all residue from their storage and handling
- Open the can from the bottom—it is less susceptible to pesticide sprays than the top
- For the safety of formula
  - Discard any concentrate after 48 hours
  - Discard all formula mixed from a powder after 24 hours
  - Discard all formula after it has been nonrefrigerated for one hour
  - Discard any unused portion when a feeding is finished to prevent contamination

9

Prenatal Considerations

Making the Decision to Breastfeed

Caregiver's Influence
- Caregivers need to adopt an attitude that assumes that all pregnant women intend to breastfeed unless they indicate otherwise
- The IBCLC can help clear up any misconceptions about breastfeeding

Facts that Correct Misconceptions about Breastfeeding
- Breastfed babies seem to display more independence because their needs are met
- Breastfeeding is less work than bottle feeding
- A well-nourished woman produces the amount of milk her baby needs
- The breastfeeding experience of the woman's mother has no bearing on her own ability to breastfeed
- Every mother's milk is ideally suited to her own baby
- Breast size has no bearing on the ability to produce sufficient milk
- Breastfeeding can be calming to a high-strung woman
- A breastfeeding baby generally tolerates the same foods his mother tolerates

- Mothers who deliver by cesarean birth have the ability to breastfeed
- All mothers find caring for their newborn infant tiring, regardless of the feeding method used
- Breastfeeding enables a mother to relax during feeding times, and she actually gets more rest than a mother who bottle feeds her baby
- Breastfeeding seems to be nature's way of ensuring that a mother gets the rest she needs postpartum
- The caloric demands of breastfeeding can help mothers control their weight
- Breastfeeding involves much more than human milk—it is a dynamic process that provides a bonding relationship between a mother and her baby
- Mothers who are separated from their babies have many options for breastfeeding

Preparation for Breastfeeding

Learning about Breastfeeding

- A woman's attentiveness and retention of information may be greater in the later months of her pregnancy
  - Focus early discussions on the decision-making processes
  - Discuss practical aspects of breastfeeding management closer to the time that she will deliver
  - See Figure 9.1
- Encourage women to attend breastfeeding classes
  - Keep classes simple
  - Address attitudes and expectations
  - Mothers recall the impressions they gain in class:
    - Health benefits
    - Ease of breastfeeding
    - Risks of not breastfeeding
  - Encourage parents to trust their instincts and to respond to their baby's cues

- How does she feel about the prospect of breastfeeding?
- What practical knowledge does she have about breastfeeding?
- What prior experience or exposure does she have to breastfeeding?
- How many friends or relatives have breastfed?
- What reading has she done on breastfeeding? What videos has she seen?
- Has she attended a breastfeeding information class?
- Is she attending prepared childbirth classes?
- What has her physician discussed with her about breastfeeding?
- What has she done to prepare for breastfeeding?
- Has she checked for inverted nipples?
- What has she learned about breast care?
- What clothing does she have that will allow her baby easy access to her breast?
- What arrangements has she made for help at home
- Does she plan to have rooming-in if she is delivering in a hospital?
- Is she interested in attending group discussions with other breastfeeding mothers?
- What are her specific concerns or questions?

Figure 9.1 Questions to ask pregnant women about breastfeeding

- Teach parents that there are no rules in breastfeeding except the following:
  - Babies must gain weight appropriately
  - Mothers must be comfortable in the process
- Reinforce learning with handouts and visual aids
- Invite breastfeeding parents to class to talk about their recent experiences

- Help parents focus on the positive aspects of breastfeeding—consider it a learning process for both mother and baby
- Advertise the class as an infant feeding class rather than a breastfeeding class
  - Makes it clear that the class is open to everyone
  - Encourages fathers to attend
- See Figures 9.2 and 9.3

Prenatal Breast Care

- Determine whether the mother's nipples will need assistance for a good latch
- Perform the pinch test near the beginning of the third trimester (see Chapter 19, "Breastfeeding Techniques and Devices")
- Decide on and discuss nipple correction as follows:
  - Discuss with a physician his advice on nipple preparation, breast foreplay, and intercourse
  - If the mother has a history of premature delivery, tendency toward miscarriage, or severe false labor, nipple stimulation may induce labor
  - Discuss the use of breast shells and inverted syringes (see Chapter 19)
  - Discuss the following aspects of removing colostrum prenatally
    - Colostrum acts as a barrier to bacteria and viruses
    - Removing it leaves the breasts susceptible to invasion and possible infection and may deprive the baby of colostrum
    - Removing it may cause the breasts to become uncomfortably full with colostrum (infrequent)
    - Women can gently express only to the point of comfort
  - If the breasts leak, the woman can gently blend the colostrum into areola
  - Moisten the bra with warm water before removing it if colostrum causes the bra to stick to the nipple

- Welcome and Introductions (5 minutes)
- Risks to the mother and baby of not breastfeeding (class discussion—15 minutes)
- What is Infant formula? (15 minutes)
  - Its use and overuse (lecture and discussion)
  - What our culture says about formula (class discussion)
  - What our culture says about breasts (class discussion)
- How we were fed (15 minutes)
  - Our parents and grandparents did their best at that time (lecture and discussion)
  - Guilt for us and those around us (lecture)
  - How guilt helps us (lecture)
- Break (10 minutes)
- Our babies (10 minutes)
  - Speaking their language (lecture)
    - Sleep states
    - Feeding cues
  - What the human baby needs (lecture and discussion)
    - Relating the baby's nutritional needs and growth to adult eating patterns
    - Relating baby's nighttime needs to the adult's needs
- Breastfeeding basics (30 minutes)
  - Milk supply (lecture)
    - Milk removed is replaced
    - Getting started, rooming-in, and the first week
    - How to know the baby is getting enough nourishment
    - Feeding diary
  - Positions for the mom and baby (lecture and video)
    - Basics: How to achieve good position and why it is important
    - Options
    - Comfort
  - Attachment and suckling (lecture and video)
    - Why it is important
    - How good positioning helps
    - Steps to a good latch
    - Normal suckling
- Breastfeeding myths you may hear (lecture and discussion—10 minutes)
- How to find breastfeeding help and why you may need it (lecture—10 minutes)

Used with permission of Debbie Shinskie

Figure 9.2 Sample Outline for a Prenatal Breastfeeding Class

- Welcome and Introductions (5 minutes)
- Breastfeeding's continued importance (lecture and discussion—15 minutes)
  - Review of the risks of not breastfeeding
  - AAP breastfeeding recommendations
- A growing baby's milestones and issues (lecture and discussion—20 minutes)
  - Growth spurts
  - Crying
  - Sleep
  - New abilities
  - Teething
- New parents' issues (lecture, discussion and video—20 minutes)
  - Resuming activities, prioritizing, and not overdoing
  - Ideas for including the baby
  - Staying healthy—rest, diet, and exercising
- Break (10 minutes)
- Returning to work or school (lecture, hands-on, and discussion—30 minutes)
  - Options
  - Planning ahead—talk with the employer and prioritize needs
  - How you will feed the baby in your absence
  - Pumps and other devices
  - Troubleshooting and realistic expectations
- The family table and weaning (lecture and discussion—10 minutes)
- Where to find breastfeeding help (lecture—10 minutes)

Used with permission of Debbie Shinskie

Figure 9.3 A sample outline for a postpartum breastfeeding class

Practices to Avoid for Healthy Breasts

- Using soap or other drying agents on the nipples and areola
- Using plastic liners in breast pads
- Using artificial lubricants (unless needed)

- Using lubricants that do not enable skin to breathe or that cannot be washed off (read labels on lotions and creams carefully)
- Expressing colostrum prenatally
- Rubbing the nipples with a towel or washcloth
- Wearing tight, restrictive clothing

Practical Planning Suggestions for Breastfeeding

- Suggestions for a nursing area
  - Choose a quiet spot where the mother can relax undisturbed for 20 minutes or more at a time
  - Have several pillows available for finding a comfortable position
  - Have a comfortable chair with armrests to help support the baby during feeds
  - Have a footstool to raise the mother's knees for additional support
  - Have a small table within arm's reach
  - Have a location for beverages, snacks, and reading materials
- Clothing suggestions
  - Tops that cover the mother's upper torso and enable the baby easy access to the breast (the baby will cover the mother's lower chest and abdomen)
    - Outfits that are loose-fitting and opened midway
    - Two-piece outfits
    - Pullovers
    - Sweaters
  - Dresses with front or side openings
  - Blouses that button in the front with the bottom unbuttoned
  - A sweater, jacket, blanket, or diaper draped over the exposed area
  - Half slips
  - Front-opening gowns or pajamas
  - Dark-patterned materials that will hide milk leakage
  - Natural fiber materials for comfort

- Suggestions for a nursing bra
  - Select one during the last trimester of pregnancy
  - Select one that provides support and does not bind
  - Underwires and elastic around the cups can prevent sufficient drainage by pressing on milk ducts
  - Seams need to be situated well past the front of the breast, toward the underarm
  - Should be a cotton or cotton-polyester blend
  - Breast pads, handkerchiefs, or diapers can be placed inside the bra to absorb leaking
  - Should provide easy access for feeds with simple cup fasteners
  - Practice unfastening and fastening the bra to see if it is manageable with one hand
  - Velcro fasteners, although convenient, are sometimes noisy
  - Initially buy only one to decide whether it meets her needs
- Planning for help at home
  - Have the father at home for several days while the mother and baby get settled in
  - Clarify the roles of the potential helpers before accepting any offers of assistance
    - Help the mother relax, rest, and care for her baby
    - Understand that the parents will be caring for and bonding with their baby
    - Help with household tasks, running errands, and ensuring that the mother is well rested and well nourished
- Sleeping arrangements
  - Keeping the baby in the parents' bed or in a separate bed in the same room facilitates nighttime feeds as follows:
    - The mother will need to make only minor adjustments for her baby to latch on
    - Limits the disruptions so that the mother and baby will quickly return to sleep

- If parents do not wish for the baby to remain in their bed, they may do the following:
    - Place an extra bed or mattress on the floor in the baby's room
    - When the baby falls asleep after nursing, the mother can return to her own bed
- See Chapter 11, "Infant Assessment and Behavior," for further discussion

Physician for the Mother and Baby

Factors to Explore When Selecting a Physician

- Parents need to be comfortable and secure in their decision
    - They should be confident in their physician's abilities
    - The parents and physician should be able to develop an adult working relationship
    - The physician must be willing to listen, respond to questions, and demonstrate flexibility
    - The parents must be able to form a partnership with their physician in order to develop a health plan for the most favorable outcome
- The physician's background can be explored in the following ways:
    - Contact local hospitals
    - Request information from the physician's receptionist
    - Call the county medical society
    - Question friends who use the physician's services
- The physician's continuing education
    - Materials present in his office such as recently published books and information about breastfeeding management
    - Any continuing education in breastfeeding
    - Any other activities the physician takes part in such as teaching at a nearby hospital or medical school
- Hospital affiliation

- Physician's accessibility
  - Can parents' questions be answered by a phone consultation
  - Who handles phone questions
  - For pressing medical concerns, can parents speak directly with the physician after describing the problem to the nurse
  - Is coverage provided by someone who is acceptable to the parents
- Standing orders
  - What are the physician's standing orders for all newborns
  - If developing a plan different from standing orders or nursing protocol, a physician should do the following:
    - Ensure the parents' wishes are observed by putting it in writing
    - Have a copy of their wishes signed by both the parents and physician
    - Have copies available to the parents, physicians, and hospitals
- The physician's relationships with patients
  - Does the physician genuinely listen to patients
  - Does the physician give understandable explanations
  - Does the physician welcome all questions
  - Does the physician return calls
  - Does the physician openly discuss alternatives
  - Does the physician welcome second opinions

Recommending Physicians

- Give the names of at least three physicians, when possible
- Give factual and practical information, not personal opinion
- Provide pertinent questions to ask a prospective physician

Questions to Ask the Baby's Physician

- How soon after birth will the first office visit be scheduled
- How many times does the physician expect to see the baby for health maintenance
- Does the physician have staff privileges at the hospital where the baby will be delivered
- What is the degree to which parents are encouraged to make nonmedical decisions
- What is the physician's treatment of jaundice in a newborn
- What is the physician's viewpoint on circumcision
- What is the hospital's policy regarding delaying the placement of antibiotic ointment in the baby's eyes in order to enhance the initial bonding between the parents and their baby
- What is the physician's policy on vitamin, iron, and fluoride supplements
- What is the physician's percentage of breastfeeding babies in the practice and the average duration of their breastfeeding
- What is the hospital's policy regarding how soon a mother can breastfeed her baby after delivery
- Does the hospital encourage rooming in
- What is the breastfeeding protocol in the hospital
- Is there a policy on water and formula supplementation
- Is the physician willing to allow the mother to determine her breastfeeding management
- What is the physician's management of breastfeeding problems
- Is there a person who can answer breastfeeding questions
- Is there an International Board Certified Lactation Consultant (IBCLC) on staff
- Are mothers referred to an IBCLC if there is not one currently on staff
- What are the physician's criteria for starting solid foods

- What are the physician's criteria for weaning
- Does the physician have a relationship with any breastfeeding support groups in the community

Working with the Physician

- It is is never too late to discuss a concern with a physician
- A mother may need help in order to formulate questions and clarify a physician's responses
- Encourage mothers to talk tactfully with their physicians in the following ways:
  - Share any confusion
  - Communicate her feelings about the importance of breastfeeding
  - Appeal for support through difficulties

When the Physician's Advice Seems Detrimental to Breastfeeding

- Suggest that the mother work with the physician who is the most supportive and knowledgeable about breastfeeding (if speaking of a medical team)
- Provide the mother with a solid basis of information before her physician visits
- Give the mother literature to help educate her physician or herself about breastfeeding
- Physicians should advise; they do not command
- Patients can decide whether or not to act on a physician's advice
- Physicians cannot make patients comply unless there is a clear and definite danger to the child
- Help mothers work through conflicts
  - Prepare the mother before a visit
  - Remind the mother of the typical breastfeeding management at her baby's present stage of development
  - Encourage the mother to prepare specific questions prior to a visit

- With seemingly detrimental advice, ask why the physician gave the advice and whether an alternative treatment is possible
- Help the mother work out solutions with her physician
- Never encourage a mother to go against a physician's medical advice
- Help the mother adapt advice to breastfeeding when possible
- Ask for a consultation
  - A mother's difficulty may be resolved if she seeks a consultation with another physician
  - The decision to change physicians must be initiated by parents
  - Do not suggest that a mother change physicians
  - Suggest the names of three local physicians if the mother requests a referral

10

Hospital Practices that Support Breastfeeding

Setting the Stage Prior to Birth

Establish Supportive Breastfeeding Policies
- Develop breastfeeding policies that are based on current scientific knowledge
- Keep the number of policies to a minimum and cover the salient points
- Post these policies where they can be frequently reviewed by staff
- Communicate these policies to all health care staff who come into contact with breastfeeding mothers and infants

Teach Breastfeeding Management to Staff
- Educate the health care staff on how to implement breastfeeding policies (see Chapter 24, "Professional Considerations")
- Understanding rationale and scientific basis behind policies increases their acceptance
- Teaching basic breastfeeding management frees up the International Board Certified Lactation Consultant (IBCLC) to concentrate on more difficult cases
- Ensure that mothers receive appropriate and consistent help when an IBCLC is not available

Educate Pregnant Women

- All women need to know about the benefits and management of breastfeeding
- Help mothers make informed decisions and dispel any myths they may have
- The classes will reach women who may not otherwise receive this information
- You can work in cooperation with childbirth education classes
- You can work with obstetrics, family practice physicians, and prenatal clinics to ensure they give correct and consistent information

Labor and Delivery Practices that Support Early Breastfeeding

Provide Labor and Delivery Support

- It results in fewer medications, less anesthesia, and fewer complications
- Mothers who were supported are more likely to be breastfeeding at six weeks than those who were not
- After an unmedicated birth, babies are more alert, responsive, and better able to begin breastfeeding within one to two hours after birth
- The presence of a doula results in fewer interventions for both mother and baby

Limit Interventions

- It is difficult to superimpose normal breastfeeding over interventionist labor and delivery practices
- Policies that routinely separate mothers and babies interfere with the process of breastfeeding, are not in the best interest of mothers and babies, and need to be changed
- Caregivers need to acquaint themselves with techniques that are least likely to interfere with breastfeeding

- Medications that a mother receives during labor may cause babies to become drowsy and have difficulty suckling, and may make the mothers less responsive to their babies—the following are some examples:
  - Analgesia—Mothers who are medicated during labor are more likely to leave the hospital without having established breastfeeding
  - Epidural anesthesia
    - Women who receive epidural anesthesia in labor are given significantly more pitocin in labor, have more forceps deliveries, and spend less time with their babies while in the hospital
    - The babies of mothers who had epidurals have poorer behavioral outcome and recovery, are less alert, have less of an ability to orient over the first month of life, and are less mature in their motor functions
    - Traces of bupivucaine from epidurals are found in babies' cord blood and in their blood up to three days after their delivery
    - Mothers who receive epidurals during labor have an increased incidence of intrapartum fever, which may result in the baby being worked up for sepsis, receiving antibiotics, and being transferred to the Neonatal Intensive Care Unit (NICU)
    - The earlier an epidural is given, the higher the risk of a cesarean birth
  - Episiotomy
    - It is difficult to get comfortable afterward, particularly when a mother sits upright
    - The pain can inhibit the milk ejection reflex
  - Deep suctioning and visualization of the larynx
    - The staff may be inclined to put the baby to breast immediately to soothe him
    - The baby may then associate breastfeeding with pain

- Forceps and vacuum extraction
  - Creates an increased risk of bruising and sensitivity to the infant's head
  - Creates an increased risk of jaundice, sleepiness, and lack of interest in feeding
- Pitocin to induce or stimulate labor
  - Edema is a possible result, particularly in extremities such as breast and nipple tissue
  - Its use can result in "meaty" and "flat" nipples
  - Women who receive several liters of IV fluids in conjunction with epidurals and pitocin seem to experience a delay in milk production
- Babies often are placed in radiant warmers
  - Warmers are unnecessary if the mother and baby remain together in skin-to-skin contact
  - Babies who are snuggled skin to skin with their mothers warm faster, stay warm longer, and have less risk of dehydration
  - When held skin to skin with their mothers, infants breathe warm, humidified air, rather than breathing dry hospital air when placed in radiant warmers

Promote Bonding

- The bonding between a mother and her baby is strongest in the first one or two hours
- Bonding is enhanced even further with skin-to-skin contact
- A newborn's rooting and sucking reflexes are particularly strong in the first hour or two after an unmedicated delivery
- A mother's normal body bacteria will colonize her baby's body only if she is the first person to hold him
- Laws in the United States require that all newborn infants' eyes be treated with an antibiotic; this treatment can be delayed at least one hour to enable uninterrupted bonding time for the parents and their baby

- The positive results of bonding are as follows:
  - Behavioral and developmental advantages for the child during the early years
  - A higher incidence of breastfeeding
  - More caressing and face-to-face contact with the child
  - At three months, mothers perceive their infants to be at ease and have fewer problems with nighttime feeds, and the babies and their mothers smile and face one another more often
  - At five years, children have significantly higher I.Q.s and better-developed skills

Help Mothers Initiate Breastfeeding

- Mothers who breastfeed in the delivery room are more likely to breastfeed longer than those who initiate breastfeeding 12 to 16 hours later
- The increased oxytocin secretion from suckling contracts the uterus more quickly and controls bleeding
- Colostrum clears meconium from a baby's gut and provides the needed immunologic factors
- The delay of the first bath enables the vernix to soak into the baby's skin and prevents temperature loss
- Women should be allowed to labor in any position they choose, rather than being required to labor lying down to facilitate birthing
- Let the baby lead the way
  - A mother and her unwrapped baby can be left alone with a warmed blanket placed over both of them to prevent heat loss
  - A mother should be allowed to remain quietly in skin-to-skin contact until her baby is ready to breastfeed
  - Babies typically work through prefeeding behaviors such as bringing their hands to their mouths and making sucking motions
  - This is an excellent time to teach feeding cues and encourage a mothers' response (see Chapter 11)

- Hospital practices need to allow mothers and their babies to stay together for at least two hours without any interference
- Every mother should be helped with the first breastfeed
  - Birth attendants can place her baby in skin-to-skin contact with the mother's abdomen or chest immediately after birth
  - The mother can make her breast available by placing it close to her baby's mouth and by allowing him to lick and explore it
  - Caregivers should be available to help if the baby wishes to breastfeed and has not started spontaneously within one hour
- Breastfeeding after a cesarean delivery
  - A mother can breastfeed as soon as all physical repairs are completed and she has been moved to the recovery room
  - If a mother received general anesthesia, she may breastfeed as soon as she is awake and able to respond
  - Lying on her side with the baby placed next to her will help a mother avoid incisional pain in the first hours
  - Pillows can be placed under a mother's top knee, under her abdomen and behind her back to facilitate her comfort during a feed
  - A mother can lie flat with her baby lying on top of her during the feed
  - If a mother feeds in a sitting position, a pillow placed over the surgical incision will cushion it from the pressure of the baby's body

Creating a Supportive Postpartum Climate

Eliminate Negative and Unnecessary Practices

- Help mothers limit interference by encouraging them to request that visitors wait until they are at home to visit

- Encourage mothers to give nothing but their own milk to the baby
- Give a baby a supplement only in rare instances of a specific medical need—offer it in small amounts and only after a breastfeed has taken place
- Supplements should not be given routinely
- Never leave the supplements with a mother without specific usage instructions
- See the section titled "Acceptable Medical Reasons for Supplements" in Chapter 23 for further discussion
- Do not give any artificial nipples to an infant
  - Babies suckle differently on an artificial nipple than at the breast
  - If a supplementary feed is required, use an alternate feeding method (see Chapter 19)
  - Use nipple shields appropriately (see Chapter 19)
- Do not place any restrictions on feeds
  - Babies should breastfeed frequently beginning immediately after their birth
  - Mothers should feed their babies every two to three hours or in response to a baby's feeding cues
  - A rigid schedule ignores a baby's natural feeding cues in the following ways:
    - Does not help a mother learn how to respond to her baby's feeding cues
    - Often does not enable a baby to begin feeding until he becomes frantic
    - Slower milk production results
    - Mothers experience increased breast engorgement
    - Increases the incidence of jaundice and hypoglycemia in the baby

Promote Practices that Support Breastfeeding

- Encourage rooming in for the following reasons:
  - Increases a mother's self-confidence in handling her baby

- Mothers learn to recognize hunger cues
- Is reassuring to a mother to have her baby close to respond to him
- Does not interfere with sleep—mothers who room-in with their babies and take no pain or sleep medication sleep just as well as those who take medication and leave their babies in the nursery
- Promotes longer breastfeeding duration
- Incorporates the baby into a family unit immediately after birth
- Promotes frequent feeds
- Reduces breast engorgement
- Encourages early milk production
- Enables babies to become better breastfeeders
- Promotes greater infant weight gain
- Promotes less crying and movement, which conserves the baby's energy
- Promotes higher blood glucose levels due to lack of crying

- Teach mothers feeding cues for the following reasons:
  - Enables the baby to nurse whenever he demonstrates feeding cues
  - Ensures an early establishment of milk production
  - Helps avoid milk stasis that can lead to engorgement or plugged ducts
  - Encourages early milk production and decreases uncomfortable breast fullness by enabling frequent feedings day and night
  - Most babies show feeding cues (see Chapter 11) for up to 30 minutes before sustained crying
  - Observing the number of feeds within 24 hours rather than timed intervals between feeds is more normal
- Show mothers how to breastfeed for the following reasons:
  - A mother needs a knowledgeable caregiver present for the first feed to assist her and answer questions

- Every breastfeeding mother needs to be taught basic breastfeeding management
- Teach mothers breast care in the following ways:
  - Following a feed, a mother can leave her breasts exposed to air until any moisture has dissipated
  - If a mother plans to apply a lubricant to her nipples, always recommend air drying them first
  - Note that nipples require no treatment unless they are tender or sore
  - Advise the mother to not allow drying agents such as soap or shampoo to touch her nipples
  - It is sufficient for a mother to stand in a shower and allow water to stream over her breasts for cleansing
- Provide discharge planning for the following reasons:
  - This is a time in a mother's parenting experience when she is eager to listen and learn
  - Before discharge, a mother should be taught basic breastfeeding management, how to assess her baby's needs, the typical patterns of feeding, and breastfeeding milestones
- Provide follow-up care through the following ways:
  - Anticipate a mother's immediate needs when she returns home
  - Help her plan realistically
  - Provide referrals to community resources such as an IBCLC, breastfeeding support group, or local WIC agency
  - Provide a warm line to support mothers after they go home
  - Contact a mother early and provide a telephone follow-up from knowledgeable caregivers
  - Do a weight check on the baby within 48 hours of discharge
  - Place a follow-up phone call at least two days after discharge
  - Perform a home visit around day three if it is covered by the mother's insurance plan

Forty-Eight Hour Plan of Care for Breastfeeding Management in the Hospital

Labor and Delivery
- Teach the positioning and management of a first feed
- Show the mother feeding cues her baby is exhibiting at this time
- If the baby is not interested in feeding, place him skin to skin with mother

Hours One to Eight
- Review the baby's positioning and observe his latch
- Observe a breastfeed and point out the difference between a nutritive and non-nutritive suck
- Review the baby's feeding cues (see Chapter 11) and put him to breast according to these cues
- Keep the baby and mother together
- A baby may feed only once or several times during the first eight hours

Hours Nine to Sixteen
- Review basic nutrition—eating a normal healthy diet and drinking when thirsty
- Baby should breastfeed two or more times during the next eight hours
- Feed the baby expressed milk with an alternative feeding method if he is not breastfeeding
- Review the risk factors for breastfeeding problems and take appropriate action (see Figure 10.1)

Hours Seventeen to Twenty-Four
- Mothers should be able to demonstrate correct positioning and latch-on techniques
- Observe a feed, and ask the mother to point out nutritive and non-nutritive sucking
- Babies should breastfeed two or more times during this time period

- There should be a total of at least six feeds in the first 24 hours
- If the baby is still not latching on, a mother should continue to express her milk two or three times during this shift, feed expressed milk to the baby, and notify the IBCLC

Hours Twenty-Five to Thirty-Two

- Teach mothers the appropriate number of feeds, wet diapers, and stools that should occur in a 24-hour time period
- Give mothers printed materials that include a breastfeeding diary to record feeds, voids and stool, how to know when breastfeeding is going well, and warning signs that indicate a problem (see Figure 10.2)
- Teach mothers the prevention of nipple soreness and engorgement, and when to call an IBCLC
- Babies should be breastfeeding two or more times during this shift

Hours Thirty-Three to Forty

- Make sure the mother can position and latch her baby on by herself
- Observe a complete feed, and document the findings
- Teach the mother about cluster feeds, the father's role, the avoidance of artificial nipples, and the hazards of formula use
- Discuss cosleeping with the mother
- Provide the mother with anticipatory guidance for the first few nights at home

Hours Forty-One to Forty-Eight

- Mothers should be able to observe nutritive sucking and swallowing during feeds
- Teach mothers that crying is the last sign of hunger—feeding cues are in place for 20 to 30 minutes before sustained crying—and that crying compromises and disorganizes the baby's suck

Maternal Factors
- Gained less than 18 pounds during pregnancy
- Previous breast surgery or breast trauma
- Little or no breast change in size or color during pregnancy
- History of low milk supply or breastfeeding "failure" with previous infants
- Flat or inverted nipples or taut, tight breast tissue
- Primipara
- Epidural in labor
  - In place longer than three to four hours before delivery
  - Put in more than one time
  - Received more than one bolus of epidural medication
- Induction of labor with pitocin
- Received excessive intravenous fluids; on magnesium sulfate; edema present in ankles that was not present before labor
- Pain medication in labor more than one hour before delivery
- Breastfeeding initiated more than one hour after delivery
- Sore nipples throughout the feed at the time of discharge from the hospital

Infant Factors
- Less than 37 weeks' gestation
- Weighs less than seven pounds
- Male infant

- Vacuum or forceps used for delivery
- Baby has ankyloglossia (tongue tie) or cleft lip or palate, or both
- Fetal distress; meconium during delivery
- Insult to the oral cavity (laryngoscope and deep suctioning)
- Baby is kept in nursery instead of with mother
- SGA or LGA
- Feeding restrictions placed on infant (timed feeds, NPO)
- Multiple bottles given during hospitalization
- Jaundice
- Sleepy, difficult to wake; doesn't give clear feeding cues
- Difficulty latching on consistently; has not established effective breastfeeding by hospital discharge
- Seven percent or greater weight loss at time of hospital discharge

All factors can contribute to problems with breastfeeding. Some are more significant than others. Multiple factors indicated that the dyad must be followed after discharge from hospital. The goal of this checklist is to identify potential dyads who may have problems establishing either an adequate milk supply or positive milk transfer. The health worker can work with them while they overcome their problems and in a manner that is both safe and supportive of the breastfeeding experience.

LGA, large for gestational age; SGA, small for gestational age.

Printed by permission of Jan Barger and Linda Kutner.

Figure 10.1 Red flags and risk factors for breastfeeding problems

- Babies should be latching on and feeding well at this time
- Mothers should appear comfortable when holding, dressing, and diapering their infants

Discharge

- Make sure that the mother understands the signs of adequate milk production (see Chapter 14, "Breastfeeding in the Early Weeks")
- Provide the mother with contact information for community resources, including pump rental stations if necessary
- Notify the baby's physician of potential problems based on any risk factors
- Ask the mother to confirm when she will take the baby to her physician for a weight and skin color check

Baby-Friendly Hospital Practices

- Evaluate the degree to which the hospital promotes and supports breastfeeding (see Figure 10.3)
- Assist hospital staff and administrators in establishing supportive policies and practices

Baby's birth date and time _____
Your baby will be 4 days old on _____
Baby's birth weight _____
Baby's discharge weight _____
Baby's first week weight _____
Baby's second week weight _____

Lactation Consultant's name _____

Telephone Number _____

BREASTFEEDING IS GOING WELL IF:

- Your baby is breastfeeding at least 8 times in 24 hours.
- Your baby has at least 6 wet diapers every 24 hours.
- Your baby has at least 4 bowel movements every 24 hours.
- You can hear your baby gulping or swallowing at feeds.
- Your breasts feel softer after a feed.
- Your nipples are not painful.
- Breastfeeding is an enjoyable experience.

Remember! If you go home from the hospital in less than 48 hours, your baby should be seen by a physician 2 or 3 days after discharge and again at 10 days to 2 weeks of age. Generally, these visits are for physical assessments and color and weight checks. It is your responsibility to contact the clinic or doctor to schedule these visits, and to notify them and/or your board certified lactation consultant if at any time you feel breastfeeding isn't going just right for either you or your baby.

(continues)

Figure 10.2 Warning signs that breastfeeding is not going well

WARNING SIGNS!
CALL YOUR BABY'S DOCTOR OR LACTATION CONSULTANT IF:

- Your baby is having fewer than 6 wet diapers a day by the 6th day of age.
- Your baby is still passing meconium (black, tarry stools) on the 5th day of age or is passing fewer than 4 stools by the 6th day of age.
- Your milk supply is full but you do not hear your baby gulping or swallowing frequently during breastfeeding.
- Your nipples are painful throughout the feed.
- Your baby seems to be breastfeeding "all the time."
- You do not feel that your milk supply has become full by the 5th day.
- Your baby is gaining less than 1/2 ounce a day, or has not regained his birth weight by 10 days of age.

Printed by permission of Breastfeeding Support Consultants.

Figure 10.2 Warning signs that breastfeeding is not going well (continued)

Step 1. Have a written breastfeeding policy that is routinely communicated to all health care staff.

1.1 Does the health facility have an explicit written policy for protecting, promoting, and supporting breastfeeding that addresses all Ten Steps to Successful Breastfeeding in maternity services?

1.2 Does the policy protect breastfeeding by prohibiting all promotion of and group instruction for using breast milk substitutes, feeding bottles, and teats?

1.3 Is the breastfeeding policy available so all staff who take care of mothers and babies can refer to it?

1.4 Is the breastfeeding policy posted or displayed in all areas of the health facility that serve mothers, infants, and/or children?

1.5 Is there a mechanism for evaluating the effectiveness of the policy?

Step 2. Train all health care staff in skills necessary to implement this policy.

2.1 Are all staff aware of the advantages of breastfeeding and acquainted with the facility's policy and services to protect, promote, and support breastfeeding?

2.2 Are all staff caring for women and infants oriented to the breastfeeding policy of the hospital on their arrival?

(continues)

Figure 10.3 Ten steps to successful breastfeeding: A self appraisal tool

2.3 Is training on breastfeeding and lactation management given to all staff caring for women and infants within 6 months of their arrival?
2.4 Does the training cover at least eight of the ten steps?
2.5 Is the training on breastfeeding and lactation management at least 18 hours in total, including a minimum of 3 hours of a supervised clinical experience?
2.6 Has the health care facility arranged for specialized training in lactation management of specific staff members?

Step 3. Inform all pregnant women about the benefits and management of breastfeeding.

3.1 Does the hospital include an antenatal care clinic or an antenatal in-patient ward?
3.2 If yes, are most pregnant women attending these antenatal services informed about the benefits and management of breastfeeding?
3.3 Do antenatal records indicate whether breastfeeding has been discussed with the pregnant woman?
3.4 Is a mother's antenatal record available at the time of delivery?
3.5 Are pregnant women protected from oral or written promotion of and group instruction for artificial feeding?
3.6 Does the health care facility take into account a woman's intention to breastfeed when deciding on the use of a sedative, an analgesic, or an anaesthetic (if any) during labor and delivery?
3.7 Are staff familiar with the effects of such medicaments on breastfeeding?

3.8 Does a woman who has never breastfed or who has previously encountered problems with breastfeeding receive special attention and support from the staff of the health care facility?

Step 4. Help mothers initiate breastfeeding within a half-hour of birth.

4.1 Are mothers whose deliveries are normal given their babies to hold, with skin contact, within a half-hour of completion of the second stage of labor and allowed to remain with them for at least the first hour?
4.2 Are the mothers offered help by a staff member to initiate breastfeeding during this first hour?
4.3 Are mothers who have had caesarean deliveries given their babies to hold, with skin contact, within a half-hour after they are able to respond to their babies?
4.4 Do the babies born by caesarean delivery stay with their mothers with skin contact at this time, for at least 30 minutes?

Step 5. Show mothers how to breastfeed and how to maintain lactation, even if they should be separated from their infants.

5.1 Does nursing staff offer all mothers further assistance with breastfeeding within 6 hours of delivery?
5.2 Are most breastfeeding mothers able to demonstrate how to position and attach their babies correctly for breastfeeding?
5.3 Are breastfeeding mothers shown how to express their milk or given information on expression or advised of where they can get help, should they need it?

(continues)

Figure 10.3 Ten steps to successful breastfeeding: A self appraisal tool *(continued)*

5.4 Does a woman who has never breastfed or who has previously encountered problems with breastfeeding receive special attention and support from the staff of the health care facility?

5.6 Are mothers of babies in special care helped to establish and maintain lactation by frequent expressions of milk?

Step 6. Give newborn infants no food or drink other than breast milk, unless medically indicated.

6.1 Do staff have a clear understanding of what the few acceptable reasons are for prescribing food or drink other than breast milk for breastfeeding babies?

6.2 Do breastfeeding babies receive no other food or drink (other than breast milk) unless medically indicated?

6.3 Are any breast milk substitutes including special formulas that are used in the facility purchased in the same way as any other foods or medicines?

6.4 Do the health facility and all health care workers refuse free or low-cost supplies of breast milk substitutes, paying close to retail market price for any? (Low-cost = below 80% open-market retail cost. Breast milk substitutes intended for experimental use or "professional evaluation" should also be purchased at 80% or more of retail price.)

6.5 Is all promotion for infant foods or drinks other than breast milk absent from the facility?

Step 7. Practice rooming in allows mothers and infants to remain together—24 hours a day.
7.1 Do mothers and infants remain together (rooming-in 24 hours a day, except for periods of up to an hour for hospital procedures or if separation is medically indicated)?
7.2 Does rooming in start within an hour of a normal birth?
7.3 Does rooming in start within an hour of when a caesarean mother can respond to her baby?

Step 8. Encourage breastfeeding on demand.
8.1 By placing no restrictions on the frequency or length of breastfeeds, do staff show that they are aware of the importance of breastfeeding on demand?
8.2 Are mothers advised to breastfeed their babies whenever their babies are hungry and as often as their babies want to breastfeed?

(continues)

Figure 10.3 Ten steps to successful breastfeeding: A self appraisal tool *(continued)*

Step 9. Give no artificial tests or pacifiers (also called dummies or soothers) to breastfeeding infants.

9.1 Are babies who have started to breastfeed cared for without any bottle feeds?
9.2 Are babies who have started to breastfeed cared for without using pacifiers?
9.3 Do breastfeeding mothers learn that they should not give any bottles or pacifiers to their babies?
9.4 By accepting no free or low-cost feeding bottles, teats, or pacifiers, do the facility and the caregivers demonstrate that these should be avoided?

Step 10. Foster the establishment of breastfeeding support groups, and refer mothers to them on discharge from the hospital or clinic.

10.1 Does the hospital give education to key family members so that they can support the breastfeeding mother at home?
10.2 Are breastfeeding mothers referred to breastfeeding support groups, if any are available?
10.3 Does the hospital have a system of follow-up support for breastfeeding mothers after they are discharged, such as early postnatal or lactation clinic check-ups, home visits, telephone calls?
10.4 Does the facility encourage and facilitate the formation of mother-to-mother or health care worker-to-mother support groups?
10.5 Does the facility allow breastfeeding counseling by trained mother-to-mother support group counselors in its maternity services?

Used by permission from UNICEF/WHO

Figure 10.3 Ten steps to successful breastfeeding: A self appraisal tool (continued)

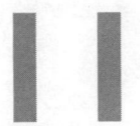

Infant Assessment and Behavior

Assessment of the Newborn

Performing Infant Assessment
- Obtain a complete history of the mother and infant as it pertains to breastfeeding
- Perform an infant assessment, which is generally recommended with any initial contact
- Perform the assessment with the baby completely undressed
- Conditions that require an infant assessment are as follows:
  - Concern about weight gain
  - Food intolerance
  - Irritability
  - Lethargy
  - Sucking difficulties

Posture
- The posture of a healthy newborn is generally one of flexion—in a fetal position
- When awake, the baby will resist having his extremities extended and may cry
- As the baby matures, he will remain in a fetal position less often and will spend more time comfortably in a semi-extended position

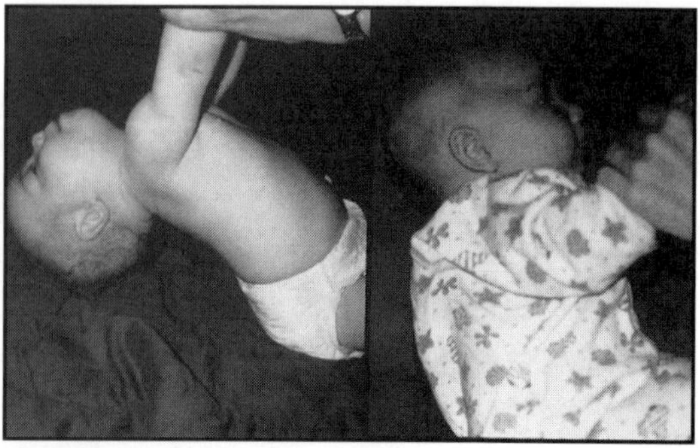

Figure 11.1 A hypotonic baby compared with a baby with good muscle tone

Printed by permission of Kay Hoover.

- When held in a ventral position (the infant on his abdomen draped over the hand of the examiner), the baby will alternate between trying to bring his head up and putting it down again

Hypotonia

- The infant's extremities are in extension (see Figure 11.1)
- There is little resistance to passive movement
- The infant appears to be floppy, sluggish, flaccid, and perhaps even lazy
- The infant may have difficulty latching on or maintaining intraoral negative pressure even on the examiner's finger, due to weak suck
- The infant frequently nurses with his shoulders elevated to just beneath his ears in an effort to support his neck and chin
- In a ventral position, the infant lays over the examiner's hand with his head hanging down, unable to bring it up

Hypertonia

- The baby is often in hyperextension (see Figure 11.2)

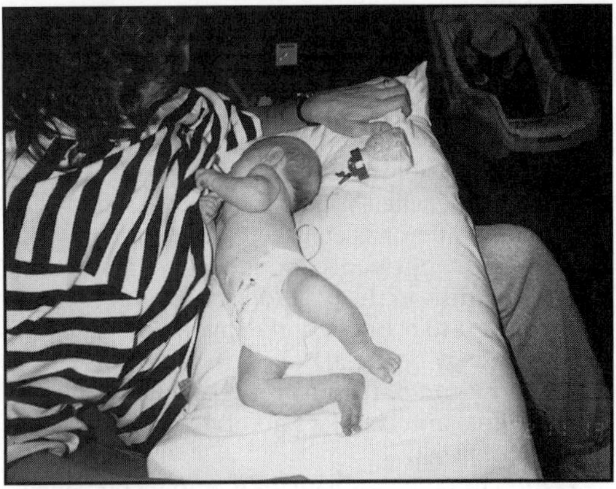

Figure 11.2 Example of a hypertonic infant whose body arches away from the mother

Printed by permission of Linda Kutner.

- He may be difficult to comfort
- He cannot tolerate being handled
- He arches away from the breast and away from the mother
- He pulls his head and face away from contact
- He does not snuggle into the mother's chest or neck
- He holds his head erect from a prone position or on the shoulder
- He is virtually straight, lifting both head and buttocks and maintaining them on a horizontal plane when held in a ventral position

Skin

- Healthy newborn skin is warm and dry, with a pink or ruddy appearance
- Acrocyanosis may be present after birth
  - Caused by poor peripheral circulation
  - Usually disappears after a few days

- **Hydration**
  - Turgor
    - Test skin turgor on the baby's chest, abdomen, or thigh by gently grasping the skin between your finger and thumb
    - Skin should spring back to its original shape when you let go of the tissue
    - Skin that has an indentation, fold, or wrinkled appearance or loose skin that slowly returns to the position level with the tissue next to it is a sign of dehydration
  - Skin may be dry, flaky, or peeling, especially by the end of the first or second week—this is normal and is not a sign of **dehydration**
- Skin color
  - In natural light, blanch the skin by pressing it with your index finger and noting the color when your finger is lifted
  - Yellowing of the skin is caused by an increased level of bilirubin (see Chapter 20, "Temporary Breastfeeding Situations," for further discussion)
- Diaper rash
  - Is a rash that does not go away after appropriate treatment—may be caused by a yeast infection (see Chapter 14, "Breastfeeding Issues in the Early Weeks")
  - If excoriated or has pustules, the infant's skin needs to be seen by a physician to rule out bacterial infection

Head

- May appear asymmetric due to molding from the birthing process
- **Caput succedaneum**
  - Is a collection of fluid between the newborn's skin and cranial bone that usually forms during labor as a result of the presentation of the head in the cervical opening
  - Occurs in 20 to 40 percent of vacuum extractions
  - May be red or bruised discoloration
  - May be sensitive to pressure on that area

- **Cephalhematoma**
  - Is swelling caused by the pooling of blood between the bones of the head and periosteum
  - May begin to form during labor and slowly becomes larger in the infant's first few days of life
  - Causes the baby's bilirubin levels to increase due to blood reabsorption
  - Takes about six weeks to completely resolve
  - Is usually a result of trauma, often from delivery with forceps
  - May cause sensitivity on that area
- **Fontanels**
  - The anterior fontanel remains soft until the baby reaches about 18 months
  - The posterior fontanel closes at about two months
  - May be soft and sunken when he is lying down
- **Facial asymmetry**
  - Results from injury to nerves due to birth trauma
  - Causes a baby's tongue to not be centered in his mouth
  - Position the nipple over the center of the baby's tongue rather than the center of his mouth

Oral Cavity

- It is not necessary to perform an oral digital exam on all babies
- A visual inspection of the mouth assesses the extension of the tongue over the lower alveolar ridge
- The tongue should extend up to the middle of the baby's mouth when it is open wide
- **Frenulum**
  - Ankyloglossia—short frenulum—may cause a heart-shaped appearance to the tip of the tongue (see Figure 11.3)
  - Can interfere with breastfeeding if the baby is unable to extend his tongue over the alveolar ridge

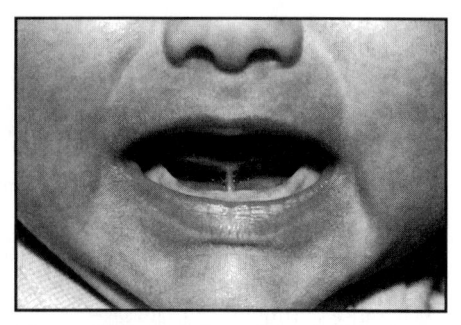

Figure 11.3 A baby with a tight frenulum

Printed by permission of Kay Hoover.

- Can cause chronic nipple soreness
- Can make it difficult for a baby to stay attached to the breast during feeding
- May result in poor weight gain
- **Buccal pads**
  - Help decrease the space within the infant's mouth
  - Can increase the negative pressure
  - Facilitate milk transfer
  - May not be present in an infant who is malnourished or born preterm
  - May need to position the infant at the breast so the mother can use her finger against the infant's cheeks to compensate for the lack of these fatty pads of tissue
- **Palate**
  - High, arched, or bubble palate may cause the nipple to get "caught" in the groove causing the following to occur:
    - The nipple cannot elongate as it should
    - Difficult for the infant's tongue to compress lactiferous sinuses adequately
    - The mother possibly experiences nipple soreness and inadequate milk transfer

- Cleft of the soft palate that escapes initial diagnosis
  - May cause an infant to choke and gag while nursing
  - May cause milk to escape from the infant's nose during letdown
- See Chapter 23, "Mothers and Babies with Long-Term Special Needs," for more information on clefts
- **Thrush**
  - Is often characterized by white patches that cannot be removed without causing bleeding
  - Can appear between a baby's gums and lips, on the inside of his cheeks, and on his tongue
  - See Chapter 14 for a discussion about yeast as a cause of nipple soreness

Clavicle

- Fractured clavicles are a fairly common birth trauma
- The baby may restrict the use of his arm and resist breastfeeding in a position that places pressure on the fractured area
- Treatment for the fracture consists of immobilizing the arm by pinning it in a t-shirt
- Clavicles heal quickly—within about three weeks

Reflexes

- The moro (or startle) reflex encourages more gentle handling of the baby
- A grasp reflex is encouraging to parents because they see their baby responding to them
- **Arching**
  - Indicates a need for different positioning or a pause from activity
  - May cause the baby to arch backward if pressure is exerted on the back of his head or if his face is pushed into a surface (i.e., against the breast during a feed)

- **Bauer's response**
  - Is the spontaneous crawling effort and extension of a baby's head
  - Is elicited by pressure on the soles of a baby's feet
  - Ensure that the baby's feet do not come into contact with the back or side of the couch or chair when positioning him for a feed—this could cause him to extend away from the breast
- **Rooting**
  - Stroking the baby's cheek lightly will cause him to turn his head in the direction of stimulus
  - Causes the baby's mouth to open and his tongue to come forward
- **Sucking**
  - Any object will elicit sucking when it is placed far enough back into the baby's mouth and it reaches the juncture between the hard and soft palates
  - High-flow nutritive sucks are long, deep, suck-swallow-breathe patterns with about one suck per second
  - Low-flow non-nutritive sucks are a light suck of about two sucks per second—almost a flutter—with short jaw excursions and little or no audible swallowing

Digestion

Spitting Up

- Many babies spit up quite often during the early months of life
- The passage between a baby's stomach and mouth is very short
- Muscle valves at the upper end of the baby's stomach (the cardiac sphincter) are not as efficient as they will be later in life
- The causes of frequent spitting up are as follows:
  - Overfeeding
  - An overactive letdown reflex

- Waiting too long between feeds
- Mucus present in the baby's stomach—more common directly after birth or whenever the baby is congested from an upper respiratory infection
- Milk allergies or nicotine use
- The following reduces the incidence of spitting up:
  - Burping the baby more often during a feed to bring up air bubbles
  - Burping the baby before a feed to enable tiny bubbles that have coalesced into one big enough to come up
  - Feeding more frequently
  - Limiting the baby to one breast at a feed to avoid overfullness
  - Laying the baby on his right side after a feed to aid gastric emptying

Projectile Vomiting

- Is distinguished from spitting in terms of the force with which it is expelled
- Is a violent expulsion of milk that travels five to ten feet
- The following may require a physician's attention:
  - The baby violently expels his stomach contents more than once or twice a day
  - The baby suddenly begins vomiting when he is several weeks old
  - The baby's vomiting gets progressively worse with a decreasing number of wet diapers
- Is possibly due to **pyloric stenosis**—where the stomach's outflow valve will not open satisfactorily to permit its contents to pass through
- Can also indicate an obstruction of the intestines or a strangulated hernia

Gastroesophageal Reflux (GER)

- Is the backflow of the stomach's contents into the esophagus
- Is often caused by the failure of the lower esophageal sphincter to close

- Brings up acidic gastric juices that produce a burning pain in the esophagus
- Causes infants to spit up several times after a feed and some to spit up even during the feed
- Teaches some infants to limit their intake as they associate a full stomach with the pain that may accompany reflux
- Results in poor infant weight gain
- Regurgitating human milk is not as irritating as with artificial baby milk (ABM)
- Human milk is digested more quickly than ABM and more can be absorbed in same amount of time
- Breastfed infants have a lower pH in their stomachs
- It is not appropriate to treat GER by switching a breastfed infant to ABM feeds
- Form a feeding plan
  - Feed the infant in an upright position so gravity helps the milk stay down
  - Feed the infant frequently
  - Nurse from only one breast at a feed
  - In the past, physicians frequently requested that mothers mix their milk with cereal to see if the thicker fluid would stay down better; however, it has not been shown to have a positive impact on GER and is not commonly recommended today

Elimination

- Current recommendations for newborn voiding and stooling are based on clinical observation and bits of information from unrelated research:
  - Are often based on infants who have had birth and postpartum interventions
  - Do not allow for exclusive, uninterrupted breastfeeding in the early days of life
- Mothers can record the baby's intake and output to evaluate his pattern (see Table 11.1)

- **Voiding**
  - Urine should range from a pale yellow to clear in color
  - Pink (copper or brick dust) stains that appear with urination are generally not significant in the first one to three days of life
  - An assessment of the baby's hydration status is warranted if stains appear after this time period
  - In the first week of life, a baby should have an increasing number of voids each day
  - By the time the baby is six days old, he should be voiding at least six times every 24 hours
- **Stools**
  - A newborn's first stools are black, tarry meconium and should be passed within the first 24 to 36 hours
  - Transitional stools are greenish black to greenish brown as the meconium gives way to a brown golden or mustard yellow color at about 48 to 72 hours of age
  - Stool texture may range from watery, to seedy yellow, to a toothpaste consistency
  - There is virtually no odor to a newborn's stools
  - In the first month of life, a baby should have at least four or more soft yellow runny stools a day
  - A baby who has less than four stools in a 24-hour time period and is over five days old may have an insufficient caloric intake
  - Babies' bowel habits change with age
  - Exclusively breastfed infants frequently decrease the number of stools they have each day
  - After one month of age, a baby may begin going for longer periods between bowel movements
  - In older infants, the number of stools produced may range from several stools every day to only once every three or four days
  - For examples of the variations in stools, see Table 11.2

TABLE 11.1 MY BREASTFEEDING RECORD FOR THE FIRST WEEK

Use this record when you breastfeed and when your baby needs a diaper change during the first week. This record will help you keep track of how well your baby is breastfeeding. Look at the sample.

1. Circle the hour closest to when your baby starts each breastfeeding.
2. Circle the W when your baby has a wet diaper.
3. Circle BM when your baby has a bowel movement.

It is ok for your baby to have more wet diapers or more bowel movements than the goal. Call your breastfeeding helper if your baby has less than the goal on the record.

Birth Date: ____ / ____ / ____   Time: _____ AM PM

Birth Weight _____   Discharge Weight _____

Sample for Day One

12 1 2 3 4 ⑤ 6 ⑦ 8 9 10 ⑪ Noon ① 2 3 4 5 ⑥ ⑦ 8 9 ⑩ 11
Ⓦ Ⓑ Ⓜ Ⓑ Ⓜ
Wet diaper.
Black tarry bowel movement.
On the first day, this baby fed seven times, had wet one diaper, and had two bowel movements. The mother wrote in the extra BM.

	GOAL (at least)
	6 to 8 or more
	1
	1

Day One

																								GOAL (at least)
12	1	2	3	4	5	6	7	8	9	10	11	Noon	1	2	3	4	5	6	7	8	9	10	11	
Wet diaper.																		W						6 to 8 or more 1
Black tarry bowel movement.																				BM				1

Day Two

																								GOAL (at least)
12	1	2	3	4	5	6	7	8	9	10	11	Noon	1	2	3	4	5	6	7	8	9	10	11	
Wet diaper.															W		W							6 to 8 or more 2
Brown tarry bowel movement.															BM			BM						2

Day Three

																								GOAL (at least)
12	1	2	3	4	5	6	7	8	9	10	11	Noon	1	2	3	4	5	6	7	8	9	10	11	
Wet diapers.															W	W		W						8 or more 3
Green bowel movement.															BM		BM							2

(continues)

TABLE 11.1 MY BREASTFEEDING RECORD FOR THE FIRST WEEK (continued)

Day Four

	GOAL (at least)
12 1 2 3 4 5 6 7 8 9 10 11 Noon 1 2 3 4 5 6 7 8 9 10 11	
Wet diapers. W W W	8 or more
Yellow bowel movement. BM BM BM	4
	3

Day Five

	GOAL (at least)
12 1 2 3 4 5 6 7 8 9 10 11 Noon 1 2 3 4 5 6 7 8 9 10 11	
Wet diapers. W W W W W	8 or more
Yellow bowel movement. BM BM BM	5
	3

Day Six

	GOAL (at least)
12 1 2 3 4 5 6 7 8 9 10 11 Noon 1 2 3 4 5 6 7 8 9 10 11	
Wet diapers. W W W W W W	8 or more
Yellow bowel movement. BM BM BM BM	6
	4

Day Seven

12	1	2	3	4	5	6	7	8	9	10	11	Noon	1	2	3	4	5	6	7	8	9	10	11
Wet diapers.													W	W	W	W	W	W	W	W	W
Yellow bowel movement.													BM	BM	BM	BM			BM			

	GOAL (at least)
Wet diapers	8 or more
Yellow bowel movement	6 or more
	4 or more

Baby's weight at 1 week _____

Questions to ask when baby is 1 week old.

If you can answer "yes" to each of these questions when your baby is one week old, then you know breastfeeding is going well. If you answer "no" to any of these questions, call your baby's doctor or a breastfeeding helper. Getting help early is best for enjoyable breastfeeding.

1. Is breastfeeding going well?
2. Does your baby breastfeed at least eight times each 24 hours?
3. Does your baby have at least six very wet diapers each day?
4. Does your baby have at least four large yellow bowel movements each day?
5. Is your baby getting only your milk? (no formula or water)
6. Do you let your baby finish the first breast before you offer the other side?
7. Is your baby happy or sleepy after breastfeeding? (not in need of a pacifier)
8. Are your breasts and nipples comfortable?

You may copy this paper written by Kay Hoover, M Ed, IBCLC, Lactation Consultant.
1101 Market Street, 9th Floor, Philadelphia, PA 19107
Phone 215-685-5282 or 215-685-5237
Name and telephone number of a breastfeeding helper

Printed by permission of Kay Hoover (9/98).
Neifert M: Early assessment of the breastfeeding infant. *Contemporary Pediatrics* 13(10): 142–165; 1996.

TABLE 11.2 STOOL PATTERNS OF A BREASTFED BABY

Characteristics	Normal Stool	Variations	Possible Causes
Color	A newborn's stool is black, brown, or green in the first 3 days. This is meconium. Later, color ranges from brown or green to mustard yellow.	Unexplained color changes.	Mother's or baby's diet.
		Black, brown, or red spots.	Mother's cracked nipples (possible bleeding—there is no harm to the baby). Bleeding from the baby's rectum. If no known cause, the mother should consult the physician.
Consistency	Ranges from a toothpaste-like texture to a liquid with curds.	Very watery.	Foods in the baby's diet other than the mother's milk, antibiotic or illness.
		Hard pellets.	Foods in the baby's diet other than the mother's milk, insufficient fluids, or baby tense or ill.
		Mucous.	Newborn mucus, cold, congestion, or allergy to the mother's or baby's diet.

Odor	Very little, not unpleasant.	Fibrous. Unpleasant.	Bananas and cereal present in the baby's diet. New foods in addition to the mother's milk, antibiotics, or illness.
Frequency	Ranges from one with every feed to four a day under one month of age. Decreases in frequency after the first month of life.	Sudden change in frequency. Watch carefully and look for other symptoms.	Foods, maturity, or illness.
Volume	Varies with frequency. More frequent stools mean less volume per diaper.	Any sudden change. Watch carefully and be alert to other symptoms.	Foods, maturity, or illness.
Ease of expulsion	Easy and semicontrolled with some straining by the baby.	Flows out continually. Very difficult with extreme straining.	Foods other than the mother's milk, illness, or antibiotics. Foods other than the mother's milk or insufficient fluids.

- **Constipation**
  - Constipation is diagnosed by the consistency of the infant's stools, not by the frequency
  - As long as an infant's stool is soft, he is not constipated
  - Neither a lack of a daily bowel movement nor straining at stooling indicates constipation
  - Constipated stools are molded and firm to the touch—like pellets or marbles—generally due to iron supplements or solid foods being given
  - Treatment of constipation
    - In young infants, more frequent feeds will solve most constipation problems
    - A mother should not treat her infant with suppositories unless a physician prescribes them
- **Diarrhea**
  - A mother can mistake typical loose stools for diarrhea, especially if she has been supplementing the infant's feedings with formula and has returned to exclusive breastfeeding or if her previous children were not breastfed
  - Diarrhea stools are much looser than normal, are very watery, and may be foul smelling
  - Diarrhea may indicate the beginning of illness, food allergy, or reaction to antibiotics taken by either the mother or baby
  - Diarrhea removes the valuable intestinal bacteria that helps the digestion of food
  - Such intestinal bacteria can be built back up with human milk
  - If diarrhea is suspected, mothers can continue breastfeeding
  - A mother should contact the infant's physician immediately if the infant's diarrhea does not improve quickly or if the infant appears sick or dehydrated
- **Infrequent stooling**
  - Infrequent stooling in the first month of life almost always occurs due to the insufficient intake of milk

- A baby who is voiding but not stooling or gaining weight may not be receiving enough high fat hindmilk
- **Hirschsprung's disease** is a cause of infrequent stooling
  - It occurs because part of the infant's intestines lacks the proper nerve innervation
  - These infants frequently have large bloated abdomens from the collection of stools and gas
  - A breastfed infant with this condition may escape detection until solid foods are added to his diet that cause the stools to become more bulky and have less liquid

Infant Communication

Feeding Cues and Stages of Alertness
- Feeding cues will help parents know when their baby is ready to be put to the breast
- If parents wait until their baby cries, the baby will already be exhibiting the final signs of hunger
- A baby's interest in feeding is influenced by his level of alertness
- See Table 11.3

Knowing When to Attempt a Feed
- The following feeding cues may be evident when the baby is in light sleep, drowsy, and quiet alert states:
  - He will begin to wriggle his body
  - His closed eyes will exhibit rapid eye movement (REM)
  - He will pass one or both of his hands over his head and will bring his hand to his mouth
  - He will make sucking motions
  - If his cheek or mouth is touched at this stage, he will begin to root
  - Soon, more vigorous sucking will begin
  - Finally, he settles back into a less active state

TABLE 11.3   THE SIX INFANT STATES

Infant State	Description
Deep sleep	Characterized by limp extremities, a placid face, quiet breathing, no body movement, and no rapid eye movement (REM) (eyes flutter beneath the eyelids). The baby lies very still, with an occasional twitch or sucking movement. He cannot easily be aroused.
Light or active sleep	Resistance in the extremities when moved, mouthing or sucking motions, body movement, and facial grimaces. The baby is awakened more easily and is likely to remain awake if disturbed. Most of the baby's sleep is spent in this state, with less regular breathing and rapid eye movement. Although he may stir and move about, he can return to sleep if left undisturbed.
Drowsy	The baby is aroused easily and may drift back to sleep. His eyes may open and close intermittently, and he may murmur, whisper, yawn, and stretch.
Quiet alert	The baby looks around and interacts with others. This is an excellent time to breastfeed. The baby is extremely responsive. His body is still and watchful, his eyes are bright, and his breathing is even and regular.
Active alert	The baby moves his extremities and plays. He is even more attentive, and is wide-eyed with rapid and irregular breathing. He may become fussy and is more sensitive to the discomfort of a wet diaper or any excessive stimulation.
Crying	The baby is agitated and needs comforting.

- The baby may show feeding cues several times in the span of 20 to 30 minutes
- If his signals remain unheeded, he may become very frustrated and cry
- When a newborn begins to cry, he can easily become disorganized:
  - It may take several minutes for him to settle enough to breastfeed
  - The newborn may be unable to breastfeed at all until he has slept again for a while

If the Baby Needs to Be Awakened for a Feed
- He will be most responsive when he is in a light sleep or a drowsy state
- Most babies will move from deep to light sleep in approximately 20- to 30-minute cycles

Infant Behavior Patterns

Average Baby
- Nurses 6 to 14 times in a 24-hour time period
- Sleeps 12 to 20 hours daily

Easy Baby
- Has the same breastfeeding pattern as the average baby
- Has longer sleep periods and is less demanding
- Mothers must take care not to overexert themselves due to more free time
- A mother should devote her free time to her baby even though he does not make many bids for attention

Placid Baby
- May request as few as four to six feedings a day
- Sleeps 18 to 20 hours daily
- Makes very few demands for attention
- The mother should make sure that the baby is not becoming undernourished

- She must meet her baby's needs without receiving several cues from him
- She can place a noise device—a rattle, bell, or squeaky toy, for example—in the baby's crib to be triggered when he awakes and moves about
- She can set an alarm clock for herself to remind her to check on the baby every two to three hours
- When she finds her baby awake, she can pick him up, stimulate him, and encourage him to nurse
- Always avoid any pacifying techniques such as pacifiers, cradles, or swings
- If her baby sucks his thumb, a mother can encourage him to satisfy his sucking needs on her breast instead of his thumb

Active and Fussy Baby

- May nurse more frequently and sleep fewer hours than an average baby
- May seem insatiable at the breast and be impatient waiting for the milk to let down
- May respond well to being allowed to nurse, doze, and play at the breast for generous periods of time
- May spit up often from being overly full
- Has a greater need to use the breast for calming and comforting
- Mothers can try limiting him to one breast at a feed
- This baby may do well when placed in a sling and worn by a parent

Infant Growth

Caloric Intake

- An infant's energy needs per day decrease as the baby gets older

WEIGHT GAIN

- An infant's caloric needs are as follows:

At birth	115 kcal/kg/day
At one month	110 kcal/kg/day
At two months	105 kcal/kg/day
At three months	100 kcal/kg/day
At four months	95 kcal/kg/day
At six months	82 kcal/kg/day (then rises slightly)

- Calories are needed to prevent the reabsorption of bilirubin from the meconium
- A breastfed infant's energy intake is lower than a formula fed infant's intake throughout the first 12 months of life
- For every ounce of sugar water that a baby takes in, his caloric intake is reduced by two-thirds
- Sterile water has no calories, sugar water (D_5W) has 6 kcal/oz, while colostrum has 18 kcal/oz
- Compared to formula fed infants, breastfed infants have lower sleeping metabolic rates, rectal temperatures, and heart rates
- Caloric intakes may account for the differences in energy intake and expenditure
- The gain in lean body mass is greater in breastfed infants

Weight Gain

- Initially after birth, a baby may lose up to seven percent of his birth weight due to the following:
  - Loss of fluids
  - Passage of meconium
  - The mother received excessive intravenous fluids, which causes a fluid shift to the infant that artificially increases the baby's birth weight
  - Exposure to medications during labor
- An infant's weight loss of more than seven percent needs evaluation and the mother needs assistance with breastfeeding

TABLE 11.4 A BABY'S WEIGHT GAIN PATTERN

Baby's age	Baby's weight
First month	5–10 oz/week
1–3 months	5–8 oz/week
3–6 months	2.5–4.5 oz/week
6–12 months	1–3 oz/week

Source: Dewey K et al. Growth of breast-fed and formula-fed Infants from 0 to 18 months: The DARLING study. *Pediatrics* 89: 1035-141: 1993

- Weight loss is stabilized by the end of the first week
- Weight should be regained by 10 to 14 days after birth
- Infants who are not back to their birth weight by this time need to be evaluated
- See Table 11.4 for an example of a baby's weight gain pattern
- See also Chapter 15, "Breastfeeding Beyond the First Month"

Sleeping Patterns

Parental Issues
- In a 24-hour time period, babies can sleep from eight to twenty hours
- Many parents have voiced concerns about their babies' sleeping habits
- You can help a mother determine whether she has realistic expectations
- A mother can increase her rest by doing the following:
  - Sleeping when her baby sleeps
  - Taking several naps
  - Going to bed early in the evening and taking her baby to bed with her

- Having the baby's father bring the baby to the bed for feedings, enabling the mother to stay in bed at night

Encouraging a Baby to Sleep

- Establish a bedtime ritual with quiet, soothing activities directly before bedtime
- Darken the room for the baby at bedtime
- Warm the bed with a heating pad or a hot water bottle before putting the baby in it
- Use flannel sheets to avoid waking the baby with the initial coolness of cotton sheets
- If the baby sleeps for longer periods during the day, gradually condition him to reverse his schedule by waking him every two to three hours during the day

Breastfeeding Issues with Sleep

- Nursing directly before bedtime will help soothe the baby and give him a full stomach
- Nurse lying down in the middle of the bed and leave him there when he falls asleep, remaining attentive to safety issues
- Stimulate the baby as little as possible when he wakes in the middle of the night to nurse
- Place a night light in the baby's room to avoid turning on a bright light
- If his diaper needs to be changed, change it before he is put to the second breast
- Both the baby and the mother need to be kept warm so that they can return to sleep more easily

Cosleeping

- Cosleeping infants arouse more often and in synchrony with their mothers than do separate sleepers
- Cosleeping may reduce the risk of Sudden Infant Death Syndrome (SIDS)
- More frequent arousal promotes nighttime breastfeeding

- Mothers who cosleep with their babies nurse them three times more frequently than those whose babies sleep in a separate room
- Routinely bedsharing and breastfeeding mothers and infants receive more total sleep than routine solitary sleeping and breastfeeding mothers
- Routine bedsharers evaluate their sleep more positively than solitary sleeping and breastfeeding mothers
- Some parents are uncomfortable with cosleeping; these parents are concerned that:
  - It is emotionally unhealthy for an infant to share the same bed as parents
  - It is difficult to break the habit after it has been established
  - The mother can harm her baby by inadvertently rolling over onto him while she is asleep
- Most mothers instinctively recognize their babies' presence and respond accordingly
- A baby would most likely cry out and wake his mother if she were to roll too close to him
- Cosleeping is inappropriate at times when parents may not be as responsive to the baby's presence, such as in the following situations:
  - Illness
  - Under the influence of medications, alcohol, or recreational drugs
  - It is not advisable to cosleep in a water bed

Sudden Infant Death Syndrome (SIDS)

- Not breastfeeding a baby may place him at a greater risk for SIDS and he does not receive immunologic protection from human milk
- Placing the baby in a supine position (on his back) rather than in a prone position (on his stomach) reduces the incidence of SIDS substantially
- Breastfed babies almost always exclusively sleep next to their mothers in a supine position
- Breastfeeding and bedsharing mothers almost always put their babies on their backs to facilitate reaching the breast to feed

- Statistically, the babies of bedsharing, low income mothers have an increased risk for SIDS—these mothers also smoke in conjunction with bedsharing, put their babies in a prone position, and fail to breastfeed
- The two most significant risk factors for SIDS are sleeping in a prone position and maternal smoking
- Another risk factor is the baby's inhalation of passive smoke

Crying and Colic

Purpose of Crying

- Infant crying is a cause-and-effect relationship
  - Teaches the baby he has the ability to make things happen through crying
  - Elicits his parents' response
  - Shows his needs will be met
- Premature infants have different crying patterns than full-term infants:
  - Different rhythm, pause, and inhalation-exhalation patterns
  - Cry is a full octave higher, signaling greater urgency
- Enables the baby to form greater attachment to his parents
- Develops his trust more readily, which causes him to cry less

Effect of Infant Crying

- The following are the effects of crying on the infant:
  - Causes difficulty breastfeeding
  - Often causes an inability to organize themselves and their behavior for a period of time after a crying spell
  - Increases blood pressure
  - Increases intracranial pressure

- Flows poorly oxygenated blood back into systematic circulation rather than into the lungs
- Increases the cerebral blood volume and decreases cerebral oxygenation—such a fluctuating pattern of cerebral blood flow is associated with intracranial hemorrhage
- Obstructs the venous return in the inferior vena cava and re-establishes fetal circulation to the heart
- Increases the alveolar distention within the lungs where it is not needed, which may, in the extreme, lead to a pneumothorax
- Leads to increased glucose expenditure, which results in hypoglycemia in the immediate postpartum period
- Increases gastric distention, which results in a very discontented baby due to gas pain
- Teaches those babies repeatedly left to cry alone to ultimately learn to give up and tune out the world
- The effects of crying on the mother are as follows:
  - Causes her heart to beat faster
  - Increases her blood pressure
  - Increases her breast temperature

Identifying the Cause of Crying

- If the baby is crying from hunger
  - Learn to recognize his hunger cry
  - Consider the length of time since the last feed, how well he nursed at the previous feed, his general disposition, and whether he can be soothed easily
  - Note that mothers who respond to hunger cries by nursing have more contented babies
- If the baby is crying due to body discomfort, check for the following:
  - Wet or soiled diapers that cause a drop in temperature
  - Too much heat
  - State of undress, even when temperature is controlled

- Skin irritations such as a texture of cloth that touches his body
  - Heat rash
  - Diaper rash
  - Internal discomfort such as gas or overfeeding
- External stimuli—anything that happens to the baby suddenly or the baby being overhandled

Comforting a Crying Baby

- Provide a background of constant rhythmic stimulation
- Hold the baby
- Swaddle the baby (unless he indicates he does not like to be swaddled)
- "Wear" the baby in a sling
- Encourage parents to focus on the cues their baby gives
- Encourage a baby's positive response to a technique
- Try a new approach if the baby exhibits withdrawal or avoidance behaviors

Distinguishing Crying from Colic

- Definition of colic
  - Is the spasmodic contraction of smooth muscle, causing pain and discomfort
  - Is unconsolable crying for which no physical cause can be found
  - Lasts more than three hours daily
  - Occurs at least three days a week
  - Continues for at least three weeks
- Signs of colic
  - Is any unexplained fussiness, fretfulness, and irritability
  - Is when a baby appears to suffer from severe discomfort most of the time
  - Is shown by cries that are piercing and explosive attacks
  - Can be a rumbling sound that is audible in the baby's gut

- Causes the baby to swallow air and further aggravate discomfort through continuous crying
- The following are a baby's possible responses to colic:
  - Draws his legs up sharply into his abdomen
  - Has apparent abdominal pain
  - Clenches his fists
  - Appears intense, energetic, excitable, and easily startled
  - Grimaces and stiffens
  - Twists his body
  - Awakens easily and frequently

Occurrence of Colic
- As many as 16 to 30 percent of all infants experience colic-like symptoms
  - In a majority of infants, the symptoms subside by 16 weeks of age
  - There seems to be no distinction between bottle-feeding and breastfeeding infants
  - It seems to be more common when solid foods are introduced in the diets of infants younger than three months of age
- Its exact cause has not been determined medically, however it could possibly be caused by the following:
  - Immature gastrointestinal and/or neurologic systems
  - A lack of muscle tone causing food to move up out of the stomach
  - Intrauterine and birth-related problems such as prematurity, small for gestational age (SGA), birth trauma or anoxia
  - Maternal hypertension coupled with epidural anesthesia
  - A prenatal intake of street drugs
  - A smoking parent
  - Food sensitivity (see Chapter 15)

Cow and Soy Milk Intolerances

- The protein in cow's milk is a common cause of allergies in infants
- Immunoglobulin G (IgG) is higher in the milk from mothers of colicky babies than in mothers of noncolicky babies
- It is estimated that 30 percent of colic-like behavior in breastfed infants is due to the intolerances of protein found in cow's milk
- A mother can try to cure a colicky baby by eliminating dairy foods from her diet for two weeks
- If cow's milk was the cause of the infant's colic-like behavior, she may see improvement within 48 hours to several days
- A mother should gradually reintroduce dairy slowly into her diet after two weeks of a dairy-free diet
- It is recommended that the mother start with hard cheeses or yogurt during Week 1, add soft cheeses during Week 2, butter and ice cream during Week 3, and cow's milk in small quantities during Week 4
- Any time the symptoms return, the mother can once again reduce her dairy product intake

The Diet of the Mother and Infant

- The mother needs to remove all possible sources of intolerance from her diet and from her baby's diet
- Feed the baby nothing but his mother's own milk
- Vitamins, fluoride, and iron supplements may be a source of discomfort
- Infants who receive antibiotics may be at greater risk for food allergies
- A mother should monitor her food intake, which includes any medications, vitamin supplements, caffeine, high-protein foods, milk, wheat, chocolate, eggs, and nuts

Lactose Overload

- Colic-like symptoms can occur when an infant consumes too much lactose and not enough fat
- Causes of lactose overload include the following:
  - Overactive letdown
  - Overabundant milk production
  - Insufficient hindmilk intake
  - Limits placed on the baby's time at the breast
  - Prolonged antibiotic therapy of the mother or baby
- Lactose ferments in a baby's gut, which leads to gassiness and fussiness
- Stools may be green, frothy, loose, and frequent in addition to the infant having poor weight gain, a bloated abdomen, and a great deal of gas
- To avoid lactose overload, allow the baby to feed without restrictions, staying at the first breast until he has received the fatty hindmilk

Treatment of Colic-Like Symptoms

- Infant massage is the most effective soothing method
  - The mother holds the naked baby on her lap with his head on her knees
  - She gently massages his stomach, shoulders, head, hands, and feet
  - She then turns him over to massage his back
  - Finally, she holds him against her shoulder and soothes him until he is calm
  - The infant will likely cry throughout the massage but is usually calm by the end
  - If massaged regularly, the colic-like symptoms may disappear within one or two weeks rather than the usual three to six months
- See Figure 11.4 for examples of other interventions
- If all comfort measures fail, the parents may want to consult the baby's physician to rule out any illnesses

Supporting Parents of a Baby with Colic-Like Symptoms

- Suggest the following helpful reading materials:
  - *The Fussy Baby* and *The Baby Book*, both by Sears (1992, 1993)
  - *Curing Infant Colic* by Taubman (1990)
  - *Crying Baby, Sleepless Nights* by Jones (1992)
- A baby's disposition can be affected by his mother's emotional state
  - The baby may be comforted immediately when another person picks him up
  - This may further add to the feelings of guilt that the mother feels
- Parents need a great deal of emotional support
  - Frequent close contact with a support person
  - Time away from the baby to maintain perspective

- **Holding techniques**

  "Wear" the baby around the house in a cloth baby sling, walking and dancing in a soothing manner.

  Hold the baby upright against the parent's shoulder near the neck.

  Place the baby on his stomach across the parent's lap or knees.

  Carry the baby against the parent's hip.

  Lay the baby face down on the parent's chest.

  Lay the baby face down on the inside of the parent's forearm with the baby's head held in the crook of the parent's hand. The pressure on the stomach feels good and the parent can use the free hand to pat and rub the baby's back.

  Pick up the baby as soon as he starts to fuss. This will decrease the length of time he is fussy and prevent it from escalating.

- **Sounds and motion**

  Provide a steady noise from a vacuum, clothes dryer, music, humming, or tapes of the mother's heartbeat.

  Play a recording of the baby's own cry.

Parents speak closely and softly in whispers.
Baby looks at the mother's and father's face.
Provide an unexpected distraction to startle the baby to cease crying.
Take the baby for a car ride to provide soothing, rhythmic motion.
Bounce, swing, rock and walk in slow, rhythmical movements.

- **Security and warmth**

Place the baby in a warm bath.
Check for any rashes which could indicate reaction to the fiber or detergent in clothing or blankets.
Swaddle the baby to provide closeness and security, or unswaddle him if the blanket seems too constricting.
Check the diaper for dampness and keep the baby warm with sweaters or blankets.
Place a warmed hot water bottle against the baby's stomach area to help him release tension and thereby encourage the passing of gas.

Figure 11.4 Measures for comforting a colicky baby

12

Getting Breastfeeding Started

Encouraging Baby-Led Feeds

Allow the Baby to Set the Pace
- Begin each feed on the side that received the least stimulation at the previous feed
- Continue nursing on that breast until the baby removes himself
- Unlatch the baby for burping or due to discomfort—resume nursing on that breast again
- Allow the baby to feed at one breast at a feed if he wishes to do so

Place No Restrictions on the Length of Feeds
- The use of restrictions confuses and frustrates the mother and baby
- Restrictions alter a baby's natural regulation of foremilk and hindmilk intake
- Restrictions may lead to colic-like symptoms in babies
- Mothers should be encouraged to watch their babies, not the clock
- In addition, see also Chapter 11, Infant Assessment and Behavior

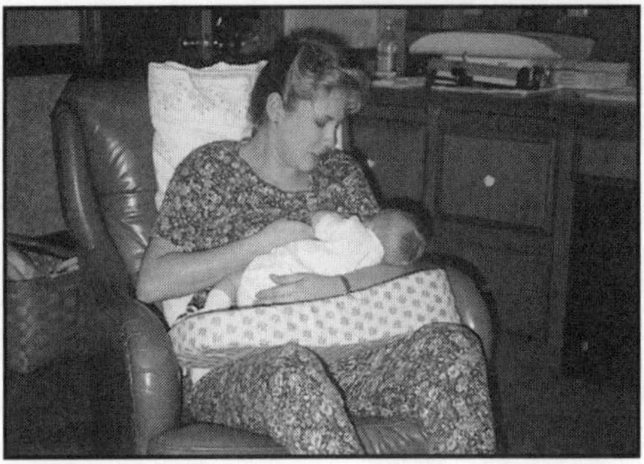

POSITIONING

Figure 12.1 A mother positioned with pillows to help with comfort and positioning of the baby

Printed by permission of Linda Kutner.

Positioning for Feeding

Mother's Body: Zone One

- Place pillows where necessary (see Figure 12.1)
- Support the mother's back and arms
- Raise the baby to a level near the breast
- Rest the mother's feet comfortably on the floor or a footstool with her knees higher than her hips when sitting
- The following are options for breastfeeding after a cesarean birth:
  - Place a pillow on the mother's lap to protect her abdominal incision
  - Position the baby at the mother's side in a clutch hold

Mother's Breast: Zone Two

- Weight of the breast may cause it to be pulled slightly from the baby's mouth
- Pulling of the breast from the baby's mouth causes the baby to nipple suck rather than to breastfeed
- For the first few weeks, the mother should support her breast during feeds

Latch-On

- Use the C-hold to support the breast (see Figure 19.3 in Chapter 19)
- Some babies benefit from the Dancer hand position (see Figure 19.4 in Chapter 19) due to the following problems:
  - Prematurity
  - Weak muscle development
  - Difficulty holding the jaw steady while they suck

Baby's Body: Zone Three

- The baby is well supported, is held chest to chest by the mother, and is level with her breast
- The baby's ears, shoulders, and hips are aligned
- The baby's body is flexed
- Both of the baby's cheeks are the same distance from the mother's breast
- The baby is held closely enough so that the tip of his nose and chin indent the mother's breast
- If breathing becomes obstructed by the mother's breast, place the baby as follows:
  - Pull the baby's lower body inward toward the mother's body
  - Angle the baby's head slightly away from the breast

Baby's Mouth: Zone Four

- The baby's mouth is wide open
- The baby's mouth is positioned slightly below the center of the breast
- The baby's lower lip covers more of the areola than does the upper lip
- The baby's tongue is extended over the lower gum (alveolar ridge)
- Rooting reflex
  - The baby instinctively turns his head toward the stimulation source
  - Touching other parts of the baby's face can confuse and frustrate him
  - Forcing the baby to the breast can disturb the rooting-tongue-reflex system

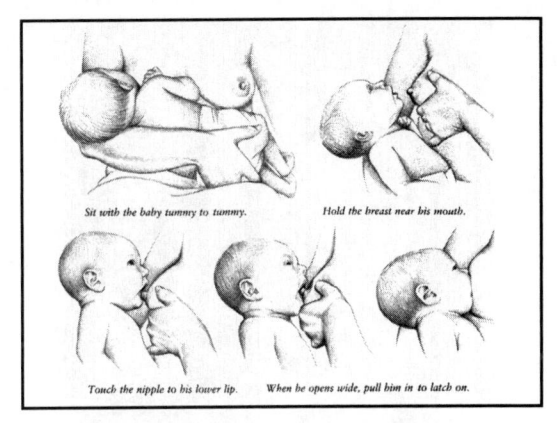

Figure 12.2 The process of a latch-on
Source: Huggins K. *The Nursing Mother's Companion*, the Harvard Common Press, 1986.

- When crying, a baby places his tongue up toward the palate
- If forced to the breast (even with gentle force), the baby may remember the forced situation and defend himself by placing his tongue in the palate at subsequent feeds
- See Figure 12.2 for the process of a latch-on
- In addition, see Chapter 13, Infant Attachment and Suckling for a discussion about latch-on

Using a Variety of Breastfeeding Positions

Cradle Hold
- See Figure 12.3 for an example of a cradle hold
- The mother has limited control over the movement of the baby's head
- The mother cannot assist or guide her baby to a better latch
- A cradle hold is not a good position if there are problems with latching on or milk transfer

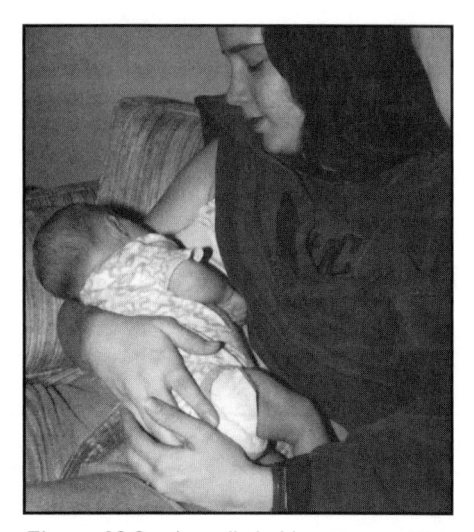

Figure 12.3 A cradle hold nursing position
Printed by permission of Debbie Shinskie.

Clutch (Football) Hold
- See Figure 12.4 for an example of the clutch hold
- The mother is able to hold the baby's entire body on her arm
- The mother can control the baby's body movements better
- This hold encourages a baby to nurse on the breast even if he refuses to nurse in the traditional sitting position
- This hold is an effective nursing position for the following types of infants:
  - Premature infants
  - Infants who have difficulty latching
  - Twins

Dominant Hand Position
- See Figure 12.5 for an example of the dominant hand position
- It is also referred to as the cross cradle hold

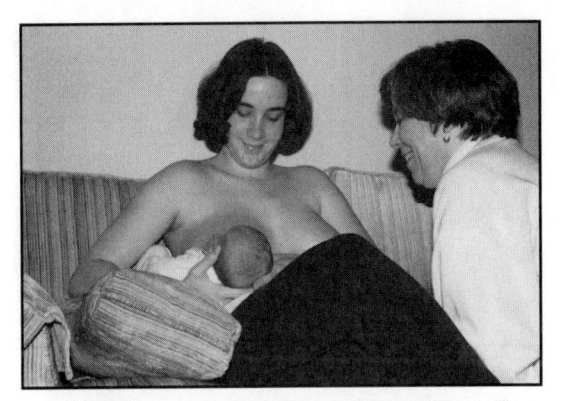

Figure 12.4 A clutch (football) hold nursing position
Printed by permission of Debbie Shinskie.

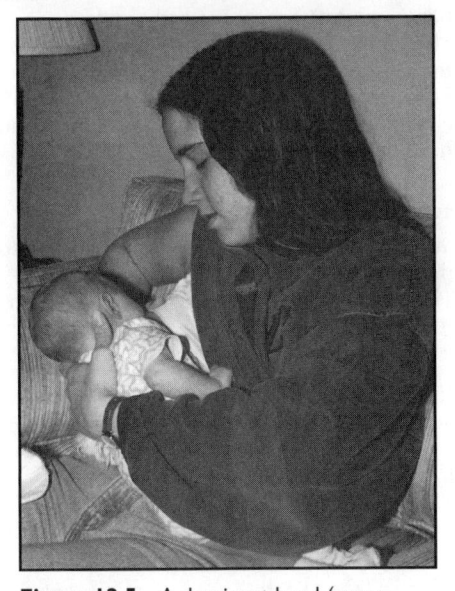

Figure 12.5 A dominant hand (cross cradle) nursing position
Printed by permission of Debbie Shinskie.

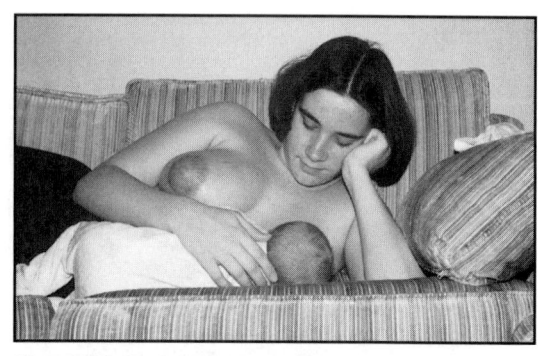

Figure 12.6 A lying down nursing position
Printed by permission of Debbie Shinskie.

- This position enables a mother to control her baby's movements during early feeds
- The mother can switch breasts without repositioning her hold on the baby
- The mother can begin a feed at one breast in a clutch hold and end the feed with a cross cradle hold on the opposite breast

Lying Down Position
- See Figure 12.6 for an example of the lying down position
- This position helps a mother get her necessary rest

Posture Feeding
- See Figure 12.7 for an example of posture feeding
- The mother begins in a sitting position, puts her baby to breast, and then lies down
- The mother may need to support her baby's forehead with the heel of her hand to help him hold his head up and away from her breast
- Gravity assists feeding
- This hold prevents excessive amounts of milk from gushing into the baby's mouth

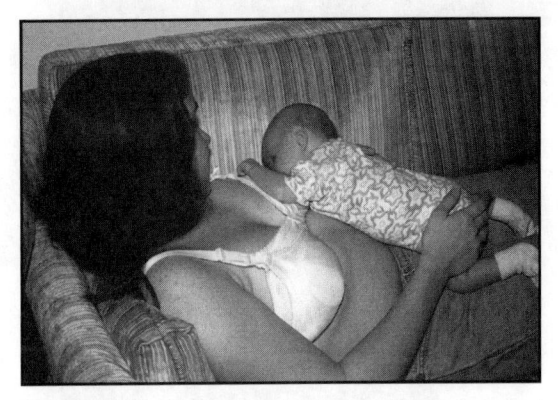

Figure 12.7 The posture feeding position
Printed by permission of Debbie Shinskie.

- This hold encourages the baby's jaw to fall forward by gravity
- It is useful for
  - A mother with an overabundant milk supply
  - A baby who bites or retracts his tongue

Unconventional Nursing Positions

- Special nursing positions are useful when conventional nursing positions do not work, such as in the following situations:
  - The nipple has a sore spot that is aggravated during feeds
  - A plugged duct cannot be cleared
  - The baby is in traction or post surgery
- Nursing over a baby on all fours
  - See Figure 12.8 for an example of nursing over a baby on all fours
  - The mother places her baby on a bed, leans over him on her hands and knees, and positions her breast in his mouth by rotating his body
  - To avoid back strain, the mother can raise the baby by placing pillows or blankets under him

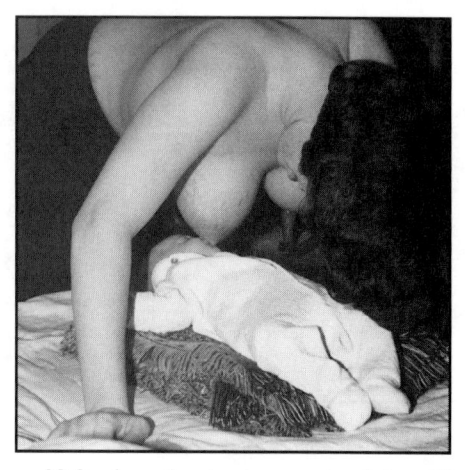

Figure 12.8 A mother leaning over her baby while on all fours

Printed by permission of Debbie Shinskie.

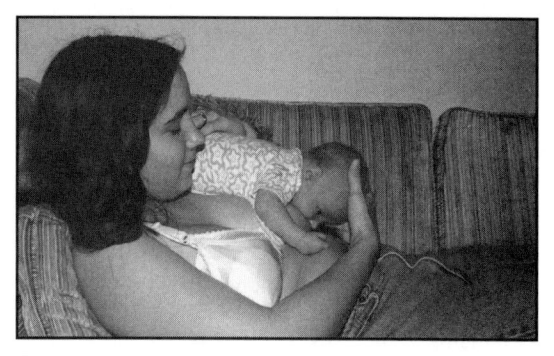

Figure 12.9 A baby lying over a mother's shoulder

Printed by permission of Debbie Shinskie.

- Nursing a baby over the mother's shoulder
  - See Figure 12.9 for an example of nursing over the mother's shoulder
  - The mother lies on her back and places her baby on his stomach with his feet over her shoulder

Assisting at a Feed

Observe the Mother
- Is the mother comfortable and is her back supported?
- How does she hold the baby?
- How does she hold her breast?

Observe the Baby
- What is the position of his body?
- What is the position of his mouth?
- What is the placement of his tongue?
- Are the baby's lips flanged out?
- Are the baby's cheeks smooth and equally distant from the breast?

Observe the Baby Feeding
- Nutritive sucking
  - The baby suckles about once per second
  - A large quantity of milk is flowing
- Non-nutritive sucking
  - The baby suckles about two times per second
  - There is little milk flow
  - May indicate that a baby is not attached well, or that there is little milk available, if observed during an entire feeding

Assisting a Sleepy Baby
- The following are possible causes of a baby's sleepiness:
  - Medications taken during labor
  - Traumatic birth, caused by a long labor or a long second stage labor
  - Usual sleepy period
  - Delayed first feeding
  - Overlooked feeding cues
  - Sensory overload (for example, a loud nursery)

Sleepy Baby

- - Crying related to interventions, particularly circumcision
  - Jaundice
  - Schedule-imposed feeds
  - Cesarean delivery
  - Hypothermia
- The following are acceptable parts of a care plan for a sleepy baby:
  - 24-hour rooming in
  - Skin-to-skin contact
  - Attempting a feed when the baby shows signs of a light sleep state
  - Responding to the baby's feeding cues
  - Putting the baby to breast every 30 minutes to one hour
- Until feedings are established, a mother should do the following:
  - Pump or hand express milk
  - Feed the baby her expressed milk by cup

Techniques Used to Rouse a Baby

- Talking to the baby and trying to make eye contact
- Loosening or removing the baby's blankets
- Holding the baby upright in a sitting or standing position
- Partially or fully undressing the baby
- Changing the baby's diaper
- Stimulating the baby through increased skin contact, massage, or gently rubbing his hands and feet
- Stimulating the baby's rooting reflex
- Bringing the baby close to the breast so the baby can detect the scent of the mother's skin
- Stimulating a baby's sense of taste by expressing milk onto a nipple or into his mouth
- Wiping the baby's forehead and cheeks with a cool moist cloth
- Manipulating the baby's arms and legs by playing pat-a-cake or by doing baby exercises

RESISTING BREASTFEEDING

- Providing increased skin-to-skin contact—giving the baby a bath or having the mother take a bath with him
- If the baby takes the breast but does not maintain a rhythmic suck-swallow-pause pattern, stroke the baby under his chin from front to back, and compress the breast as with manual expression

Assisting a Baby Who Cries and Resists Going to Breast

- The following are the possible causes of fussiness:
  - The baby has been handled too much by caregivers
  - The baby is in pain or has experienced pain
  - The mother received medication during labor that was transmitted to her baby
  - The baby has discomfort from the use of forceps, vacuum extraction, or an internal monitor lead; or he has a cephalhematoma
  - The baby is experiencing oral aversion as a result of deep suctioning
  - The baby is irritable
  - The baby was given artificial nipples or pacifiers, which resulted in a nipple preference
  - The mother's lack of confidence causes her to hold her baby tentatively
  - The baby needs to be swaddled to provide boundaries, or needs to be soothed by being cuddled skin to skin with parents
  - The baby has shut down due to too much intervention, such as someone attempting to push him on the breast
  - The mother and infant have been separated, which resulted in missed feeding cues
- The following are parts of a care plan for a fussy baby:
  - Limiting the invasive procedures to minimize crying
  - Providing skin-to-skin contact

- Cuddling without pushing the baby to breastfeed
- Working with a baby in short cycles
- Being sensitive to and respecting the baby's cues
- Building the mother's confidence
- Using slow, calm, deliberate movements in caring for the baby
- Cuddling, holding, and walking with the baby
- Talking or singing to the baby in a soft voice
- Swaddling the baby
- Nursing in a dark, quiet room
- Rocking in a rocking chair in order to relax both the mother and baby
- Burping the baby often
- Carrying the baby in a position that puts gentle, firm pressure on his abdomen (on the mother's hip or shoulder)
- Playing music, creating monotonous noise (noise from a vacuum cleaner or dishwasher, for example), or using a recording of such sounds
- Changing a baby's diaper when it becomes damp or soiled
- Having the mother and baby sleep or nap together so the baby is comforted by the mother's body warmth and heartbeat
- Massaging the baby for 10 to 15 minutes (the baby may fuss during the massage and become quiet afterward)
- Using a sling to carry the baby close to the mother's body
- Using a baby swing for times when individual attention is not possible
- Removing the baby's clothes to expose his body to the air for limited amounts of time (only acceptable when the baby is full term and has established good temperature control)
- Lying the baby on his stomach on his mother's lap and having the mother gently bounce her knees or move her knees back and forth

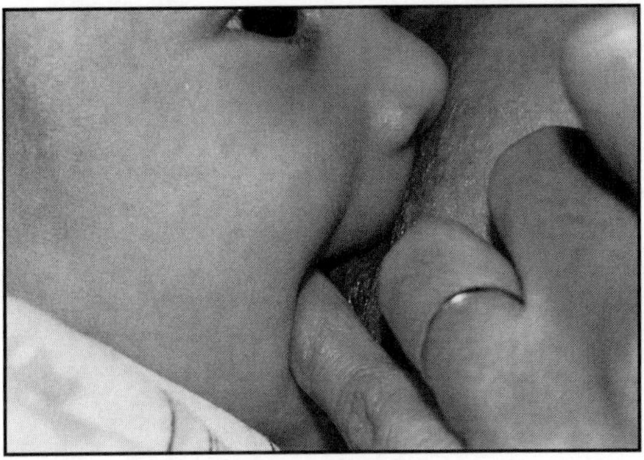

Figure 12.10 A finger placed in the corner of the baby's mouth between the gums helps break suction so that the breast can be gently removed.

Printed by permission of Kay Hoover.

- Having the mother and baby take a bath together
- Providing monotonous movement by giving a carriage or car ride
- Removing all allergens from the mother's diet

Ending the Feed
- The mother should allow the baby to determine the length of the feed
- His mouth will gently release her breast when he is finished
- If the mother needs to remove the baby from her breast (see Figure 12.10), she should do the following:
  - Break the suction by inserting her finger gently into the corner of his mouth between his gums
  - Press a finger against her breast near the corner of the baby's mouth enabling her breast to slip easily out of her baby's mouth

Infant Attachment and Suckling

Sucking and Suckling

Effects of Sucking on a Baby
- Stimulates saliva, which contains enzymes that help predigest food before the stomach enzymes begin to work on it
- Stimulates gastrointestinal secretions, hormones, and motility
- Releases certain hormones that promote satiety and sleepiness in a baby
- Has a calming effect on the baby and helps him to pass gas and move his bowels

Effects of Sucking on a Mother
- Activates the release of prolactin that stimulates milk production and feelings of yearning for her baby
- Releases oxytocin, which causes cuddly and warm feelings in a mother, enables her milk to let down, and helps her uterus to return to its prepregnant size

Sucking

Infant's Sucking Pattern
- Process of sucking
  - The baby draws the breast into his mouth
  - Maintains a negative pressure to keep it there
  - Actively suckles milk out with peristaltic action of his tongue
- Nutritive sucking
  - Increases the rate of milk flow
  - Is a slower sucking rate of about one suck per second
- Non-nutritive sucking
  - Increases in rate as milk is removed
  - Reaches about two sucks per second
  - Occurs when milk removal is minimal

Factors That Affect Sucking
- Nutritive sucking is adversely affected by central nervous system depressant drugs when they are given to a mother in labor
- Letting a baby cry can compromise the baby's innate sucking behavior, which creates a disorganized suck
- Full-term neonates younger than 24 hours old have less rhythmic sucking than older full-term infants
- Normal sucking is a partly learned behavior
- Babies who exhibit short suckling bursts and shorter overall suckling times have more feeding difficulties at six weeks of age than those who have longer, continuous bursts and spend more of their time suckling

Physiology of Suckling and Milk Transfer
- The baby uses his tongue to draw the nipple and areola into his mouth
- This forms a cone-shaped extension of the breast that conforms to the shape of the baby's mouth
- The baby's tongue ripples in a rhythmic, wavelike motion from the front toward the back of the mouth

- The areola and nipple are pressed upward progressively against the upper gum, hard palate, and soft palate at the back of the mouth, which moves milk through the lactiferous sinuses and out the nipple (see Table 13.1)
- The baby's jaw drops and creates negative pressure, which allows milk to move from the nipple to the baby's mouth
- Swallowing cannot occur simultaneously with breathing
- A pattern of more sucks per minute is associated with fewer swallows, more breaths, and higher oxygen saturations
- Figure 13.1 shows an infant suckling at the breast

Sucking on a Bottle
- The baby draws the nipple into his mouth (see Figure 13.2)
- The baby must alter his mouth to accommodate the shape of an artificial nipple
- The baby must generate enough suction pressure so that the milk flows freely from the bottle (whereas in breastfeeding, milk is released through negative pressure)
- The baby breathes less often while feeding than does one who breastfeeds
- A baby who is bottle-fed is more likely to experience a decreased heart rate
- Use of an artificial nipple may do the following:
  - Alter the proper development of swallowing, the alignment of teeth, and the shaping of the hard palate
  - Weaken the baby's suck
  - Reduce the strength of the masseter muscle
  - Increase the strength of orbicularis oris muscles
  - Cause the facial muscles to develop in an exact opposite pattern from which they were intended to develop

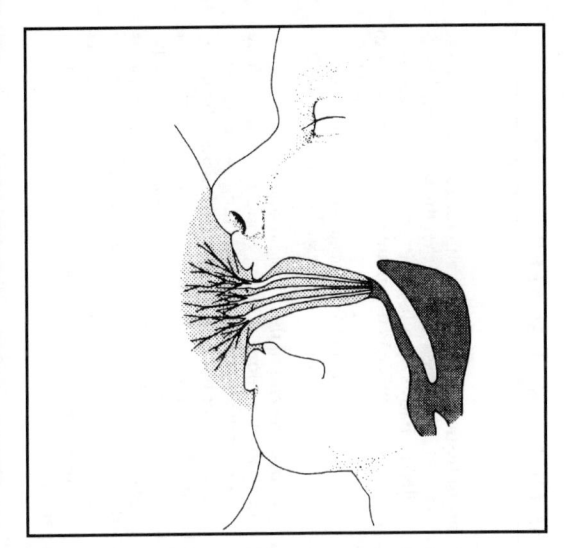

Figure 13.1 Infant suckling correctly at the breast

Woolridge M. The anatomy of Infant sucking. *Midwifery* 2:164–171; 1986. Reprinted with permission.

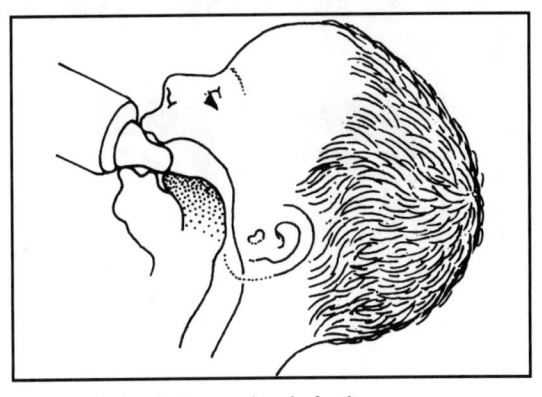

Figure 13.2 Sucking in bottle feeding

Illustration by Marcia Smith.

TABLE 13.1 THE PROCESS OF MILK TRANSFER

Step		Description
One	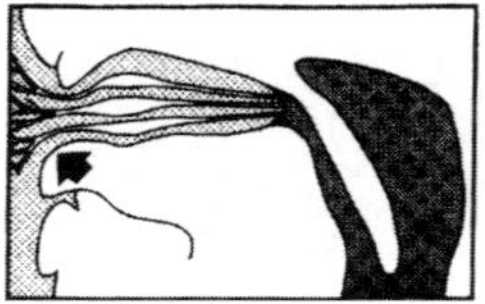	The baby takes the breast tissue into his mouth and forms a teat from the mother's nipple, areola, and breast tissue. (Note that the teat formed by the breast and nipple fills the baby's mouth, leaving no room for movement of the breast within the mouth.) As the infant draws the teat far into his mouth, his tongue cups around the teat to form a trough for the milk. The baby's tongue stays cupped along the sides of the breast and nipple teat, and covers the alveolar ridge throughout the suckling cycle.
Two		The cycle of suckling begins. The end of the nipple is drawn back to the soft palate by a combination of suction and compression. When it is fully extended, the nipple is approximately three times as long as it is at rest. This suggests that the baby cannot traumatize the breast tissue if he has a good mouthful of breast. The nipple is compressed for only a fraction of a second and will not look flattened or compressed when the feeding ends if the baby was attached correctly. When the nipple touches the soft palate at the back of the oral cavity, it elicits the baby's suckling reflex. The baby then raises his lower jaw to pinch off milk that has collected in the lactiferous sinuses. At the same time, the anterior tip of his tongue begins to push upward against the breast tissue.

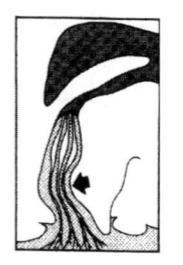

214

Three

The baby strips the milk from the lactiferous sinuses. A peristaltic wave of compression moves along the underside of the teat. The baby's tongue then pushes against his hard palate, thus compressing the sinuses. A bolus of milk is then squeezed from the teat. (Note that when the sinuses are compressed, milk flows from the breast. The baby does not get milk from the breast by suction.)

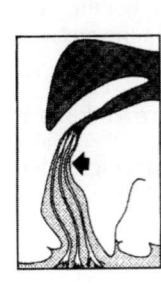

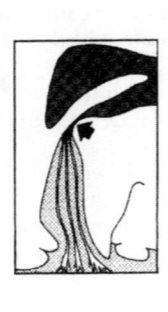

Four

This wave of compression continues to the back of the tongue, which pushes against the soft palate and rises to seal the nasal cavity. The trachea and vocal chords are closed off by the epiglottis, and milk is propelled into the esophagus. This, in turn, initiates the baby's swallowing reflex.

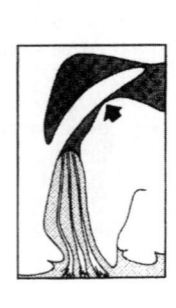

Five

The compression ends at the posterior base of the infant's tongue. The back of the tongue depresses, which creates negative pressure. The breast is then drawn back into the baby's mouth to begin another cycle.

Source: Woolridge MW. The Anatomy of Infant Sucking. *Midwifery* 2: 64–171; 1986. Reprinted with permission.

A Good Latch

- The baby may develop a preference for an artificial nipple over the mother's breast
  - Milk flows easier and quicker from a bottle nipple
  - When a baby returns to the breast, he must suckle actively to receive milk

Latching the Baby On

Signs That the Baby Is Latched Well

- Audible swallows are heard
- Long, drawing, nutritive, high flow sucks occur
- In the first 24 to 48 hours, the following occurs:
  - Swallows can be heard that often sound like little puffs of air after three to four high-flow, nutritive sucks
  - The mother may report a tugging or pulling sensation, yet is free of pain both during and after the feed

Principles of a Good Latch

- Lips
  - Are flanged out and open wide at an angle of at least 140 degrees (see Figure 13.1)
  - The bottom lip covers most of the areola, while the top lip covers a lesser degree of it
  - Ensures an adequate compression of the lactiferous sinuses that lie deeper in the breast
- Tongue
  - Is positioned under the breast
  - Extends outward far enough to cover the alveolar ridge
- With his mouth open wide and lips flanged, the baby does the following:
  - Takes in a large mouthful of breast tissue
  - Forms a trough with his tongue
  - Draws the nipple into the center of his mouth or tongue

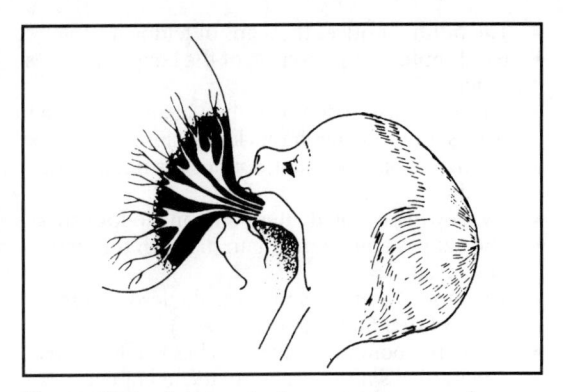

Figure 13.3 A baby who has not taken enough breast tissue into his mouth

Source: King FS. Helping mothers to breastfeed, revised edition, p. 14. Nairobi, Kenya: AMREF. Reprinted with permission.

- The baby then positions his jaws behind the lactiferous sinuses and
  - Compresses them rhythmically
  - Continues to hold the breast in his mouth
  - Establishes a pattern of repeated bursts of suck/swallow/pause . . . suck/swallow/pause
- If the baby does not take enough breast tissue into his mouth (see Figure 13.3), the following could occur:
  - He will have difficulty extracting milk
  - He will compensate by increasing his suction and compressing his lips to hold the nipple securely
  - His intense suction and lip compression could result in nipple soreness
  - He cannot draw breast tissue back to his soft palate
  - He may fail to gain weight

Signs of Good Milk Transfer

- The baby moves from short, rapid sucks to slow, deep sucks early in the feed

- The mother notices the signs of letdown
- No dimpling or puckering of the baby's cheeks is noted
- The breast tissue does not slide in and out of the baby's mouth when he sucks or pauses
- No smacking or clicking sounds are noted with sucking
- Swallowing is noted after every one to four sucks
- The baby is able to maintain his latch throughout a feed
- The mother's breast softens as the feeding progresses (after Stage II lactogenesis)
- The baby spontaneously unlatches and is satiated
- The mother's nipple is not blanched or compressed when the baby unlatches
- The baby is content between most feeds
- The baby's voiding and stooling are appropriate for his age

Problems Getting the Baby Latched onto the Breast

When a Poor Latch Occurs

- Keep the attempts to breastfeed very short—about ten minutes
- When a baby demonstrates withdrawal or avoidance behavior
  - The baby cries, pushes away, hiccoughs, coughs, gags, or sneezes
  - First calm the baby and then try again
  - If the baby rejects the breast after three such attempts, stop all efforts for that feed
  - Snuggle skin to skin with the baby in a relaxed manner
- Watch for the return of approach behaviors
  - The baby will extend his tongue, bring his hand to his mouth, and root
  - Gently put him to the breast and try again

- Give the baby expressed milk until an effective latch is achieved
- See Table 13.2

Possible Signs of a Poor Latch
- The baby is unable to stay on the breast for more than several sucks
- Pain is reported by the mother during or after feeds
- Dimpling or puckering of the baby's cheeks is noted
- The breast slides in and out of the baby's mouth throughout sucking
- Clicking or smacking noises can be heard when the baby suckles
- Little or no swallowing is noted during the feed
- The baby is discontented during or after feeds
- The mother's nipple appears flattened, creased, or blanched after the baby unlatches
- Little or no breast changes occur from the beginning to the end of a feed after Stage II lactogenesis occurs
- The baby has inadequate voiding or stooling, or both

Feeding Adjustments to Improve Latch
- Provide lots of skin-to-skin contact without attempting to put the baby to breast
- Have the mother lie on her back, with her baby between her breasts
- If the baby begins to root for the breast, help guide him, making sure to not push him onto the breast
- Have the mother hold her baby in the position where her dominant hand is in control
- Tickle the baby's lower lip with your finger when the baby is content, awake, and happy
  - Talk to the baby all the time, saying slowly, "o...p...e...n...w...i...d...e"

TABLE 13.2 THE BABY WHO CANNOT GET ATTACHED

CAUSE	SUGGESTIONS FOR MANAGEMENT
The baby is being held in a position that requires him to twist his neck in order to breastfeed.	Help the mother hold her baby closely, and have the baby directly facing and slightly lower than the center of the breast.
The baby does not open his mouth enough.	Tease the baby with the nipple by gently touching his lower lip until he opens his mouth wide before attaching.
The baby has been given an artificial nipple and has developed a sucking preference. He may thrust or hump his tongue when he tries to attach and suckle.	Do not give artificial nipples to the baby; only allow him to suckle at the breast. If supplementation is necessary, use a small cup or a tube at the breast.
The mother's nipples are flat because of engorgement.	Be sure the mother's breasts do not become too full due to limited feedings. If her breasts are engorged, express milk to help the nipple protrude and to soften the areola.
The mother's nipples are inverted to the point that the baby cannot get attached.	Draw out an inverted nipple with mild suction before the feeding using an inverted syringe or pump. (Note that most inverted nipples do not interfere with breastfeeding. Babies attach to the breast, not to the nipple.)

- When the baby responds, put your finger into his mouth, pad side up, to suck on as a reward
  - The mother can demonstrate a wide mouth by opening her mouth wide
- Alternative feeding methods can be helpful to a mother who is frustrated to the point of weaning (see Chapter 19, Breastfeeding Techniques and Devices)
- See Table 13.3

Consequences of a Poor Latch

- An incorrect latch is the primary cause of nipple soreness
- Pain or the anticipation of pain can inhibit a mother's milk ejection reflex
- The baby is unable to remove milk from the mother's breasts adequately
- The mother is at risk for engorgement, plugged ducts, and mastitis
- Milk production is seriously compromised
- The mother's decreased milk ejection reflex causes the baby to receive foremilk primarily and the following to occur:
  - Increased hunger, increased fussiness, and colic-like symptoms
  - Low urine and stool output (possible jaundice)
  - Failure to gain weight or even weight loss
  - In the absence of any intervention, lactation failure is likely to result

Babies Who Have Difficulty Suckling

Causes of Suckling Difficulty

- Most feeding difficulties are caused by improper or incorrect attachment and faulty positioning of the baby at the breast

TABLE 13.3 THE BABY WHO CANNOT STAY ATTACHED

CAUSE	SUGGESTIONS FOR MANAGEMENT
The baby must reach or twist his neck to keep the breast in his mouth.	Be sure that the mother is holding her baby closely. The mother should place him directly facing and slightly lower than her breast, with his nose and chin touching the breast, and his ear, shoulder, and hip in alignment.
The baby is unable to breathe when he is at the breast.	Avoid flexing the baby's head forward in such a way that his nose is pushed against the breast. His head needs to be slightly extended so that his chin and nose are just touching the breast. Pull his bottom in more, and his head will angle out.
The mother is moving either her breast or her baby, or is not supporting the baby enough so that the breast falls away.	Hold the baby in a side-sitting position with his head cradled in the mother's hand for greater head control (avoid pushing at the back of his head). Help the mother identify a good attachment and focus on what it feels like so she can recognize if the baby gradually slips off the breast. Put pillows or blankets under the mother's arm so that a fatigued arm muscle will not

	let the baby slip. Help her check during the feed for good attachment, and to learn trauma-free unlatching and relatching so that both the mother and baby develop the habits of a wide-open, mouth-full attachment. If you can see the problem but the mother cannot, she will continue doing the wrong thing.
The mother's milk is flowing too forcefully.	Be sure that the mother's breasts do not become too full because of limited feeds. If the breasts are engorged, expressing milk will help the nipple to protrude. Suggest that the mother express her milk before a feed so that the flow is less forceful. In addition, the mother should allow her baby to feed on only one breast per feed, without time limitations, until the initial oversupply has diminished. The mother may need to express milk from the other breast for comfort. If she has an overabundance of milk, she may want to nurse the baby on the same side two or three times before changing to the other breast.

- In many cases, suckling difficulties can be alleviated through patience, practice, and the proper positioning of a baby's body and mouth on the breast
- Mothers and caregivers need to recognize the difference between a disorganized suck and a dysfunctional suck
- Babies may exhibit an uncoordinated suck in the first few days of life due to the following:
  - Sucking habits in utero
  - Birth interventions
  - Early artificial nipple feeds
  - Some cases are unexplained
- Most uncoordinated sucking can be resolved with the passage of time or increasing the baby's caloric intake
- See Table 13.4

Assisting the Baby

- Intervention in the hospital for a healthy term infant is rarely indicated
- A baby's oral cavity is extremely sensitive with many complex innervations
  - Too much inappropriate manipulation can result in an aversion to anything going into his mouth, including the breast
  - A finger should be inserted into a baby's mouth only in special circumstances, and it should only be done very carefully by trained personnel

Levels of Intervention for Suckling Difficulty

- Proceed to the next level only if the present measures are unsuccessful (see Chapter 19)
- Noninterventive techniques
  - Determine the probable cause of the suckling difficulty
  - Consider whether the situation will improve with time

TABLE 13.4 ISSUES THAT MAY CAUSE PROBLEMS WITH LATCH-ON OR SUCKLING

CAUSE	SUGGESTIONS FOR MANAGEMENT
Medication received by the mother during labor.	Encourage childbirth educators to focus on labor support issues. Encourage labor and delivery staff to focus on nonpharmacologic comfort measures for labor.
Forceps delivery or vacuum extraction.	Watch the positioning of the infant to avoid putting pressure on the infant's head.
Post birth interventions such as deep laryngeal suctioning or circumcision.	Avoid putting the baby to breast immediately following deep suctioning or any other oral insult until the baby demonstrates readiness. Delay circumcision until the baby has fed well at the breast at least three times.
Prolonged crying, especially due to interventions.	Prevent prolonged crying by helping the mother with her baby. Comfort the baby before putting him to the breast. Teach the mother and staff the importance of feeding on cue rather than when the infant cries. Keep the mother and baby together (rooming in) rather than having the baby in the nursery.
Baby has a fractured clavicle or cephalhematoma.	Position the baby in a manner that prevents pressure on the affected area.

(continues)

TABLE 13.4 ISSUES THAT MAY CAUSE PROBLEMS WITH LATCH-ON OR SUCKLING (continued)

CAUSE	SUGGESTIONS FOR MANAGEMENT
Mother has tight, taut breast tissue with flat or inverted nipples.	Massage the breast before a feed. Use a hold that enables the mother to maintain control over her baby's head movement (clutch hold or cross cradle hold). Use an inverted syringe to form the nipple (see Chapter 19). The mother may also need to use a nipple shield (see Chapter 19).
Incorrect positioning at the breast.	Correct any positioning problems. Make sure that both the mother and her baby are comfortable.
Mother's lack of confidence in handling baby and putting him to her breast.	Give encouragement to the mother and help her see that she and her baby will become more comfortable with one another with practice and time. Show the mother how to handle her baby and how to put him to her breast. Avoid doing it for her.
High-arched or bubble palate.	Use the clutch hold. Take the infant off the breast after 30 to 60 seconds and then re-attach. The second latch helps draw more tissue farther back into the infant's mouth.

Short or tight frenulum.	Contact the pediatrician, dentist, oral surgeon, or ear-nose-throat specialist for evaluation and possible clipping of the frenulum.
Cleft lip.	The lip usually molds around the breast to form suction. If this is not the case, the mother can cover the cleft area with her breast or finger. Massage the breasts before and during the feed.
Cleft palate.	Nurse in a semi-upright position. Hold the breast in the baby's mouth during feeds. Interrupt feeds as necessary to enable the baby to burp or breathe. If the baby cannot obtain sufficient milk through suckling, express and feed the baby milk in a tube feeding device or cup. An obturator—a feeding plate placed over the cleft—may be helpful. The mother will need a referral to a cleft palate team if one is available in your area.
Hypoglycemia in the infant.	Feed the baby. Give the baby expressed colostrum via cup or spoon. Use an artificial baby milk if the mother's expressed milk is not sufficient for the baby's needs. Make sure that the baby is fed at regular intervals. Wake him for a feed if necessary.

(continues)

TABLE 13.4 ISSUES THAT MAY CAUSE PROBLEMS WITH LATCH-ON OR SUCKLING (continued)

Cause	Suggestions for management
Baby is hypotonic or hypertonic.	Positioning is the key. Some hypertonic babies may need to find their own comfortable position. A hypotonic baby will need to be supported well. The mother may need to use a tube-feeding device if the infant does not feed well. Decrease external stimulation for the hypertonic infant. Use rousing techniques for the hypotonic infant, starting with infant massage. Use gentle massage to calm the hypertonic infant. Short and very frequent feeds (every 1 1/2 to 2 hours) will be more effective than longer feeds at longer intervals. Condition the baby by establishing a routine for latching on the breast, especially if the baby's rooting reflex is not well developed. Supplement feeds with expressed milk in a cup or bottle after nursing if the infant is unable to obtain enough milk through use of a tube-feeding device at the breast. Express milk, and supplement the baby's feeds until the condition improves.
Baby engages in tongue sucking or tongue thrust.	A baby who consistently sucks his tongue has been doing so in utero for months. Have the baby learn to suck progressively on the mother's small finger, middle finger, and then thumb to gradually increase his comfort level with larger object sizes in his mouth. Use finger feeding until the baby can latch on.

- Minimal level of intervention
  - Place an index finger in the baby's mouth to pacify him or to initiate rhythmic sucking
  - Use a supplemental feeding device at the breast for a baby who attaches and does not suckle adequately, to help the infant get his necessary calories and to stimulate sucking at same time (this is not helpful if the baby is not latching on to the breast)
- Low-level intervention
  - Insert an index finger into the baby's mouth
  - Evaluate his oral cavity and his suck
- Moderate-level intervention
  - Place an index finger into the baby's mouth to organize his sucking
  - Place slight pressure on the midline of the tongue
  - Pull the finger out slowly to encourage the baby to suck it back in
- High-level intervention
  - The highest degree of intervention is suck training
  - This type of intervention is beyond the scope of most nurses and IBCLCs
  - If there is a need for suck training, often other neurological problems exist and sucking is often the first area in which these problems present
  - A baby who needs suck training must be referred to a professional who is trained and skilled in this field—a physical therapist, a speech therapist, or a neurodevelopmental therapist

14

Breastfeeding Issues in the Early Weeks

Establishing Milk Production

Signs of Sufficient Milk Intake

- Urine output soaks at least six or more regular diapers in the absence of supplemental fluids (fewer if super absorbent diapers are used)
- Stooling four or more times each day after day five through the first month
- Regular intervals of wakefulness, sleep, and feeding
- Healthy skin tone and color
- Fat creases in the baby's arms and legs
- Filling out of clothing
- Increases in length and head size
- Regular weight gain

One Breast or Two

- In the first few days when feeding times are shorter, a baby may nurse on only one breast at each feed, and then drift off to sleep
- A mother should not be concerned about her baby's refusal of the second breast

- Drowsiness occurs in part due to the release of cholecystokinin (CCK) in the baby's system during suckling—a gastrointestinal hormone that enhances digestion, sedation, and the feelings of satiation and well-being
- As days pass and the baby is more alert, feeding times increase and the baby is more likely to feed at both breasts during a session
- Let the baby be the guide if milk production is plentiful and the baby is gaining weight well

Duration of Feeds

- In general, the length of a feed should be determined by the baby's needs
- Limiting the time a baby spends on the breast can result in the following:
  - Baby receives foremilk from both breasts
  - Baby becomes too full to obtain a significant amount of hindmilk from either breast
  - A high-volume, low-fat feed results in poor weight gain
- As the baby matures, he becomes more efficient at extracting milk, and the time spent at the breast decreases
- Unlimited suckling time beginning directly after birth improves breastfeeding
- Mothers may experience some initial nipple discomfort that peaks between the third and sixth day postpartum, lasting until her breast tissue becomes accustomed to suckling
  - Nipple soreness is caused primarily by improper positioning
  - Decreasing the time or frequency of feeds will not prevent this tenderness

Frequency of Feeds

- During the first month
  - Feeding frequency for a healthy, fully developed baby may range from eight to fourteen feeds daily—most babies require eight to ten feeds

- Babies may nurse every one to two hours for part of the day and space other feeds four or five hours apart
- A mother does not need to wake her baby at night for feeds unless he has nursed fewer than eight times in the past 24 hours or is gaining weight slowly
- Babies typically feed as often as every hour or hour and a half during the day and several times during the night
- By six weeks of age, the baby has usually developed a pattern
  - Feeds every two to three hours
  - Has a longer stretch at night
  - Feeding frequency may be balanced by a period of almost constant wakefulness and suckling, generally in the early evening

Increases in Feeding Frequency

- All babies experience periods of sudden growth during their early months
- Babies react to these growth spurts by feeding more frequently
- Mothers have a reserve of milk to carry through until this growth spurt passes
- During the first month of life
  - Patterns of milk intake are established that will continue through the following five months
  - Avoid strictly scheduling feeds and allow the baby to lead his feeds
- During the first few days at home
  - If nursing was restricted at the hospital, the baby will nurse more frequently when he has the ability to establish his own pattern at home
  - The baby may react to dramatic differences between hospital and home, particularly at night

- A baby who has the ability to nurse uninterrupted may not exhibit an increase in the frequency of his feeds
- At ten to fourteen days
  - The baby experiences his first growth spurt and will want to nurse more often
  - The mother also loses the initial fullness in her breasts
- At three to six weeks
  - The baby may nurse more often
  - Increased nursing may be a response to an increase in the mother's activity level
- At three to six months
  - The baby will periodically nurse more frequently to increase milk production in order to meet his needs
  - The mother may incorrectly interpret this increase as a sign of the baby's readiness to begin eating solid foods
- The following are other reasons why there are increased feeds where the baby turns to the breast for security and comfort:
  - Illness
  - Overstimulation
  - Emotional upset
  - Physical discomfort

Decreases in Feeding Frequency

- Often occurs when the baby reaches about three months of age
- Is usually the result of having become a more efficient nurser
- Is a sign that the baby is well-nourished, and there is no cause for worry if the baby does the following:
  - Appears content
  - Is voiding and stooling appropriately
  - Is increasing in weight and body length
  - Has good skin tone

Leaking

Causes of Leaking
- The mother's milk lets down:
  - In response to hearing a baby cry
  - In response to picking up her baby to nurse
  - In response to thinking about breastfeeding or her baby
  - During sexual intercourse, oxytocin is released when the mother experiences an orgasm, and this release produces the letdown
- Overfull breasts
- Overuse of breast shells
- Frequent milk expression
- Clothing that rubs against the nipples
- An overproduction of milk
- A hormonal imbalance

When Leaking Poses a Problem
- Press the heel of the hand over the breast or cross your arms and press
- Wear absorbent breast pads and change them often
- Feed the baby before lovemaking and use absorbent towels over bedding
- Decrease the pressure on the breast from elastic in the bra cup; loosen the bra or wear a larger size
- Discontinue any practices that may stimulate nerves in the nipples, such as the rubbing of clothing on the nipples, holding or cuddling the baby in a particular manner, sexual foreplay, or the overuse of breast shells
- Express or pump milk when feeds are missed or delayed
- Wear dark, patterned clothing or a sweater to conceal any moist spots
- Check for the use of medication that may stimulate milk production, and discontinue its use

Excessive or Inappropriate Leaking—Galactorrhea

- Is excessive or inappropriate milk production—also referred to as spontaneous lactation
- Milk production that greatly exceeds a baby's needs
- Continues after the baby has been weaned
- Occurs at times not related to birth or breastfeeding
- Inappropriate milk production of a nonlactating breast may be due to the use of the following drugs:
  - Thyrotropin-releasing hormones
  - Theophyllines
  - Amphetamines
  - Tranquilizers
- Nerves can be stimulated enough in the following ways to induce significant milk production:
  - Through chest or breast surgery
  - By a fibrocystic breast
  - By herpes zoster
- Hyperprolactinemia that results in galactorrhea can be caused by:
  - Hypothyroidism
  - Hyperthyroidism
  - Psychosis and anxiety medications
  - Chronic renal failure
  - Pituitary tumors
  - Uterine and ovarian tumors

Nipple Soreness

Initial Tenderness—Transient Nipple Soreness

- Is part of the typical postpartum course for a majority of mothers
- Is described as a tenderness during the initial latch and first few sucks
- Peaks in the first week postpartum, particularly between the third and sixth days
- Is associated with the breast becoming accustomed to its use in breastfeeding a newborn

Assessment of Sore Nipples

- The following information should be gathered:
  - Age of the baby and when the nipple soreness began
  - Mother's description of the pain—how it feels and at what times it feels a certain way
  - Any maternal chronic conditions as well as her medication usage
  - Mother's use of soaps, creams, lotions, laundry products, and perfumes
  - Baby's growth and development
  - Possibility of another pregnancy
- An assessment of sore nipples requires an in-person evaluation of the following:
  - Baby's attachment and positioning during a feed
  - Baby's alignment and closeness to the breast
  - Mother's position
  - Connection of mouth to breast
  - Appearance of the nipple before and after a feed—blanching and flattening of the nipple may be clues to a poor latch
  - Mother's technique for ending the feed (observe)
  - Visually assess the baby's oral cavity, especially his tongue and frenulum
  - If no obvious cause can be found by observing the mother and baby during a feed, it may be necessary to perform a digital exam of the baby's oral cavity (see Chapter 19, Breastfeeding Techniques and Devices)

Treatment and Care Plan

- Determine the cause and correct it (see Table 14.1)
- Provide palliative care
  - Pain medication
  - Apply ice in a wet cloth to the nipples prior to a feed
  - Start a feed with the least sore breast
  - Initiate the milk ejection reflex before putting the baby to the breast

TABLE 14.1 SORE NIPPLES

Causes	Actions for the Mother
Soreness from newborn suckling.	• Check to ensure that the baby is put on and comes off the breast properly. • Check to ensure that the nipple is back far enough in the baby's mouth. • Hold the baby closely during nursing so the nipple is not constantly being pulled.
Dried colostrum or milk.	• Moisten the bra or pads before taking the bra off so keratin will not stick to the bra or breast pads when removed.
Poor positioning.	• Bring the baby close to nurse, so he does not pull on the breast. • Bring the baby to the breast so that he has a big mouthful of breast tissue.
Baby chewing or nuzzling onto the nipple.	• Form the nipple for the baby. • Set up a pattern of getting the baby onto the breast, using the rooting reflex.

(continues)

TABLE 14.1 SORE NIPPLES (continued)

Causes	Actions for the Mother
Baby is nursing on the end of the nipple.	• Ensure that the nipple is way back in the baby's mouth by properly latching the baby onto the breast. • Check for flutter tongue. • Check for an inverted nipple. • Check for engorgement.
Baby is chewing his way off the nipple or the nipple is being pulled out of his mouth at the end of the feed.	• Remove the baby from the breast by placing a finger between the baby's gums to ensure the suction is broken. • End a feed when the baby's sucking slows, before he has a chance to chew on the nipple.
Baby is overly eager to nurse.	• Respond to feeding cues promptly. • Pre-express milk to hasten letdown and avoid vigorous sucking.
Inadequate letdown.	• Use massage and relaxation techniques before feeds. • Condition a letdown by setting up a routine for latching the baby onto the breast.

Nipples are not allowed to dry.	- Check for leaking milk. - Check that there are no plastic liners in the breast pads. - Eliminate synthetic fabrics in bras and clothing; wear only cotton or cotton blends. - Air dry the breasts completely after feeds. - Change breast pads frequently.
Improper use of a nipple shield.	- Use shields only to draw the nipple out, then have the baby nurse on the breast. - Avoid shields with inner ridges that irritate the nipples.
Inadequate milk supply; baby is tugging or sucking with no milk removal.	- Nurse more frequently (every 1 to 1 1/2 hours). - Nurse long enough to facilitate good milk production.
Nipple skin is not resistant to stress.	- Improve your diet, especially by adding fresh fruits and vegetables and vitamin supplements. - Eliminate or decrease the use of sugary foods, alcohol, caffeine, and cigarettes. - Check for the use of cleansing or drying agents.

(continues)

TABLE 14.1 SORE NIPPLES (continued)

CAUSES	ACTIONS FOR THE MOTHER
Natural oils are removed or keratin layers are broken down by drying agents (soap, alcohol, shampoo, or deodorant).	• Eliminate irritants. • Wash the breasts with water only. • Apply a lubricant after air drying, if necessary.
Nipple is irritated by going braless under rough clothing or by rubbing against the bra during vigorous exercise.	• Wear a bra or change to one with more support (a jogger's bra, for example). • Wear a softer fabric blouse.
Residue of laundry products is on the clothing.	• Use less detergent, and rinse wash loads twice. • Try different laundry products.
Teething causes increased feeds, chomping down on the nipple, irritation by a change in the baby's saliva, or medication used for the baby's gums.	• Wash the breast after every feed in plain, warm water to remove the baby's saliva or other irritants. • Breastfeed before giving solid foods rather than after. • Use soothing techniques instead of nursing to comfort the baby. • Stop feeding after the first incident of biting and resume when the baby is more hungry.

240

Baby falls asleep and clamps down on the breast.	• Keep a finger ready to break suction and stop feeding when the sucking pattern changes. • Remove the baby before he falls asleep.
Teeth marks on the breast (not usually a cause for soreness, but the mother may say the baby is biting).	• Alternate the nursing positions.
Irritation from food particles in the toddler's mouth.	• Check the toddler's mouth before feeds. • Offer the toddler a sip of water or wipe his mouth with a clean, moist cloth before nursing. • Breastfeed before offering solid foods.
Mother is menstruating or pregnant.	• If menstruating, the discomfort will last only a few days. • If pregnant, discuss plans for continued nursing or weaning.
Thrush (a yeast-like infection; see discussion of thrush).	• Have a physician check and prescribe medication for both mother and baby. • Discard or boil any items that the baby puts in his mouth.

(continues)

TABLE 14.1 SORE NIPPLES (continued)

Causes	Actions for the Mother
Sensitivity to a topical ointment applied to the breast.	• Discontinue its use.
Improper use of a breast pump or nipple shield.	• Use items correctly or discontinue their use.
Baby bites down reflexively.	• Support the baby's head, use prone positioning, support the baby's chin, press gently under the chin.
Baby does not flange his lips.	• Help the baby flange either or both of his lips.
Baby clenches his jaw, causing nipple vasospasms (nipple blanches and becomes painful).	• Use warm compresses to help heal the nipple. • Increase intake of calcium and magnesium in the mother's diet. • Vasospasms of the nipple have also been identified with a Raynaud-like phenomenon. • Refer to a qualified neurodevelopmental (NDT) therapist if the baby has oral-motor difficulties.
Frenulum is tight and the tongue cannot extend over the lower lip.	• Clip the frenulum.
Poor positioning.	• Baby's body must be in alignment with his head. • Baby's head must be facing and level with the breast.

- Eliminate prolonged, non-nutritive sucking at the breast
  - Try alternate massage
  - Help sustain sucking and swallowing
  - Relieve long periods of negative pressure
  - Apply expressed milk to the sore area and allow for air drying of the areola
  - Apply a topical cream or ointment; research on the use of topical agents on sore nipples is inconclusive (see Chapter 19)
  - Pump the breasts with a quality electric breast pump while healing, and provide the expressed milk to the baby with an alternative feeding method if sucking cannot be tolerated
- Topical creams and ointments
  - Research on the use of topical agents on sore nipples is currently inconclusive
  - See Chapter 19 for further discussion

Interruption of Breastfeeding

- When treatment provides little or no relief, breastfeeding may need to be interrupted to avoid weaning
- Stop breastfeeding from several feeds to several days
- Use a hospital-grade, electric breast pump to maintain milk production, preferably double pumping on a low setting for 10 to 15 minutes every two to three hours
- Closely match pumping to the baby's feeding frequency
- Dab a bit of olive oil on the areola before pumping to lessen the pulling on the areola within the flange
- Cup feed the expressed milk to the baby until breastfeeding resumes

Alternating Breastfeeding Positions

- Avoid further irritation to a sore spot
- Point the baby's chin, and thus his tongue, away from the sore part
- Thinking of her breast as a clock, the mother can describe the location of the sore spot

YEAST

Cracked Nipple
- A crack or fissure can occur on the nipple when soreness persists
- Appears either crosswise or lengthwise along the nipple
- Infrequently the nipple folds over, causing a stress point at the fold
- See Table 14.2

Yeast Infections
- Yeast infections are associated with the following:
  - Diabetes
  - Illness
  - Pregnancy
  - Oral contraceptive use
  - Poor diet
  - Antibiotic therapy
  - Steroid therapy
  - Immunosuppression
  - Local factors such as obesity or excessive sweating, which provide constantly warm, moist areas where Candida can thrive
  - Vaginal yeast infection
  - Nipple damage early in lactation
  - Mastitis
- A yeast infection in the baby's mouth is called thrush—it presents as white patches that look like milk curds
- Yeast on the nipple does not always present with visual symptoms—it is unusual to see white patches or a redness on the nipple, although it is possible
  - The most obvious symptom is usually breast and nipple pain
  - Severely sore nipples after a period of pain-free breastfeeding
  - Pain described as intense and burning, which is radiating through the breast during or after feeds

TABLE 14.2   CRACKED NIPPLES

Causes	Actions for the Mother
All causes of sore nipples carried to the extreme.	• Consult a physician about using ibuprofen, acetaminophen, or any other pain killers. • Encourage the mother to improve her nutritional status by increasing protein, vitamin C, and zinc intakes. • Refer to all previously mentioned actions for sore nipples.
Foldover nipple (crack appears at the fold).	• Air dry breasts after a feed.
Local infection (baby with staph or other organism infected the mother's nipples).	• Have a physician check the nipples, get a culture of the baby's throat and the mother's nipples, and treat the patients accordingly.
Baby overly eager at feeds.	• Respond to feeding cues promptly. • Limit nursing times to ten minutes per breast. • Pre-express milk to hasten letdown. • Nurse in a position which does not aggravate the crack. • Soak the nipple to soften it before nursing.

- Treatment of a yeast infection
    - The mother's nipples and baby's mouth must be treated simultaneously even if only one has symptoms
    - Treat other sites of infection as well

- Treat with an antifungal topical solution
  - Nystatin—is often the first treatment suggested
  - Over-the-counter topicals that are generally more effective
    - Clotrimazole, 1 percent
    - Miconazole nitrate, 2 percent
    - Gentian violet, 0.5 percent—swabbed in the baby's mouth and when the baby latches onto the breast, the nipple is treated through direct contact—one time per breast per day for three days
  - Prescription topicals that are generally more effective
    - Ketoconazole, 2 percent
    - Ciclopirox, 1 percent
    - Naftifine hydrochloride
- Usual treatment of an oral yeast infection in a baby
  - Rinse his mouth with water after breastfeeding
  - Shake and pour an antifungal agent into a cup and apply it to all surfaces of his mouth with a cotton swab
  - Never re-use a swab—never dip twice into the original vial of Nystatin
- Treatment of the mother's nipples
  - Rinse with a solution of one cup of plain, tepid water with one tablespoon of vinegar
  - Air dry
  - Apply an antifungal cream
  - Change breast pads at least as often as every feed
- Oral antifungals such as Fluconazole and Ketoconazole may be used for a yeast infection that does not respond to topical treatments
- Stopping the spread of yeast
  - Wash hands well before and after diapering, using the toilet, and breastfeeding
  - Boil anything coming in contact with the mother's breast or the baby's mouth once a day for at least 20 minutes—includes the mother's bra, breast shells, breast pump parts, baby's pacifier, bottle nipple, and teething ring

- Discard bottle nipples, pacifiers, and teethers after one week
- Use the mother's fresh milk—do not use frozen milk because freezing does not kill Candida
- Clean toys thoroughly with hot soapy water
- Launder the family's clothing in very hot water
- Alter the mother's diet by decreasing her intake of dairy products and sugars, and increasing her intake of acidophilus, garlic, zinc, and Vitamin B if she has a persistent yeast infection

Engorgement

Physiology of Engorgement
- Is overfullness that occurs when milk is inadequately or infrequently removed from the breast
- The duct system is not sufficiently cleared of colostrum before milk accumulates
- Back pressure that results in breasts that feel firm, hard, tender, and warm or hot to the touch
- Inability of the skin to stretch any further, causing it to look shiny and transparent
- Nipples may become flattened, or even disappear in extreme cases, which results in a difficult latch for the baby and sore nipples for the mother
- Milk production and secretion begins decreasing rapidly
- Danger of permanent harm to breast tissue—some alveolar cells and myoepithelial cells begin to atrophy
- Bacteria is not removed by the lymphatic system at a normal rate, increasing the possibility of infection
- Can further inhibit letdown
- Fewer nutrients become available to make milk
- Unrelieved, severe engorgement can cause insufficient milk production by six weeks
- See Figure 14.1

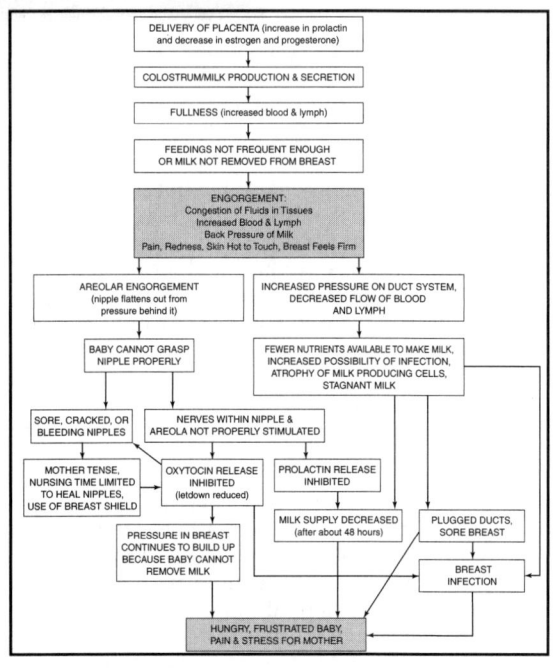

Figure 14.1 Progression of engorgement

Occurrence of Engorgement

- Is an iatrogenic entity, which is caused by medical interference with natural processes through regulations, schedules, and poor lactation management
- Occurs when breastfeeding is started and nursing patterns are irregular
- Occurs when feeds are missed
- Occurs when milk is not regularly removed from the breasts
- Occurs when the baby begins sleeping through the night
- Occurs whenever a mother and baby are separated long enough for feeds to be missed
- Occurs during weaning, especially if rapid weaning is necessary

Preventing Engorgement
- Initiate breastfeeding within the first hour of life
- Keep mothers and babies together 24 hours a day throughout the maternity stay
- Feed the baby eight or more times within a 24-hour period (including night feeds)
- Wake the baby and put him to breast for relief if fullness increases
- Express milk to maintain lactation when the baby is sleepy and not adequately nursing
- Have a caregiver assess every mother and baby for correct latch and positioning
- Avoid the use of artificial nipples

Treatment of Engorgement
- See Figure 14.2 for an example of an engorgement care plan
- See Figure 14.3 for a summary of treatment options for engorgement

Plugged Ducts

- Contain cells and other milk components that were shed within the ducts
- Are localized in the breast and do not produce systemic symptoms
- May be absorbed by the body, may appear in the milk, or may be removed by the mother
- See Table 14.4 for treatment of plugged ducts

Mastitis

Physiology of Mastitis
- An inflamed area of the breast becomes red, hot, and tender to the touch
- Produces a fever and flu-like symptoms

ENGORGEMENT CARE PLAN

As your milk supply increases, your breasts should feel heavier and full. This normal fullness should not prevent your baby from being able to latch on easily. Your breasts should also be pain-free. Breasts that become engorged are very hard, and the nipples can be flattened out because of the swelling occurring inside the breasts. The breasts may also be tender or quite painful, and the skin may appear shiny.

Engorgement, if left untreated, can cause the loss of some or all of the milk supply. It is important to treat engorgement quickly. The treatment's goal is to decrease the swelling and to enable the baby to latch on effectively. Note that heat (hot moist compresses, for example) increases swelling and that icy cold compresses and cabbage leaves decrease swelling.

Suggestions:
1. Try to breastfeed 10 to 12 times during every 24-hour time period.
2. Try to breastfeed at least 15 minutes on the first breast before offering the baby the other breast.
3. Feed your baby with just a diaper on in order to keep him awake and stimulated.
4. Hand express some milk to soften the areola before putting your baby to your breast.
5. Wear breast shells for about 20 minutes prior to feedings.
6. Wear a well fitting, supportive bra.
7. Lie flat on your back with a bra on between feedings to elevate your breasts.
8. Apply icy cold compresses to your breasts and under your arms. (Compresses can be made by pouring water onto disposable diapers and placing them in the freezer for 15 to 20 minutes. Or you can

use a bag of frozen vegetables. Do not apply the compress directly on your breast; place a towel over your breast first.) Apply compresses for _____ minutes every _____ hours.
9. Express your milk after nursing to remove the milk that comes out quickly and easily, or for _____ minutes.
10. Express between feedings for comfort if necessary, but do so only as long as the milk comes out quickly and easily.
11. Apply olive oil to your nipple and areola before pumping to help prevent pulling and soreness.
12. Take a warm shower and hand express milk in the shower. Have the water flow against your back rather than onto your breasts.

If the areola is swollen and hard, the nipple is flattened, and/or the baby will not or cannot latch-on, follow these instructions:
1. Do not breastfeed until the breast has softened enough to let the baby latch on comfortably.
2. Apply green cabbage leaves to your breasts:
   - Discard the outer leaves from the cabbage.
   - Remove the inner leaves. Rinse and dry them. They can be kept in the refrigerator.
   - Crush the leaves slightly with your hands.
   - Cover the breasts entirely with the leaves (and under your arms if needed). Put your bra on over the leaves to hold them in place.

(continues)

Figure 14.2 An example of an engorgement care plan

- Change the leaves every two hours or more frequently if they become wilted.
- Check your breasts often. As soon as you feel the milk begin to drip, or if your breasts begin to feel *different*, remove the leaves and try to express your milk.
- Express enough milk to soften the breast and areola. Put the baby to your breast.
- Reapply the cabbage as needed. You may use the icy compresses over the cabbage.
- Use only the green leaves. The white inner leaves do not work.
- As soon as your breasts become soft enough to nurse comfortably, you may stop using cabbage leaves.
3. Call _____ if you are not getting any relief or if you have any questions.

Mother's signature: _____ Date: _____

Lactation consultant's signature: _____ Date: _____

Figure 14.2 An example of an engorgement care plan (continued)
Printed with permission of Breastfeeding Support Consultants, Chalfont, PA, 1998.

- Most breast infections are located outside the ductwork in surrounding breast tissues and do not enter the milk; therefore, it is reasonably safe for a baby to nurse through an infection

Causes of Mastitis
- Fatigue and stress are the most common conditions that precede mastitis
- Organisms that cause breast infection most frequently come from the baby or the home, and the mother likely produces antibodies in her milk to fight the infection
- See Table 14.5
- The following are causes of recurrent mastitis:
  - Anemia or other deficiencies
  - The mother was treated with the wrong antibiotic
  - The mother was not treated with antibiotics long enough
  - The mother does not follow advice

Treatment of Mastitis
- Bed rest for several days
- Remove milk from the breasts efficiently in the following ways:
  - Nurse the baby with his chin pointed toward the inflamed area
  - Remove milk more effectively by the baby nursing than by expressing
  - Feed frequently to cleanse the breast and prevent milk stasis
- Apply warm, moist compresses to the inflamed area before and during a feed
- Apply crushed cabbage leaves to the breast between feeds
- Take an anti-inflammatory medication to relieve pain
- Contact the primary health provider if the mother runs a temperature higher than 100.7 or when breast inflammation has not resolved within 24 hours

TABLE 14.3 TREATMENT OF ENGORGEMENT

Causes of Engorgement	Actions for the Mother
• Missed feeds or infrequent feeds.	Room in with the baby in the hospital. Breastfeed the baby 10 to 12 times each 24 hours, or more if he is willing around the clock. Watch the baby for feeding cues and respond to them. Use rousing techniques to waken a sleepy baby. Increase skin-to-skin contact to encourage a baby to nurse. Have the mother remove her shirt and bra, and hold her baby with only a diaper on. Pump breasts with a hospital-grade, electric breast pump any time the baby is unwilling or unable to nurse.
• Milk removal not adequate at feeds.	Check that the baby's latch and position are appropriate. Stop the use of all artificial nipples. Increase skin-to-skin contact during feeds. Have the mother remove her shirt and bra and hold the baby with only a diaper on. Do breast compression during feeds to encourage the baby to suckle.

- Inadequate letdown due to edema and pain.
  - Pump the breasts after a feed with a hospital-grade, electric breast pump only to remove the milk that comes out quickly and easily.
  - Pump the breasts between feeds for comfort, if necessary, for only as long as the milk comes out quickly and easily.
  - Relax in a warm shower with water running over the mother's back, avoiding the breasts; and hand express to relieve fullness.
  - Breastfeed after the breast has softened enough to enable the baby to latch on comfortably.
  - Use relaxation techniques and gentle breast massage during feeds.
  - Lie flat on her back between feeds to elevate the breasts.
  - Apply cool compresses to the breasts and under her arms. Frozen peas or corn work well. Note: Do not apply them directly on the skin.
  - Apply green cabbage leaves to the breasts.

PLUGGED DUCT

TABLE 14.4 TREATMENT OF A PLUGGED DUCT

CAUSES	ACTIONS FOR THE MOTHER
Poor positioning to remove milk.	• Try a variety of positions for better milk removal. • Nurse the baby with his chin pointed toward the plugged duct. • If prone to plugged ducts, avoid missing feeds or pump the breasts. • If the baby does not adequately remove milk from the breasts, pump or express milk after feeds.
Breasts are overfull due to missed feeds, irregular nursing patterns, or engorgement.	• Nurse long enough on each breast for the baby to remove sufficient milk. • If the baby does not remove milk, pump or express the milk after feeds.
Incomplete removal of milk from the breast.	• While nursing on the affected side, use massage and heat to encourage drainage. • Nurse more frequently on the affected breast. • Gently roll, pull, and rub the plug down while in a warm shower. • Use moisture to remove any dried secretions that are blocking nipple pores.
External pressure on the breast.	• Avoid positions that put pressure on one spot for long periods (for example, always sleeping on one side, always holding the baby one way, or the baby sleeping on the mother's chest). • Use a larger nursing bra or a bra extender. • Avoid bunching up a sweater or nightgown under the arm during a feed. • Use a nursing bra instead of pulling up a conventional bra to nurse in order to avoid pressure on the ducts.

TABLE 14.5 TREATMENT OF A BREAST INFECTION

Causes	Actions for the Mother
Milk stasis: Breasts are overfull due to missed feeds, an irregular nursing pattern, or engorgement. The mother is too active.	• Nurse as long as the baby desires. If the breast is full after the baby is finished, express the milk for relief. • Avoid missed or delayed feeds. • When feeds are delayed, pump or hand express to remove milk from the breasts.
Low resistance to infection due to anemia or poor diet.	• Rearrange priorities and daily schedule. • Get help with all tasks. • Improve diet. • Get some exercise. • Reduce stress.
Lack of adequate sleep or fatigue.	• Take daytime naps or have rest periods (sleep rebuilds the immune system). • Nurse lying down. • Take the baby to bed at night.
Failure to clear a plugged duct.	• Work the plug down manually, if it is not too painful. • Have the baby nurse with his chin pointed toward the plug.
Infection via a cracked nipple.	• Eliminate non-nutritive sucking. • Briefly soak the breasts in a saline solution (1/4 tsp salt in 8 oz water) after feeding and air dry them.
Infection passed from the baby or another family member.	• Treat the primary infection in conjunction with the mother's infection.

- Begin antibiotic treatment immediately to reduce the severity of the infection and to protect milk production
- Follow through on the entire regimen (even if the infection seems to clear quickly)

Abscessed Breast
- Forms from a breast infection that was not treated or was unresponsive to treatment
- The symptoms are less severe than with mastitis because the abscess is walled off
- It can be a serious health hazard and should be treated immediately by a physician
  - It is usually lanced and allowed to drain
  - The infection is treated with medication
- The mother can continue to nurse using the unaffected breast depending on the location of the abscess, the pain associated with it, and the medication being prescribed
- If the mother is unable to nurse, she will need to express milk from the affected breast, or wean her baby from that breast
- If the mother still wishes to nurse on the affected breast, see the suggestions shown in Table 14.5

15

Breastfeeding Beyond the First Month

Patterns of Growth in a Breastfed Baby

Weight Gain
- During the first three months, babies usually gain 5 to 10 oz/week
- Over the next three months, their weight gain is usually 2.5 to 4.5 oz/week
- Babies will double their birth weight by the fifth to sixth months, and will triple their weight in one year
- During the first few months, a breastfed baby grows at the same rate as a formula-fed baby
- After the first few months, the weight of a formula-fed baby exceeds a breastfeeding baby's weight
- A breastfed baby is considered overweight if he:
  - Is two categories above weight for his height
  - Is much heavier than other family members were as babies
  - Often spits up or vomits from an overly distended stomach
- If the baby is overweight, suggest ways of comforting him other than through feeds
- In addition, see Table 11.2 in Chapter 11

Length and Head Circumference
- At one year, the baby should be 1 1/2 times longer than his birth length
- By the time the baby is one year old, his head should have increased by 7.6 cm (3 inches)

Breastfeeding as Baby Grows

Breastfeeding in Public
- Encourage the mother to
  - Observe other women nursing their babies and the reactions of other people
  - Practice discreet nursing in front of a mirror or another person
  - Wear loose-fitting clothes to enable easy access to her breast
  - Place a sweater, jacket, or another garment over her shoulders to conceal the view from the side
  - Place her baby in a sling for support, extra coverage, and ease in mobility
  - Feed her baby before he is overly hungry and starts to fuss
  - Inquire about a place to nurse if she is unfamiliar with her location

Teething and Biting
- On average, a baby's first tooth erupts between six and eight months of age
  - As the tooth erupts, it causes a swelling and irritation of the gums
  - When the baby sucks, blood rushes to his gums and adds to this swelling
- The following are a baby's response to teething:
  - Pulls away from the breast and cries out with pain
  - Becomes irritable
  - Drools more than usual
  - Occasionally spits up or develops loose stools

- Wakes during the night seeking comfort
- Runs a slight fever
- Rubs his jaw or pulls on his ears
• Biting while nursing
  - When there is slowing of the suck-swallow rhythm, the mother can remove her baby from her breast
  - When the baby bites, the mother can remove the baby from her breast and wait a few minutes before resuming the feed
  - If the baby bites repeatedly, the mother can end the feed
  - Biting at the end of a feed may occur as the baby falls asleep and closes his jaw
  - If the mother reacts with an outcry, she should be cautious not to respond so strongly in the future to avoid a nursing strike
• Teething pain can be reduced in the following ways:
  - The baby may chew on a cooled teething ring
  - Ice or a cold cloth can be rubbed on the baby's gums before breastfeeding
  - The baby may chew on hard foods such as toast
  - The baby can be given over-the-counter pain relievers to temporarily numb gum tissue

Breastfeeding Beyond One Year

- Most often, cultural practices set the standards for weaning times
- Women in the United States who breastfeed longer than 12 months tend to be older, better educated, and exclusively breastfeed longer
- Breastfeeding offers comfort and stability to a child
- The following are examples of the challenges of breastfeeding a toddler:
  - The toddler may not wish to be held and will assume a position that enables him to view the room, which includes standing or straddling

- A toddler's teeth may leave pressure marks on the areola until the child learns to hold the breast with his lips
- Crumbs or food particles in a toddler's mouth may irritate a mother's nipples
- The toddler may insist on nursing at inconvenient or embarrassing moments; he may fondle his mother's body in public
- The following are examples of strategies for breastfeeding after one year:
  - Breastfeed in a quiet place to limit any distractions
  - Limit breastfeeding to certain times of the day
  - Work out with the child signals and times that are acceptable for both
  - Stretch out the intervals between feeds with a drink, a treat, or other activities
  - Link the time to nurse to a special location
- If the baby's father objects to breastfeeding, learn the reasons behind the father's objections and develop a plan to resolve the situation
- If others object, breastfeed discreetly and refrain from breastfeeding in front of those people who are critical
- If siblings resent the special attention a breastfeeding child receives, set aside a special time to spend with each child

Supplementary Feeds and Complementary Feeds

- Complementary feeds are foods added to an infant's diet to meet energy and nutrient needs that are not met by the digestion of the mother's milk alone
- Supplementary feeds are foods other than human milk fed to an infant following or in place of a breastfeed
- A mother's expressed milk is considered a supplementary feed by some
- The frequency and duration of breastfeeds will continue to diminish as more foods are added to a baby's diet

- Introduce supplementary feeds so that they have little interference with a breastfeeding pattern
  - Breastfeed before offering supplemental food to the baby
  - Do not give a substantial amount of supplements
  - Delay supplementing feeds until the baby is at least three weeks old and has established nursing habits
  - Have someone other than the mother feed the child about one ounce of fluid once or twice a week
  - Cup feeding is a preferred feeding method
  - The baby's acceptance of a bottle may require several attempts
- A mother's breasts may become full as a result of the missed feed; she can do the following to reduce discomfort:
  - Nurse or express her milk just before an absence
  - Wear a larger bra to avoid pressure
  - Express milk for use while she is away
  - Nurse her baby when she returns

When to Introduce Solid Foods

- When a baby's system can handle them, and when more nutrients are needed than can be obtained solely from the mother's milk
- Mother's milk is sufficient as the only food until about six months of age
- Note that sleeping through the night is a developmental event that cannot be changed by feeding a baby cereal
- Introducing foods before a baby's body is ready can lead to the following problems:
  - Frequent digestive upsets
  - Increased upper respiratory infections
  - Poor nutrient absorption
  - Excessive weight gain from increased calories

- Watch for signs of readiness
- If a baby nurses constantly at four or five months and seems unsatisfied, he may need solid foods
- Most babies are ready for solid foods as they approach six months of age
- Signs of readiness are as follows:
  - Eruption of teeth
  - Ability to sit up
  - Disappearance of the tongue extrusion reflex
  - Improved eye-hand coordination
  - Ability to grasp objects with his thumb and forefinger
  - Intently watches others eat, imitates chewing, reaches for food, or vocalizes his desire
  - Intensified demand to nurse is not satisfied after several days of increased breastfeeds

Decrease in Milk Production

- Breastfeeding will diminish slowly as the feeding of solid foods is increased
- During the second six months, mother's milk still meets 3/4 of a baby's nutritional needs
- During the baby's second year, human milk is still nutritionally valuable
- Early solid feeders consume less mother's milk at six to nine months

Supplementing to Provide Iron

- A mother's milk will supply a baby with sufficient iron until his birth weight triples
- Lactoferrin increases the absorption of the iron that is available in milk
- Adding iron too soon to a baby's diet interferes with iron absorption and protection from lactoferrin
- A hemoglobin test will determine if iron supplementation is necessary for premature infants and the infants of anemic mothers

How to Introduce Solid Foods

- Introduce foods gradually so that the baby is not overwhelmed and his digestive system gets used to each diet change:
  - Offer foods after the baby has nursed
  - Start feeding foods at a slow pace, with one feeding every one or two days
  - Afternoon and early evening are times when a baby may accept additional foods
  - By age seven to nine months, one or two complementary feedings daily plus a regular breastfeed will satisfy a baby's nutritional needs
  - By age nine to twelve months, a baby will have three meals daily with several nutritious snacks and several separate nursing times
  - Breastfeeding can gradually be eliminated from mealtimes as a baby begins to eat balanced meals and drink from a cup
- The texture of food needs to be compatible with an infant's ability to chew and swallow
  - First, highly pureed and diluted with a liquid and fed by spoon
  - Next, decreased liquid content and a more coarse texture
  - Continue on to chunky foods, finger foods, and then table foods
  - Can start with finger foods and chunky foods if they are delayed until the eighth or ninth month of age
  - Regular table food, cut up to appropriate sizes, by one year of age
- Amount of food given
  - Begin with a teaspoon of a food of creamy consistency
  - Work up to a few tablespoons
  - Determine the rate by the baby's appetite
  - Respond to the baby's signals when he has had enough, to avoid overfeeding

Allergy Considerations
- Exclusive breastfeeding coats the baby's intestinal tract and prevents foreign proteins from entering his system and causing allergic reactions
- Children of parents with a history of allergy appear to have a more prolonged dependence on the protective factors in human milk
  - Hereditary risk is reduced with six months of exclusive breastfeeding
  - The avoidance of the most potent, allergenic foods during the first year of life reduces allergic reactions in children
  - The degree of response to foreign proteins varies widely among babies

Causes of Allergies in Infants
- Foods in the mother's diet may cause an infant's allergies
  - Cow's milk, citrus fruits, eggs, corn, and wheat are common offenders
  - Excessive amounts of a particular food can cause allergic reactions
  - There is no need to eliminate foods unless they are suspected to be causing problems
- An infant's family may have a history of allergies
  - Be especially cautious—introduce one food at a time and wait at least one week for a possible reaction
  - Avoid cow's milk and milk products, citrus fruits, juices, eggs, tomatoes, chocolate, fish, pork, peanuts and other nuts, and wheat in the first year
  - Keep the baby's room free of dust and mold
  - Keep the home free of dogs, cats, birds, and other pets for at least six months
  - Do not allow wool and lanolin products to contact the baby's skin
  - Do not permit smoking near the baby or in the home

SIGNS OF FOOD SENSITIVITY IN THE INFANT

- Calm at the beginning of the feed then pulls off the breast, stiffens his body, and cries.
- Stuffy or drippy nose without any other signs of having a cold.
- Itchy nose.
- Red, scaly, oily rash on the forehead or eyebrows, in the hair, or behind the ears.
- Eczema.
- Red rectal ring.
- Fretful sleeping or persistent sleeplessness.
- Frequent spitting up or vomiting.
- Diarrhea or green stools, perhaps with blood in them.
- Wheezing or asthma.
- Ear infections.
- Intestinal upset, gas, diarrhea, spitting, and vomiting.
- Fussiness, irritability, and colic-like behavior.
- Poor weight gain due to malabsorption of food.
- Red and itchy eyes, swollen eyelids, dark circles under the eyes, constant tearing, and gelatin-like fluid in the eyes.

Weaning

When Weaning Occurs
- Common ages for weaning are 12 to 14 months, 18 months, 2 years, and 3 years; most mothers in the United States wean their children before nine months of age
- A baby's frequent crying may cause his mother to doubt that she is satisfying his hunger
- A mother may be frustrated and fatigued by a baby's teething, biting, or illness

- A mother may be fatigued from lack of sleep due to continued nighttime feeds
  - It may be possible to simply drop nighttime feeds
  - Help explore reasons for the baby's wakefulness
  - Weaning may be the answer for an older baby
- When changes occur in the family, it may appear that weaning would make life simple
- A mother may want to resume taking oral contraceptives and does not have information about the methods that are compatible with breastfeeding (see Chapter 17, Changes in the Family, for further discussion)
- Pressure from others can undermine a mother's commitment and confidence

Baby-Led Weaning
- Is the most natural and preferred method of weaning
- Feeds are dropped gradually and the baby is put to breast only when he indicates the need
- If the baby starts to wean when the mother does not want or expect it
  - Help the mother learn to appreciate her baby's maturity by stressing his new achievements
  - Show the mother new ways of interacting with her baby

Mother-Led Weaning
- The mother ends breastfeeding without having received any cues from her baby
  - If she has begun to resent feeds, it may be time to wean
  - Be sensitive to a mother's cues, and let her know you will help her
- Babies younger than nine months to one year need to be weaned to a bottle

- Wean babies gradually
  - Eliminate the least preferred feed first and allow at least three days for the baby and the mother's breasts to adjust
  - Substitute drinks, snacks, cuddling, or a favorite activity for feeds
  - When the mother and child are comfortable with a substitution, drop another feed and continue in this manner for several weeks or months
  - The child may continue a preferred feed
  - Feeds will decrease in frequency to once every few days until he weans completely
- If weaning proceeds too quickly
  - A child may demand more attention, request more feeds, or exhibit physical changes such as allergic reactions, stomach upsets, or constipation
  - A mother's breasts may become uncomfortable—express milk to relieve discomfort, but be careful not to express so much that it increases milk production
    - Watch for symptoms of plugged ducts or mastitis
    - Wear a supportive bra that is not binding
    - Consider other comfort measures such as a pain reliever, ice packs, or cabbage leaves

Minimal Breastfeeding

- Breastfeed between one to three times a day, using complementary feeds to provide the remaining nourishment
- Minimal breastfeeding is an option when the mother and her baby are separated for regular periods of time
- Half of breastfeeding mothers use minimal breastfeeding for an extended periods as a transition to weaning

Untimely or Emergency Weaning

- Drop every other feed the first day
- Express milk to relieve any discomfort
- Eliminate the remainder of the feeds, making sure to give the baby extra cuddling and attention
- Expect about 24 hours of engorgement that will gradually subside
  - Wrap the breasts in cabbage leaves to reduce swelling (see Chapter 14)
  - Take acetaminophen to relieve pain and to help reduce swelling
  - Use ice wrapped in a towel on the breasts to reduce pain
- The mother may not want to wean and will need your acceptance and support

After Weaning

- The mother will learn new skills for comforting her baby that will replace breastfeeding
- Help her to regard weaning as another step in her child's development, and encourage her to look forward to new stages
- Most women need to adjust their diets to eliminate the calories that supported milk production in order to avoid gaining weight
- If menstruation resumes after weaning, the cycles may be irregular for a few months
- The mother's breasts may become soft, flat, or droopy for a few months
  - Should gradually return to their prepregnancy size
  - May never regain the fatty layer that was present before conception

- Montgomery glands recede
- The areola may be darker than before conception
- Stretch marks may remain
- May experience milk secretion for several months after weaning

16

Problems with Milk Production and Transfer

Identifying Problems with Infant Growth

Hospital Discharge at 48 Hours or Less
- Advise that the baby be seen by the primary care physician within two to four days of life
- Advise a second visit to the baby's physician at approximately two weeks of age for a physical assessment and weight check (or sooner if a condition warrants it)

Appropriate Growth
- A baby's birth weight should double by the fifth to sixth month and triple by 12 months of age
- A baby's body length is a significant indicator of appropriate growth and should increase by 50 percent by one year of age
- Head circumference—which indicates brain growth—should increase by 7.6 cm (3 inches) by one year of age
- If the parents are small in stature, or gained weight slowly as infants, they can expect the same pattern for their child

Signs That Breastfeeding is Going Well

- See Figure 10.2 in Chapter 10, Infant Assessment and Behavior
- By Day Six, the infant has at least six wet diapers in each 24-hour period and pale, diluted urine
- By Day Six, the infant produces four or more stools that are yellow or at least turning yellow
- The infant continues to produce at least four stools in each 24-hour period until around one month of age
- The infant routinely breastfeeds at least eight times in a 24-hour period
- The mother's breasts feel softer after a feed (for some women, there is not a dramatic difference)
- The mother's nipples are not painful during or after feeds
- The infant is gaining 5 to 10 oz/week
- The infant has regained his birth weight in 10 to 14 days
- During a feed, the infant's sucking rhythm slows as milk is released, and swallowing or gulping can be heard
- The infant is alert and active, and his skin appears healthy
- The infant is content between feeds

Symptoms of Newborn Dehydration

- Sunken fontanels
- Weight loss greater than seven percent of birth weight
- Poor skin turgor
- Dry mucous membranes
- No tears
- Lethargy
- Weak crying
- Infrequent feeds
- Infant sleeps at the breast
- Scant urinary output
- Few or no stools

Slow/Poor Weight Gain

- Before a mother is discharged, teach her the warning signs of potential breastfeeding problems (see Figure 10.2 in Chapter 10)

Differences in Infant Growth

- Give the mother a diary to document breastfeeds, voids, and stools (see Table 11.1 in Chapter 11, Infant Assessment and Behavior)
- When there is a concern about growth, assess milk transfer by weighing the infant before and after feeds
  - Do a test weight on a digital electronic scale to ensure accuracy
  - Do not weigh the infant routinely or during the first 48 hours in the hospital
  - Weighing is reserved for problems associated with milk intake
- By four months of age, the gross energy intakes of exclusively breastfed infants are significantly less than the current recommendations (which are based on an artificial feeding)
- Breastfed infants, when compared to formula-fed infants, have normal growth rates and have lower
  - Total daily energy expenditures
  - Sleeping metabolic rates
  - Rates of energy expenditure
  - Rectal temperatures
  - Heart rates
- In unfavorable environments, infants may have higher-than-usual energy requirements
- An infant's environment could explain the differences in growth, rather than a low milk intake
- An infant's caloric needs may increase if his sleep is less restful or if there are multiple care providers

Slow Weight-Gaining Infant

- The infant has a slow, steady growth over time
- This baby's growth is proportional for his weight, length, and head circumference

- This infant is appropriately developed for his age
- In the absence of any other risk factors, minimal intervention, if any, is required
- This baby should not receive pacifiers or bottles that would reduce his sucking time at the breast
- This infant's mother needs to respond to feeding cues appropriately
- Weigh this baby twice a week and record his weights to monitor his gain

Poor-Weight-Gaining Infant
- This infant is still below birth weight by several ounces at Day 14
- This can be an older infant who is not gaining or is gaining less than 3 oz/week
- The first goal in treatment is for the baby to receive calories
- The second goal in treatment is to increase the mother's milk production to a level that can sustain her infant
- Breastfeeding regimen
  - Minimum of eight to twelve feedings daily around the clock
  - Feeds should last at least 20 minutes with a lot of audible swallowing
  - Feed the cream portion of the mother's expressed milk that has been stored
  - Give no pacifiers or bottles
  - Supplement with ABM through a tube at the breast until milk production is sufficient to exclusively breastfeed
  - Record the baby's weight at least twice a week to monitor gain
  - Gradually eliminate supplements when weight gain is steady
  - Tube feeding at the breast provides the sucking needed for milk production
  - Express milk with a hospital-grade, electric breast pump
  - If the baby begins to gain rapidly and then

slows down, the infant's supplement is being decreased too quickly
- Send a detailed report of your consultation with the mother to the primary care physician

Warning Signs That a Baby Is Not Gaining Adequate Weight

- Frequently sleeps for long periods of time to conserve energy
- May fuss when removed from the breast and then go back to sleep when put back to it
- Nurses all the time because he cannot be laid down without fussing
- Often has a worried or anxious look on his face
- Holds his body in a flexed, fetal position to help maintain temperature
- Has hanging folds of skin on his thighs and buttocks
- His cry may be a high-pitched sound like the "meow" of a cat
- Has a decreased urinary output
- The urine that is passed may be concentrated
- In an older infant, urine may smell strongly of ammonia
- In an infant younger than five to six weeks of age, few stools are passed
- May still be passing meconium after the fourth day of life
- See Table 16.1 for factors that influence milk production and transfer

Failure to Thrive

Signs of Failure to Thrive

- The baby does not regain his birth weight by three weeks of age
- Weight loss of greater than ten percent of birth weight by two weeks of age

- Growth decelerates from a previously established weight gain pattern
- The baby has minimal amounts of subcutaneous fat and a wasted buttocks
- Weight is two standard deviations or more below where it should be on a standard growth chart for older infants
- The baby may be lethargic, hypertonic, irritable, and difficult to soothe
- The baby may sleep excessively or be continuously fussy

Causes of Failure to Thrive

- Failure to thrive can result from either maternal or infant causes
- See Table 16.2 for causes of failure to thrive

Issues to Address with the Mother

- Amount of weight that was gained during pregnancy
- Changes that occurred in her breasts during pregnancy (determines if she has sufficient mammary tissue)
- History of infertility
- History of thyroid dysfunction
- Previous breast surgery
- Excessive blood loss or the use of Pitocin or intravenous fluids during delivery
- Use of oral contraceptives
- Daily diet
- Smoking cigarettes
- Experiencing any engorgement or mastitis
- Typical management of breastfeeds

Interventions for an Infant with Failure to Thrive

- Assess the baby's sucking technique, and observe how he is held at the breast

TABLE 16.1 FACTORS THAT MAY INFLUENCE MILK PRODUCTION AND TRANSFER

Maternal factors
- Primipara.
- Gained fewer than 18 pounds during pregnancy.
- History of low milk production or breastfeeding problems with previous infants.
- Flat, inverted nipples or taut, tight breast tissue.
- Epidural.
  - In place longer than three to four hours before delivery.
  - Administered more than one time.
  - Received more than one bolus of epidural medication.
- Induction of labor with Pitocin.
- Received excessive intravenous fluids; on magnesium sulfate; edema present in ankles that was not present before labor.
- Received pain medication while in labor, more than one hour before delivery.
- Had a cesarean delivery.
- Breastfeeding initiated more than one hour after delivery.
- Sore nipples throughout feeds at the time of hospital discharge.
- Embarrassed or unsure of her ability to breastfeed her baby.
- Using a nipple shield for breastfeeds.
- Sleeps far from her baby, which interferes with easy access to her baby and her response to her baby's feeding cues.
- Is taking medications, especially contraceptives, that affect milk production.
- Is fatigued or ill.
- Had previous breast trauma, or either reduction or augmentation surgery.
- Has hypothyroidism (rare).

- Has hypoprolactinemia (rare).
- Has an anatomic problem with the position of the lactiferous sinuses (rare).
- Has an extremely low food and fluid intake (rare except in food crisis).
- Experienced little or no change in size or color of her breast during pregnancy, which indicates a lack of sufficient functioning breast tissue (extremely rare).

Infant factors
- Less than 37 weeks' gestation.
- Weighs less than seven pounds at birth.
- Seven percent or more weight loss at the time of hospital discharge.
- Male infant.
- Vacuum or forceps used in delivery.
- Has a tight frenulum.
- Has a cleft lip, palate, or both.
- Insult to the oral cavity occured, as with a laryngoscope and deep suctioning.
- Fetal distress; meconium expelled during delivery.
- Is small for gestational age (SGA) or large for gestational age (LGA).

Factors associated with breastfeeding management
- Is jaundiced.
- Is sleepy, difficult to wake, and fails to give clear feeding cues.
- Has difficulty latching on consistently.
- Has not established effective breastfeeding before hospital discharge.
- Has a medical condition such as a metabolic disorder, a neuromotor problem, congenital heart disease, a respiratory infection, a urinary infection, hypothyroidism, or another disorder. (The baby needs to be seen by someone who can give special care in these areas.)

(continues)

TABLE 16.1 FACTORS THAT MAY INFLUENCE MILK PRODUCTION AND TRANSFER (continued)

- Circumcision was done before the infant established an effective breastfeeding pattern.
- Feeding restrictions were placed on the infant, such as with timed feeds or not being allowed to receive anything by mouth (NPO).
- Bottles or pacifiers are given during hospitalizations.
- Other foods and drink are being given to the baby, decreasing his appetite and time spent at the breast.
- Nighttime breastfeeds were stopped too early (prolactin response is higher at night).
- Breastfeeds are not long enough; inadequate removal of milk leads to a buildup of the suppressor peptides in milk that signals the breast to reduce milk production.
- Baby is not attached at the breast for effective suckling.
- Breastfeeds are infrequent.
- Breastfeeds are short and hurried; the baby is removed from one breast too soon and is not receiving enough hindmilk.

---

[1]LGA, large for gestational age; SGA, small for gestational age

TABLE 16.2 CAUSES OF FAILURE TO THRIVE

Maternal causes
- Previous breast surgery, either reduction or augmentation.
- Hypothyroidism.
- Hypoprolactinemia.
- Anatomic position of the lactiferous sinuses.
- Insufficient mammary tissue.
- Sheehan's syndrome.
- Disrupted neurohormonal pathways.
- Use of a nipple shield.
- Retained placental fragments.
- Mismanagement of breastfeeding.

Infant causes
- Neuromotor problems.
- Tight frenulum.
- Systemic illness.
- Sleepy infant.
- Inability to compress the lactiferous sinuses.
- Mother's anatomy versus the infant's oral cavity.
- Disorganized suck.
- "Good" baby who does not exhibit hunger cues.

- Breastfeed the baby 10 to 12 times within a 24-hour period until he has four stools per 24 hours for three consecutive days
- Alternate between breasts when the baby's suckling pattern changes and his swallowing ceases
- Use alternate breast massage during feeds
- Limit feeds to 40 minutes per session
- Include a supplement of formula at every feed
- When things improve, discontinue supplements at night
- Build the mother's confidence in her ability to breastfeed her baby

- Ensure that the baby is checked frequently by a physician
- Weigh the baby frequently and record any weight changes
- Advise the mother to stay in close contact with an IBCLC and the baby's physician
- See Table 16.3 for measures to increase milk production

Supplementing the Baby
- Offer in measured amounts so the baby is not filled with supplement, which is detrimental to nursing
- Perform a feeding assessment to determine the amount of supplement the infant needs
  - In the two-hour period preceding an assessment, the infant should not nurse, and the mother should not express milk
  - Weigh the infant before and after the feed on a digital scale to determine the amount of intake during a feed
  - Have the mother pump her breasts after the feed to determine the amount of residual milk that the infant left in her breast
  - This outcome indicates the mother's milk production over the preceding two or three hours, and the amount of milk the infant took in from the breast plus the residual milk
  - Using the calculations in Table 16.4, determine the infant's total 24-hour requirement, and divide it by the number of feeds he takes or should take in a 24-hour period
  - This calculation gives a fairly accurate measurement of the amount of supplement the infant needs
  - Knowing the amount the infant took in from the feeding assessment compared to the amount he should have taken in will give a fairly accurate measurement of the supplement that is required

TABLE 16.3 MEASURES TO INCREASE MILK PRODUCTION

Actions for the mother
- Rest as much as possible, and relax during breastfeeds to help milk flow.
- Spend 100 percent of her time with the baby for 48 hours, concentrating on increasing the feeds and resting; get help with all other tasks.
- Take special precautions to prevent sore nipples.
- Use local galactogogues (foods, drinks, or herbs believed to increase milk production).
- Keep a record of feeds including both breastfeeds and any supplements—this can show how quickly milk production is increasing and help the mother find a workable feeding pattern.
- Use a hospital-grade, electric breast pump to provide additional stimulation to the breasts.
- Improve her diet by eating more protein, fresh fruits and vegetables, and Vitamin B.

Management of breastfeeds
- Encourage a letdown by using relaxation techniques and following a daily feeding routine.
- Prepare the baby so he is alert and ready to nurse by rousing or soothing him as needed.
- Make sure the baby is attached for effective suckling.
- Put the baby to each breast several times at a feed, to increase stimulation.
- Encourage the baby to feed more frequently and longer, during both day and night.
- Nurse long enough for the baby to receive hindmilk; this will vary from one baby to another.
- Nurse to comfort a fussy baby.
- Get into bed with the baby during feeds to increase skin contact.
- Resume nighttime feeds if they had been dropped.

- Divide this number of ounces among two to four feeds, depending on the amount found to be required
- Feed the infant supplements at predetermined times
- Feed the supplements in a supplementer (see Chapter 19, Breastfeeding Techniques and Devices), so that sucking on the supplementer increases milk production while it nourishes the baby
- If the mother chooses not to use a supplementer, she can nurse first and offer the supplements afterward in a cup
- Do not use feeding bottles or pacifiers
- If the baby does not take all the supplement at a feed, he may not need as much supplement in his daily diet, or he may need those few ounces sometime later within that 24-hour time period
  - If the mother's breasts feel full after a breastfeed, she should express and feed the milk to her baby
  - Watch the baby carefully for any signs of hunger and respond accordingly
  - Keep records of the following:
    - Amount of supplement the baby is receiving
    - Number of feeds
    - Number of wet diapers
    - Number of stools
    - Frequent weight checks
- When a mother's milk production improves, slowly reduce the supplements and continue to increase the frequency of breastfeeds

TABLE 16.4 DETERMINING THE NUMBER OF OUNCES AN INFANT NEEDS

Example for an infant weighing 4 lbs. 2 oz.	
Convert the infant's weight to ounces.	4 lb. × 16 oz. = 64 oz. 64 oz. + 2 oz. = 66 oz.
Divide the total ounces by the number 6.	66 oz. ÷ 6 = 11 oz. (for a 24-hour intake)
Divide the 24-hour requirements by the number of feeds per 24-hour period.	11 oz. ÷ 8 feeds = 1.375 oz. per feed 11 oz. ÷ 6 feeds = 1.83 oz. per feed

17

Changes in the Family

Acquiring the Parental Role

Emotional Adjustments to Becoming a Mother
- Baby blues
  - Are a few rough days, which are balanced by high moments (some lasting for several weeks)
  - Appear around the third day postpartum
  - More common in a primipara who feels unprepared for her new role as a mother
  - Expressed through tone of voice, unresponsiveness, a lack of confidence in her ability to breastfeed, a lack of tolerance for others, or a failure to refer to the baby by name
- Postpartum depression
  - Characterized by mood changes, sleep disturbances, fatigue, the inability to cope, abdominal pains, or headaches
  - Typically lasts from one to six weeks postpartum
  - Causes feelings of no attachment to the baby
  - Can cause a mother to occasionally entertain thoughts of harming herself
  - Risk factors include single marital status, low educational level, low income, and pregnancy complications

- Premature weaning is known to occur more frequently among depressed women
- May require professional help
- Postpartum psychosis
  - Much more intense than postpartum depression
  - Can lead to loss of control, rational thought processes, and social functioning
  - Can cause a mother to experience overwhelming confusion and hallucinations
  - Can cause a mother to attempt to harm herself or her child
  - Priority is to keep the mother and child safe and to seek effective treatment immediately

Survivors of Sexual Abuse

- One in three women has been sexually assaulted in her lifetime
- Pregnancy and childbirth are common times for a sexual abuse survivor to become aware of or be reminded of her abuse
- Memories can be triggered by the following:
  - Sounds or feelings of giving birth
  - Feeling of a baby at her breast
  - Loss of control felt in the early days of parenting
  - Sight of milk during letdown
- You can identify a sexual abuse survivor in the following ways:
  - How she positions herself when you assist her with latch on
  - Seems uncomfortable holding her baby while discussing breastfeeding
  - Feeds her expressed milk with a bottle and does not put her baby to her breast
  - Seeks late prenatal care
  - Substance abuse present
  - Mental health concerns present
  - Eating disorders present
  - Has poor compliance with self-care
  - Sexual dysfunction present

- The following are breastfeeding implications for an abuse survivor:
  - The most stressful time is early postpartum, when a mother is stressed, tired, and vulnerable
  - Nighttime breastfeeding can be difficult because assaults most often happen in the night during bedtime
  - When the infant gets older and becomes more playful, the mother may seem reluctant to continue breastfeeding
  - Some mothers find breastfeeding too uncomfortable to continue, while others find it to be healing
- The abuse survivor needs a counselor who specializes in sexual abuse—preferably one who is familiar with breastfeeding mothers

Mother's Physical Recovery Following Birth

- A protruding abdomen, loosened pelvic ligaments and stitches, full breasts, and a lack of energy are all normal
- A mother with insufficient rest may develop excessive bleeding, exhaustion, dizziness, weak pelvic floor muscles, sore nipples, or a breast infection
- Encourage the mother to get bed rest, nap when her baby naps, and to nurse lying down
- Caution the mother to minimize her household tasks and strenuous activities
- Uterus
  - Weighs about two and one half pounds by delivery, one pound by the first week postpartum, and two ounces by six weeks
  - Lochia is present during involution
    - Consists of blood, mucus, and tissue
    - Transforms from red to pink, and then to white in three weeks
    - Changes in color from pink to white and back to red again may indicate excessive physical exertion

- May increase during feeds due to uterine contractions
- Perineum
  - After vaginal delivery, there is swelling and tenderness
  - An episiotomy can increase swelling and cause pulling sensations
  - Ice packs, sitz baths, sprays, cooling cotton pads, and medications can provide comfort
  - Kegel exercises will help the mother regain her muscle tone
  - If the muscles remain weak, the uterus may tip or sink down into the vagina and the mother may have difficulty controlling urination
- Body functions
  - Frequent urination can occur due to the loss of extra fluids
  - It may be difficult to urinate, especially if the mother had a catheter
  - The mother's bowels may not move for awhile after birth—especially a mother who had a cesarean
  - Manipulation of the intestines during a cesarean causes gas and bowel dysfunction
  - Deep breathing exercises, rocking back and forth in a rocking chair, and alternating abdominal tightening and relaxation can provide relief
- Minor irritations
  - The mother may experience backaches as a result of softened or loosened sacroiliac ligaments, or due to epidural anesthesia
  - The mother may experience heavy perspiration due to a surplus of fluid accumulated during pregnancy; she can wear cool, loose clothing and take frequent showers to feel better
  - Extra large sanitary pads that are used postnatally may be irritating; as her lochia discharge subsides, she can use smaller pads

Becoming a Father
- Fathers learn their role in the following ways:
  - Society's definitions
  - Experience with their own fathers
  - Peer pressure from other men
  - Active involvement in the pregnancy and birth
- Invite fathers to infant feeding classes and encourage their participation
  - Teach them what to expect and strategies for coping
  - Teach them the realities of breastfeeding
  - Discuss caregiving tasks such as bathing, burping, diapering, helping the mother with positioning to breastfeed, and carrying the baby in a sling
  - Discuss infant cues and responsiveness
  - Address the mother and father as a couple
- Discuss being a support person for the mother in the following ways:
  - Helping her get comfortable
  - Filling in pieces of information she may have forgotten
  - Providing encouragement when she is having a bad day
  - Helping with the care of the baby and household chores
  - When encouraged by the mother, a father often becomes the best supporter and an outspoken advocate of breastfeeding
- Discuss a father's interaction with his baby
  - A father who participates in the birth is likely to respond more openly and readily to his baby than a father whose first interaction occurs after the baby is brought home
  - A father needs time alone with his baby to develop his own parenting style
  - A father needs to be encouraged in his new role

- A father is the first person in a baby's life who teaches the baby that food and love do not need to always come from the same person
- Caution mothers against criticizing fathers about the ways they do things to the point that they limit their involvement
- Babies whose fathers interact with them on a consistent basis exhibit the following:
  - Eagerness for learning
  - More confident self-image
  - More confidence in relating to males
  - Sense of humor and a longer attention span

Changes in Family Relationships

Sexual Adjustments
- Re-establishing enjoyable sexual relations is part of the total adjustment
- Effective communication and the passage of time are major factors
- When parents are fatigued, lovemaking may seem like a chore
- Emotional factors
  - Can take several months to regain desires or responses to sex
  - The mother's breasts may be oversensitive or have no sensual response
  - The mother may become sexually aroused when nursing
  - The mother may be reluctant to engage in foreplay that involves her breasts
- Physical discomfort
  - Hormones in lactation decrease vaginal secretions
  - The mother may have pain from hospital interventions
  - Either partner may not experience physical sensations
  - Overfull or leaking breasts may be uncomfortable for the mother

LACTATIONAL AMENORRHEA

- Adjusting the sexual routine
  - Adjustments in positioning can help alleviate physical discomfort
  - The mother may breastfeed immediately before the baby's bedtime or nap and allow for lovemaking when the baby is asleep and her breasts are less full
  - The couple may need to develop new patterns of foreplay that will avoid the mother's breasts

Menstruation and Fertility

- Fertility is delayed in response to the infant's suckling
- The single most important factor in the suppression of ovulation in normal lactating women is the early establishment of the frequent and strong suckling stimulus of her baby
- A link exists between the levels of growth hormones, the luteinizing hormone, the follicle-stimulating hormone, and estrogen
- The length of time that amenorrhea and infertility lasts is linked to the following:
  - Breastfeeding frequency
  - Short intervals between feeds
  - Duration of feeds
  - Presence of nighttime feeds
  - Absence of supplemental feeds in the baby's diet
- May have a scanty show before a true menstrual cycle resumes
  - Some women report they bleed around Day 42 to 56
  - May signal an end to the lochial discharge
  - May reflect a change in the mother's activity level
  - May change the taste of the milk, causing the baby to be fussy during a feed or to refuse to nurse

Contraceptive Options for Breastfeeding Women
- Lactational amenorrhea method (LAM)
  - The following three conditions must exist (see Figure 17.1):
    - A mother's menses has not yet returned
    - The baby is breastfed around the clock without any significant amounts of other foods in the diet
    - The baby is younger than six months of age
  - If any one of these conditions is not met, there is an increased risk of pregnancy, and the mother should utilize another method of contraception if she does not desire to become pregnant
  - For the LAM to be most effective, the baby should begin to breastfeed soon after birth and continue to breastfeed exclusively day and night for six months
  - The use of artificial nipples, such as a bottle or pacifier, interferes with the frequency and duration of suckling at the breast
  - As soon as there is a decline in breastfeeding, the LAM protection decreases
- Oral contraceptives should be delayed
  - Using a combination of contraceptives—estrogen and progesterone—may affect milk volume and composition
  - Progestin-only oral contraceptives do not interfere with production
  - Delay oral contraceptive use until six weeks postpartum
- Periodic abstinence (natural family planning)
  - Keep a calendar record of the mother's menstrual periods to predict her fertile days
    - Chart the mother's basal body temperature—temperature taken when waking around the same time each day—for fluctuations to aid the couple in determining fertile periods
    - Temperature is at its lowest during menses and through her cycle until ovulation
    - After ovulation, the temperature rises and

```
Ask the mother:

Is your baby less than six months old?
  ├─ NO ──→ Her chance of pregnancy is increased. She should not rely on breastfeeding alone. Use another family planning method, but continue to breastfeed for the child's health.
  └─ YES
       ↓
Are you amenorrheic? (no vaginal bleeding after 56 days postpartum)
  ├─ NO ──→ (same box above)
  └─ YES
       ↓
Are you fully or nearly fully breastfeeding your baby?
  ├─ NO ──→ (same box above)
  └─ YES
       ↓
There is ONLY ABOUT A 2% CHANCE OF PREGNANCY: she does not need a complementary family planning method at this time.

Tell the mother: when the answer to any of these questions becomes NO - - - - - - - - - →
```

Figure 17.1 Lactational amenorrhea method

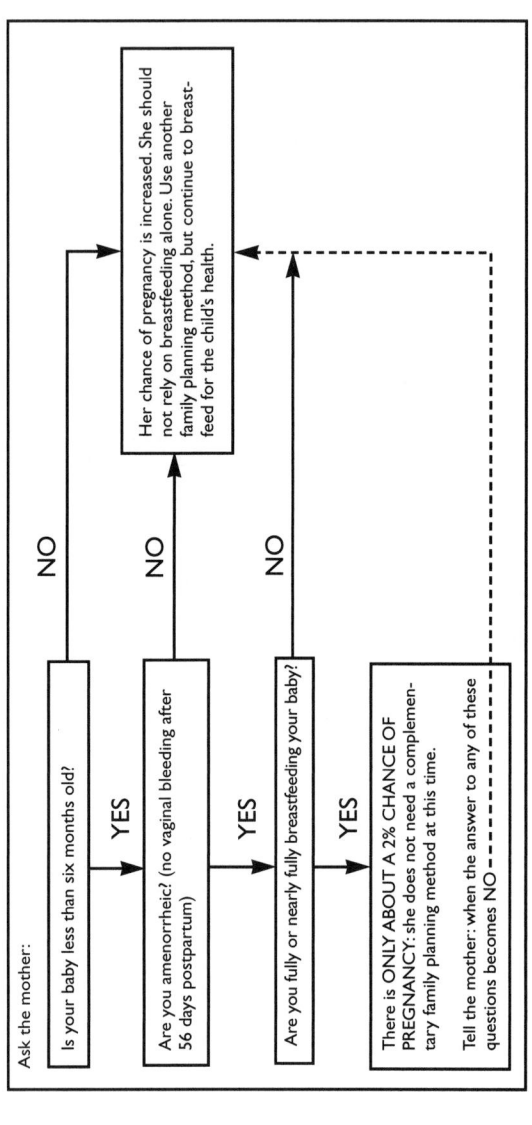

Reprinted by permission of the Institute for Reproductive Health from *Guidelines for Breastfeeding in Family Planning and Child Survival Programs,*

stays at about that level until just before the onset of menses
- Check the mother's vaginal secretions for changes in cervical mucus, which occur before ovulation, to signal the fertile period
  - Patterns during the first few months postpartum are less clearly defined than after regular cycles resume
  - Vaginal secretions change from a scant semisolid white or yellowish matter to an abundant thin, clear, watery, and slippery fluid that allows sperm to penetrate the canal of the cervix easily
- Combining mucus and temperature changes will identify the five to seven days per month when conception is possible
- This method is not to be confused with the less reliable rhythm method, which estimates the fertile period from calendar records alone
- Other contraceptive methods include the following:
  - Sterilization
  - Contraceptive foam and condom in combination
  - Diaphragm
  - Jellies and creams
  - Injectable medroxyprogesterone (Depo-Provera)
  - Implants of levonorgestrel (Norplant)

Sibling Reactions and Adjustments

Helping Siblings Prepare for the New Baby
- Share events of the pregnancy with them such as the development of the fetus, visits to the physician, and what will take place at the birth
- Involve the children in preparing for the baby by getting clothes and baby equipment ready and packing the mother's suitcase

- Explain what new babies do (such as nursing, sleeping, and crying) to the children:
  - Read books to the children that depict a new baby in the family
  - Make a booklet with magazine pictures of babies and families
  - Help children look at their own family's baby pictures
  - Have the children help care for the new baby by bringing diapers and clothing to the mother, holding the baby, talking to him, and getting him to smile
  - Visit a family with a new baby to see what a new infant looks and sounds like
  - If sleeping arrangements must be changed, do it early to ensure that older children do not feel crowded out by the new baby

Preparing Children for the Mother's Absence

- Tell the children where their mother is going, why, for how long, and what she will do while she is there
- Visit the hospital with the children so they can understand what will take place
- Arrange sibling visitation during the mother's postpartum stay
- Maintain contact with the family through phone calls, notes, and photos
- If it is appropriate and the children are prepared, have the children present at the birth

Adjusting to the New Baby

- The smoothness of the homecoming will depend on the preparation of the children and the length of time they have been separated from their mother
- Relationships will mend as the family members learn to love the baby in their own ways

- The older child was previously the "baby of the family"
- Each child needs time to understand when assuming his new role
- Siblings may want to be included during feeds
- A toddler who was weaned may ask to nurse again
- Children may exhibit the following regressive behaviors when the new baby arrives:
  - Whining
  - Baby talk
  - Bed wetting or accidents from a previously toilet-trained child
  - Waking during the night
  - Clinging to the mother
  - Hitting the baby
- Parents can handle a child's regressive behavior in the following ways:
  - Give the child more attention—this may be the child's way of asking for it
  - Often, a child will develop mixed feelings about the new baby; the mother can reassure the child that she understands and accepts his feelings
  - Help the child to adjust to his new position in the family

Special Counseling Circumstances

Opposition to Breastfeeding

Comments that Undermine the Mother's Confidence
- How long do you plan to nurse?
- Are you still breastfeeding?
- Isn't he getting a little old to nurse?
- Does he want to nurse again so soon?
- He seems hungry all the time; maybe you don't have enough milk

Opposition from Strangers
- A mother who is confident and knowledgeable about her decision to breastfeed is less likely to be affected by the opinions or remarks of strangers
- Discreet nursing in public will minimize the potential for comments

Opposition from Friends
- The mother may attempt to educate a friend who opposes breastfeeding
- The mother can develop friendships with people who are supportive or who are breastfeeding

Opposition from the Mother's Employer

- The mother should speak frankly with her employer about her plans to breastfeed
  - She can discuss any special needs she will have at work
  - She can reinforce that breastfeeding will not interfere with her performance
  - She can discuss the aspects of her job that could be compatible with breastfeeding
  - She can develop a plan within the parameters of her job (see Chapter 22, When Breastfeeding is Interrupted)
  - Note that a healthy baby means less time off and less use of medical benefits
- Discuss that negative attitudes are more a result of a lack of experience
- Help the mother re-evaluate her priorities and motives regarding working

Opposition from the Physician

- A perceived lack of support may be a result of a lack of knowledge (see Chapter 2, The Lactation Consulting Profession)
- If the physician is unsupportive, he may give misinformation to the mother
- Tell the physician how important breastfeeding is to the mother and her baby
- If the mother does not have a good rapport with her physician, she may need to consider whether that relationship is good for her
- Note that the mother will need a lot of extra contact and confidence building

Opposition from the Grandmother

- In many cultures, the grandmother has a pivotal role in the mother's breastfeeding
- The mother needs to understand the reasons for the grandmother's opposition
  - The grandmother is concerned about both the mother and the baby

- The grandmother does not want her daughter to be disappointed by failure
- The grandmother may envy that her daughter can do something she could not do
- The grandmother may be experiencing her own guilt about not breastfeeding
- Be patient and understanding with the grandmother
  - Assure the mother that her own mother (or her partner's mother) did her best when she parented her children
  - Educate the grandmother and enlist her in supporting the mother and baby
  - Accept the grandmother's view and encourage the mother to not allow it to affect her breastfeeding

Opposition from the Baby's Father

- Often, the father's views weigh greatly on the mother's breastfeeding decisions
- Fathers often worry that breastfeeding will make the baby too dependent on the mother
  - Give the father literature on child development
  - Note that meeting a child's needs makes him less dependent on parents in the future
  - Suggest ways for the father to interact with his child (see Chapter 17, Changes in the Family)
- Fathers often believe breastfeeding interferes with the couple's sex life
  - Note that a baby will interfere with parents' sex lives regardless of their feeding choice
  - Suggest that the mother spend some special time alone with the father
  - It may be difficult for a father to regard breasts as something other than sexual
- The father is concerned about the health and well-being of his partner and baby
  - Point out the positive aspects of this concern

- Note that not breastfeeding increases the health risks for both the mother and baby
- Point out that the emotional benefits of breastfeeding enhance a baby's disposition
- Give the father literature about the nutritional benefits of human milk
- Help the father recognize his baby's healthy growth and development
- A father may question the need or appropriateness of continuing to breastfeed an older baby
  - This is true, especially if the baby is male
  - The father should understand the baby's needs and the mother's desire to breastfeed
- The mother will need a great deal of support and frequent contacts
  - If the mother decides to wean, you should accept this decision and help her do so
  - Avoid getting in a conflict between the mother and her unsupportive partner
  - Refer the mother to a support group
  - Accept the father's position and help the mother cope without judging her
  - Point out the baby's positive aspects and how well he is growing

A Low-Income Mother

Characteristics of a Low-Income Lifestyle

- The mother may have a lower self-esteem, education, and occupation, and lower expectations of herself
- The mother may live in an area of overcrowding, run-down housing, crime, isolation, and inadequate community services; in addition to living among people dealing with broken families, alienation, relocation, physical and mental health problems, and language barriers
- Low-income mothers may feel they have no control over their own lives and surroundings

Psychosocial Issues
- Breastfeeding builds confidence and self-esteem
- A breastfed baby will be healthier and therefore happier
- Note that more women breastfeed now so a low-income, breastfeeding mother will not feel different
- Breastfeeding is an intelligent decision that is based on sound medical facts
- Medical personnel are seen as experts
- Your support may be critical to a low-income mother's success in breastfeeding

Breastfeeding Challenges
- A low-income mother may not take prenatal classes because of their cost, availability, or a lack of interest
- A low-income mother may receive medication during labor and delivery
- A low-income mother may lack support and accurate information
- A low-income mother may believe a human milk substitute is just as good or better ("scientific")
- The peers of a low-income mother may be uncomfortable or unsupportive of breastfeeding
- A low-income mother may distrust you because you represent the "system"
- Breastfeeding may be seen as one more stress or failure in her life
- A low-income mother may be unaware of the resources available in her community

Reaching Out to Low-Income Women
- The following factors affect whether a low-income woman will breastfeed:
  - There is a greater likelihood a low-income mother will breastfeed when she has a higher education, is married, and has a greater ego maturity
  - A low-income mother's greatest motivator seems to be a support person she respects

who has had a positive breastfeeding experience
- Access to support and accurate information play a vital role
- Those with no telephone service may need home visits
- A low-income mother will likely breastfeed when she has a good perception of her family and peer support
- The breastfeeding rates of low-income mothers increase when local health care clinics include classes, one-on-one instruction, and peer counselors
- See Table 18.1

Single Mother

Profile of a Single Mother
- Typically lives alone
- Juggles job, schooling or training, household responsibilities, and parenting
- May have no support system and no one to share concerns or parenting
- Has little time for herself
- Lacks the desire or time to prepare well-balanced meals
- Is likely to appreciate your caring and frequent contact
- See Table 18.2

Needs of Mothers Who Live with Their Parents
- Must maintain their own identity as an adult and a mother
- Must preserve the identity of a family unit for her and her baby
- May need help dealing with criticism about her parenting from her own parents
- May need some personal space due to a lack of privacy that interferes with her breastfeeding

TABLE 18.1 COUNSELING SUMMARY—LOW-INCOME MOTHER

- Listen to the mother and actively acknowledge her view of her situation.
- Determine whether the mother has any sources of support for, or any interference with, breastfeeding from a partner, family, or peers.
- Keep your instructions simple and use visual aids whenever possible.
- Praise the mother, letting her know she is making the intelligent choice, is doing the best for her baby, and is doing well at breastfeeding.
- Use outreach counseling and contact the mother frequently to help prevent problems.
- If the mother lacks support at home, encourage her to focus on major priorities, especially employment, child care, nutrition, breastfeeding, rest, and major household tasks.
- Become knowledgeable of a mother's nutritional habits and offer suggestions if any improvement is needed.
- Help the mother locate supplemental food programs and make the best use of her food dollars.
- Ensure that the mother is aware of contraceptive methods that are compatible with breastfeeding.

When Single Status Results from Death of a Spouse

- Emotional stress may cause a decrease in milk production
- The baby may tune in to the emotional state of his mother and want to nurse more
- Breastfeeding can provide comfort to both the mother and baby
- The mother will benefit from support and professional counseling

TABLE 18.2 COUNSELING SUMMARY—SINGLE MOTHER

- Become knowledgeable of the mother's nutritional habits—meal patterns, who cooks, consumption of fast foods, and so on.
- Become aware of the mother's responsibilities with her home and job.
- Become aware of the mother's living arrangements—find out whether she is living with her parents, her partner, or alone.
- Determine the mother's sources of support for breastfeeding—her partner, family, and peers.
- Refer the mother to a support group for single parents.
- Help the mother think of ways she can meet both her and her baby's needs at the same time.

Teenage Mother

Characteristics of a Teenage Mother

- Nine out of ten pregnant teenagers elect to keep their babies
- Many under the age of 18 choose not to get married
- May not complete high school
- May lack skills or income to care for their babies
- Often have no job skills and are dependent on families and society
- Wish to be treated as adults and dislike lecturing, advice, or any patronizing manner
- Sensitive to the reactions of people close to her
- Doubts her self-worth and has a poor self-image

Prenatal Issues

- Frequent pattern of inadequate prenatal care and poor nutrition among teenage mothers
- Higher incidence of premature infants, infants with low birth weight, stillbirths, and neonatal deaths

- A teen is reluctant to gain weight and may be unhappy about the changes in her body
- Pregnancy compromises the teen's health—her own growth needs compete with the growth needs of her fetus
- Needs praise for her weight gain and its benefit to her baby
- The mother's nutrition education is a primary goal
- Anxiety about the impending labor and delivery
- There is a higher incidence of prematurity, low birth weight, stillbirths, and neonatal deaths

Postpartum Issues

- Less likely to have immediate or prolonged contact with the baby
- Often feels threatened and overwhelmed by her environment
- Reluctant to ask for anything from the nursing staff
- Visitors may be more important than contact with her baby
- Needs to be encouraged to interact with her baby
- Many teen mothers accept the responsibilities of motherhood and respond in much the same way as an older mother
- May have difficulty coping with parenting and difficulty giving love and attention to the baby
- The baby may be raised as a sibling, and she may have little to do with his care
- Some mothers have a power struggle with their own mothers over the care of their baby; they see breastfeeding as one thing only they can do for their baby
- May have difficulty seeing the baby's needs beyond her personal needs

Breastfeeding Issues

- Teenage mothers have the same potential to breastfeed as older mothers
    - Try to reach teens early in their pregnancy in order to educate them on infant feeding
    - Introduce breastfeeding within their school's curricula
    - Sixty-five percent of teenage mothers breastfeed because it is "good for the baby"
    - Sixty-seven percent enjoy the "closeness" of this relationship
    - Many teenage mothers are concerned about modesty and their return to school
- Teenage mothers may lack support for breastfeeding among their family and friends
- Teenage mothers are less likely to overcome breastfeeding difficulties
- Teenage mothers find it difficult to understand that a problem will be resolved as they are living "in the moment"
- Teenage mothers may be overwhelmed by their parenting responsibilities
- Teenage mothers may fail to see the future consequences of their actions

Interactions with Teenage Mothers

- A teenage mother needs a consistent one-to-one relationship
- Discuss how a teenage mother is adjusting, how the birth went, how she feels, and what her needs are
- Many such interactions will take place in a classroom setting
    - Teach in simple, clear terms that are not overwhelming
    - Learn what teenage mothers know and what they would like to know
    - Make this time together both humorous and informative
    - Allow for nonthreatening participation

TABLE 18.3 COUNSELING SUMMARY—TEENAGE MOTHER

- Become knowledgeable of the mother's nutritional habits and influencing factors—eating with her family, body image, and so on.
- Determine whether the mother has any sources of support for, or interference with, breastfeeding—family, peers, and partner.
- Determine the mother's reactions to her pregnancy, hospital environment, and becoming a parent—self-worth, body image, and interaction with her baby.
- Determine who is the primary caretaker of the baby.
- Determine the mother's sources of emotional support.
- Refer the mother to a support group for teenage parents, when it is appropriate.
- Look for signs of adequate milk production.

- Use audiovisual aids that depict other teens breastfeeding
- Cover the breastfeeding basics whenever possible
- Make yourself available for individual time outside of class
- Encourage a teenage mother's family or friends to come classes with her
- See Table 18.3

Mothers with Cultural Differences

Becoming Immersed in a New Culture (Acculturation)

Mothers who live in a culture other than their own may do the following:
- Cling to certain values
- Replace old values with new ones as cultural differences become more diffuse, especially in succeeding generations

- The following factors influence the mother's degree of acculturation:
  - Age
  - Educational and social exposure
  - Intent to return to her country of origin
  - Contact with older relatives
  - Part of the country in which she resides
- Lower classes tend to hold onto traditional values
- Middle and upper classes incorporate other cultural practices into their own value system

Family May Be the Dominant Unit

- The decision making may be the responsibility of the eldest male or another male figure in the family
- The extended family often provides a support system for raising the child
- Take care not to interfere with the mother's family and peer support
- Provide clear, accurate information in a climate of acceptance
- A home visit may give a more complete picture of the mother's environment
- The family of the mother may be reluctant to invite strangers into their home
- Learn the customs of greeting and the inclusion of others before you visit a family

Cultural Beliefs Regarding Breastfeeding and Health

- Being ignorant of a mother's cultural differences can alienate the mother and cause you to run the risk of offering recommendations that will be irrelevant or ignored
- A mother's culture affects the way she regards health and the measures she takes to prevent or treat illnesses
- Do not try to change a mother's practices unless they are very detrimental to the mother or her baby

- Note that inappropriate advice from you may upset the mother
- Seek ways to work around culturally based practices
- Notice what is important and offer practical suggestions
- A woman who has breastfed in the culture you are encountering can assist you in learning their beliefs and can help you support the mother
- Cultural heritage and economic standing can affect how long a mother will nurse and her ability to deal with negative input from her partner, family, or friends
- Cultural values and priorities vary greatly
  - May regard health care providers and the scientific community with great respect
  - May put more faith in self-care or folk medicine
  - May regard colostrum as valueless or undesirable and discourage breastfeeding until the second or third postpartum day
  - May discourage the consumption of cold foods and beverages by new mothers for a period of time (hot teas and soups may help meet their fluid requirements)
  - May place limitations on the activity of a postpartum mother
  - May have rules about touching the baby or referring to the baby
- See Table 18.4

Language Differences May Increase Barriers

- Speak slowly and clearly, and provide simple explanations
- Find a colleague who can speak the language or ask if the mother has a bilingual friend or relative who can assist
- Contact a local school for a volunteer to serve as interpreter

TABLE 18.4 COUNSELING SUMMARY—MOTHERS WITH CULTURAL DIFFERENCES

- Investigate the mother's income level and provide suggestions if applicable.
- Become knowledgeable of the mother's cultural heritage:
    Practices relative to breastfeeding.
    Degree of acculturation.
    Religious or superstitious beliefs.
    Family support system.
    Health and illness practices.
- Bridge the language barrier by using an interpreter, visual aids, body language, and translated literature.
- Ensure that the mother has understood your message by having her summarize or demonstrate important points.
- Assess the mother's need and desire for a personal relationship with a counselor.
- Accept a mother's cultural practices if they are not detrimental to her or her baby; provide applicable information in order to eliminate harmful practices.
- Adapt your counseling approach to meet the mother's special needs.
- Include family members in your consultations with the mother.

- Note that the mother may be reluctant to share intimate information with a male other than her partner; it is best to choose a woman
- Be certain that an interpreter is communicating accurately and not adding her own opinions or values
- Note that the mother may need to converse in her own language in order to be understood and to comprehend your advice

Interpret Body Language Correctly
- Nodding and smiling may not denote understanding as it does in Western society
- Watch for nonverbal cues given by facial and body expressions
- A nod accompanied by a bland or puzzled look can imply confusion
- To ensure that a mother understands your instructions, ask her to repeat them
- Demonstrate procedures and summarize the important points at the end
- The use of listening skills is critical

Mother-to-Mother Support Groups

Meeting the Needs of Mothers
- The goal is to educate women about the options that will work for them
- Anticipatory guidance will help mothers avoid problems and obstacles
- Provide outreach assistance through childbirth classes and clinics, sharing information with professionals, phoning the mothers, and visiting high school health classes
- Develop a relationship between the IBCLC, counselors, mothers, and caregivers

Regular Group Meetings
- Provide a valuable counseling opportunity
- Encourage friendly and informal discussions
- Create a supportive environment
- Should be guided by the needs of women who are attending
- Involve the mother as much as possible

When No Support Group Is Available

- Provide ongoing support and appropriate written materials to the mothers
- Make referrals for other areas of support
- Follow-up is especially important
- Develop a group, train the group leaders, and be available as a resource

Breastfeeding Techniques and Devices

Breastfeeding Techniques

Pinch Test
- To test protractility, grasp the base of the nipple with the forefinger and thumb (as shown in Figure 19.1), and press the thumb and forefinger together several times around the base
- A nipple that moves forward is considered a normal, protracting nipple and needs no special intervention
- A retracting nipple is one that moves inward rather than forward, as shown in Figure 19.1
- See Chapter 6, The Science of Lactation, for a discussion about the differences in nipples

Breast Massage
- Oxytocin levels increase and remain high throughout breast massage
- Provides a more efficient pressure gradient for the movement of milk from an area of high pressure to an area of low pressure (the baby's mouth)
- The following are situations in which breast massage is especially useful:

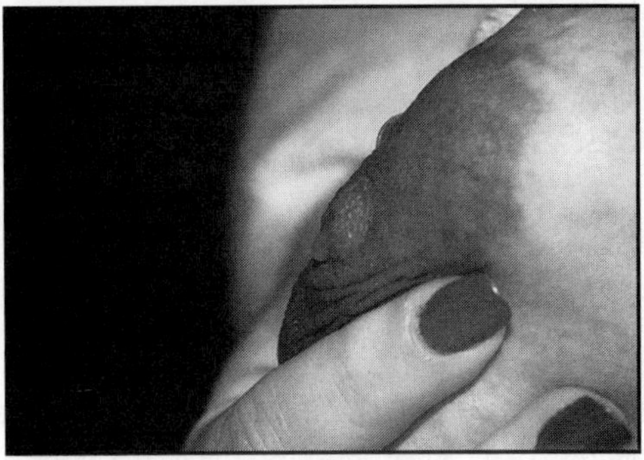

Figure 19.1 Pinch test: Nipple with compression
Printed by permission of Kay Hoover.

- When a mother is relactating or is initiating lactation to nurse an adopted baby
- When a baby seems impatient for milk to flow
- Before manual expression or pumping
- When a mother is engorged, or has a plugged duct or mastitis
- Alternate breast massage
  - Can be done when a baby pauses during a feed
  - Sustains sucking in a sleepy baby or an inefficient feeder
  - Increases the volume of fat content per feed
- Technique
  - Begin at the chest wall using the palm of the hand (not fingers) to exert gentle pressure on the breast (see Figure 19.2)
  - Massage the breast in a circular motion from the chest wall toward the nipple
  - Continue massaging in this manner, working the hand around the breast
  - Focus on the areas of greatest milk duct development—under the breast along the side under the arm

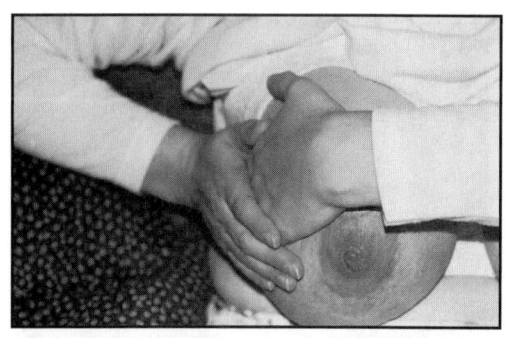

Figure 19.2 Breast massage—lifting the engorged breast to assist with lymphatic drainage

Printed by permission of Kay Hoover.

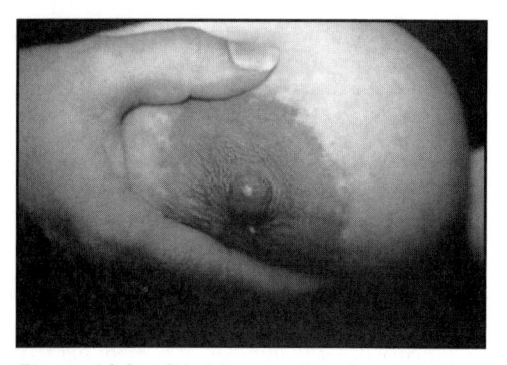

Figure 19.3 C-hold—note that this mother's fingers are NOT well behind the areola

C-Hold

- The mother cups her free hand on the breast to form the letter C
- The thumb should be on top and the fingers should be curved below the breast
- Her fingers and thumb must be placed well behind the areola
- See Figure 19.3 for an example

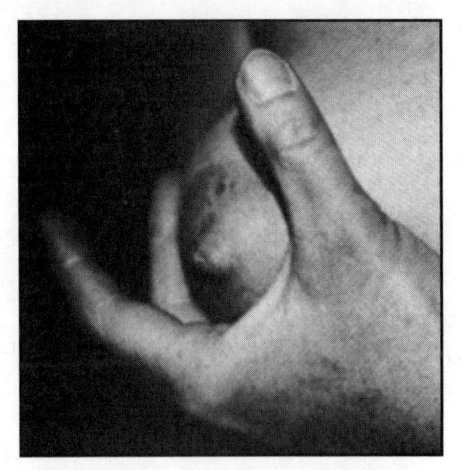

Figure 19.4 Dancer hand position
Courtesy of Childbirth Graphics, Ltd., 1985.

Dancer Hand Position

- Begin in the C-hold position
- Bring a hand forward to support the breast with the first three fingers
- Support the infant's chin with the area of the hand between the thumb and index finger
- Bend the index finger slightly
- Gently hold the infant's cheek on one side
- Hold the other cheek with a thumb
- This position decreases the space in an infant's mouth and increases negative pressure
- See Figure 19.4 for an example

Breastfeeding Devices

Breast Lubricant

- The following conditions indicate a need for an artificial lubricant:
  - Excessively dry skin, eczema, or other dermatologic condition

- Natural lubrication has been removed by the improper use of drying agents or other practices
- Nipples are sore or cracked
- The following are acceptable lubricants:
  - A mother's own milk massaged into the sore nipple
  - Hypoallergenic, medical-grade, anhydrous lanolin has been encouraged for use on sore nipples due to the following reasons:
    - Allergens and impurities of regular lanolin are removed
    - Provides a semi-occlusive moisture barrier
    - Slows down the internal moisture loss without clogging pores
    - Acts as a moist wound healer
    - Modified lanolin has an insignificant effect on nipple pain or damage during the first five days postpartum
- Topicals that are not recommended are those that:
  - Must be removed before a feed and thus delay healing time
  - Can cause irritations or allergies
  - Contain harmful substances—pesticides are found in regular lanolin
  - Do not facilitate moist wound healing—they stay on the skin's surface and do not provide the moisture necessary for healing
- Apply lubricants only after skin is thoroughly dry to avoid trapping moisture on the nipple

Using an Inverted Syringe for Flat or Inverted Nipples

- The syringe must have a barrel slightly larger than the nipple—a 10- to 20-ml syringe usually works well (see Figure 19.5)
- Procedure
  - Cut off the tapered end of the syringe
  - Reverse the plunger direction to provide a smooth surface next to the breast (the cut end should never be placed against a mother's breast)

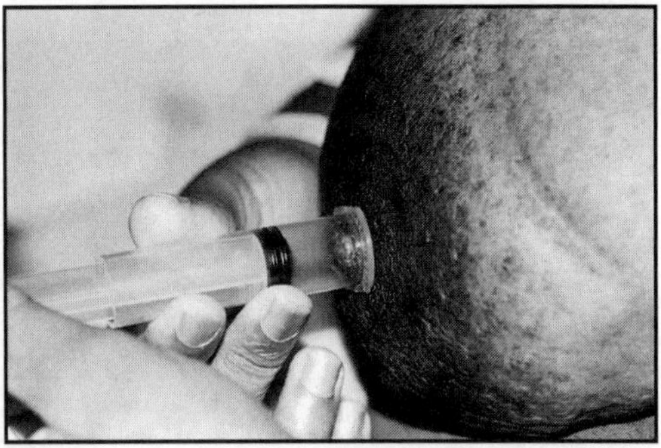

Figure 19.5 Inverted syringe
Printed by permission of Kay Hoover.

- Place the smooth end of the syringe over the nipple and pull gently on the plunger
- Hold the pressure for about 30 seconds and then release
- Repeat two or three times in each session
- Use a syringe prenatally two or three times daily until the baby is born
- It is important that the mother and not the caregiver do the pulling on the syringe

Breast Shells

- Wearing breast shells inside a bra may improve nipple protractility (see Figure 19.6)
- The shells gently place pressure on the skin
- The shells stretch and push the nipple forward
- Wearing breast shells during pregnancy has not been shown to be beneficial
- Use a bra that is one cup size larger than the shells to avoid pressing the shell too tightly against the breast
- Use a shell with several openings for air circulation
- Do not wear the shells while sleeping or for long periods of time because they may place excessive pressure on lactiferous sinuses or cause prolonged leaking

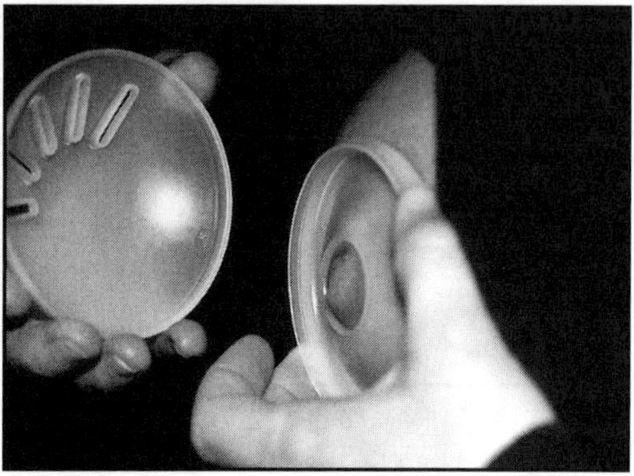

Figure 19.6 A breast shell on a breast
Printed by permission of Kay Hoover.

- If breast shells are used prenatally, intermittently wear the shells for a short time eight to ten hours or more daily until they become comfortable
- If breast shells are used after delivery, wear the shells between or for short periods before feeds to help shape the nipple

Nipple Shield
- Should not be the first choice for intervention with latching difficulties or sucking problems
- Reduces milk transfer (even modern, thinner silicon shields)
- Potential for nipple shield addiction—the baby may refuse to suckle on a soft breast because of preference for the rigid texture of the shield or other such rigid shape
- The following can indicate a nipple shield addiction:
  - Baby refuses the breast
  - Other techniques have been exhausted
  - Weaning is being considered because of difficulties

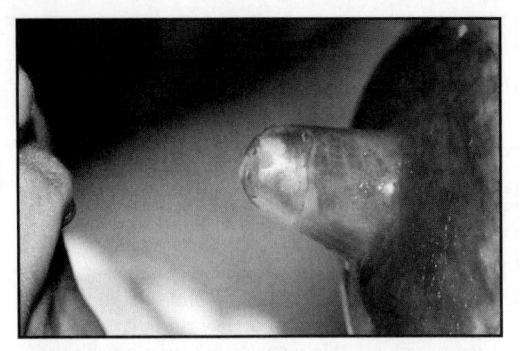

Figure 19.7 A nipple shield on a breast just after the baby has unlatched

Printed by permission of Kay Hoover.

- Always consider the following:
  - Whether the benefits of the shield's use outweigh the risks
  - Whether its use will fit in a mother's breastfeeding plan
  - Whether a mother will accept the risks and comply with careful follow-up (see the following Nipple Shield Consent Form)
- Here is the proper method for using a nipple shield:
  - Place the shield on the breast at the beginning of a feed (see Figure 19.7 for an example)
  - Remove the shield after the baby begins to suck
  - Quickly put the baby back to the breast to suckle without the shield
  - Monitor the baby's intake and output carefully, which includes a daily record of feeds, voids, stools, and frequent weight checks
  - A mother may need to pump her breasts to maintain milk production
  - Wean the baby from the shield as soon as possible

> **Nipple Shield Consent Form**
>
> I wish to use a nipple shield as a device to help my infant learn how to latch onto my breast. I understand that improper or continuous use of this nipple shield can cause a 22 percent to 50 percent decrease in my milk supply and that it may inhibit my milk ejection reflex. These effects can result in little or no weight gain for my infant. I understand that while I am using this nipple shield I must use a large, hospital-grade, electric breast pump to stimulate and maintain my milk supply. I understand that while using this nipple shield my infant's weight will need to be checked once or twice a week. I understand that the improper or continuous use of this device can lead to my infant becoming dependent on it in order to nurse from my breast. I understand that this device is to be used as a temporary breastfeeding aid and that the use of it should be discontinued as soon as possible.
>
> *Printed by the permission of Breastfeeding Support Consultants.*

- Procedure for weaning the baby from the shield
  - Put the baby to the breast periodically without a shield when it "feels right" to see if he will feed without it
  - Watch for times when the baby offers cues that he may nurse without the shield
  - A sleepy baby may be less likely to resist the change from a shield to the breast
  - Attempt to wean the baby from the shield after the initial fullness occurring at the beginning of a feed has decreased
  - Increase skin-to-skin contact with the baby
  - If the baby is particularly resistive to feeding without the shield, make it less attractive to him by stuffing a small piece of damp cloth inside the teat cavity

- A mother may need to nurse indefinitely with a shield rather than wean her baby totally
  - The mother will benefit from ongoing support
  - The mother may need to pump her breasts to ensure continued milk production
  - The baby will need periodic weight checks

Use of a Pacifier

- Pacifiers are not appropriate for a breastfeeding infant
- The risks of pacifier use are as follows:
  - Use correlates with a higher incidence of early weaning, particularly when sucking technique is incorrect
  - Increases the incidence of Candida and ear infections
  - Can cause malocclusion
  - Can suppress the central grooving of a baby's tongue
  - Does not offer a nutritional benefit to the infant; expends calories and may contribute to a slowed infant growth
  - Interferes with the natural process of a baby increasing milk production through suckling
- The appropriate and safe uses of a pacifier are as follows:
  - For meeting the sucking needs of a bottle-fed baby
  - Preterm infants have the following benefits from sucking on pacifiers during gavage feeding:
    - Accelerates maturation of the sucking reflex
    - Decreases intestinal transit time
    - Increases the rate of weight gain
  - Useful in calming infants who must undergo painful procedures
- When offering a pacifier, always tune in to the baby's cues:
  - Ascertain that the other needs are fully met—nourishment, comfort, and human contact
  - If the baby remains unsettled and roots, put him to the breast before offering a pacifier

Evaluator Techniques

Using a Finger to Pacify the Baby

- Insert an index finger very gently into the baby's mouth pad side up (see Figure 19.8 for an example)
- Wait until the baby begins sucking on the finger
- Use a finger as a pacifier in conjunction with a tube feeding system to increase the baby's calorie intake (referred to as finger feeding)

Using a Finger to Evaluate the Baby's Oral Cavity

- Attempt the evaluation when the baby is relaxed and receptive
- Insert an index finger very gently into the baby's mouth pad side up
- Evaluate the inside of the baby's oral cavity and palates
  - Is the palate normal, flat, or excessively high?
  - Does the tongue cover the alveolar ridge when the baby suckles?
  - Does the tongue cup around the bottom of the finger to form a trough?
  - Does the tongue move rhythmically from front to back?

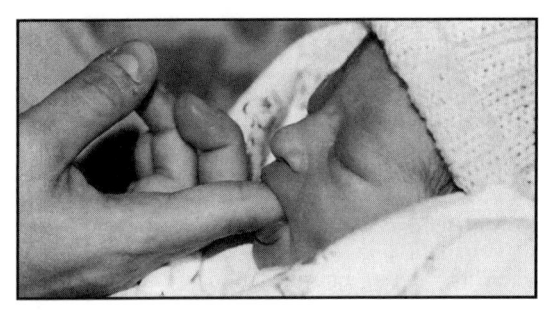

Figure 19.8 An index finger inserted pad side up into a baby's mouth with the fingertip extended to the junction of the hard and soft palate

Printed by permission of Kay Hoover.

Suck Reorganization

- Suck reorganization involves the control of a baby's sucking by a caregiver through the manipulation of a finger in the baby's mouth
- Insert an index finger very gently into the baby's mouth pad side up
- Place slight pressure on the midline of the tongue
- Pull the finger out slowly to encourage the baby to suck it back in
- Give the baby verbal reinforcement when he sucks appropriately

Suck Training

- Insert an index finger very gently into the baby's mouth pad side up
- Stimulate certain portions of the baby's oral anatomy to train him to suck
- This training is a highly active and controlling action done by the therapist
- A baby who needs suck training must be referred to a trained professional, such as a physical or speech therapist who is further specialized as a neurodevelopmental therapist (NDT)
- Suck training is beyond the scope of most nurses or IBCLCs

Milk Expression

Manual Expression

- Every mother needs to know how to hand express her milk, regardless of her breastfeeding situation
- A mother who knows how to manually express milk will be able to extract milk despite any unforeseen circumstances such as a broken pump, power failure, natural disaster, or low battery

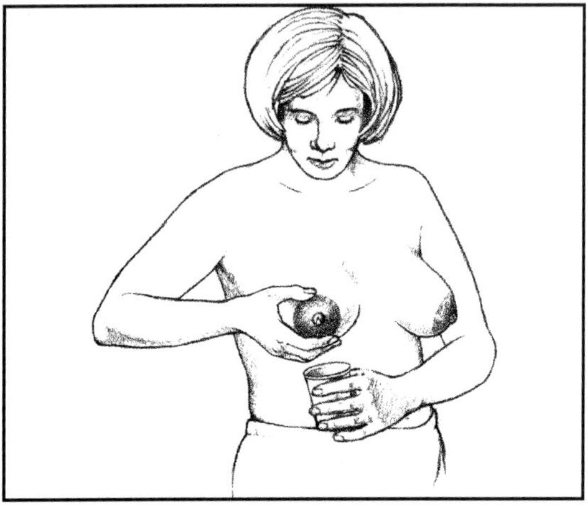

Figure 19.9 Manual expression
Illustration by Marcia Smith.

- No difference exists in milk contamination between manual expression and milk removed with a breast pump
- The following is the technique for manual expression (see Figure 19.9 for an example)
  - Begin by leaning slightly forward with the nipple aimed at the collection container
  - Grasp the breast with the C-hold
  - Place the thumb behind the areola above the nipple
  - Place the first finger behind the areola below the nipple
  - Press the thumb and first finger inward a short way toward the chest wall
  - Firmly press on the lactiferous sinuses beneath the areola between the finger and thumb to squeeze the milk out
  - Rotate the thumb and forefinger around the areola to compress all lactiferous sinuses
  - Do not squeeze the nipple itself and do not move the fingers along the skin

Criteria for Selecting a Breast Pump

- Factors to look for when selecting a breast pump include:
  - Is manufactured by a company whose primary mission is to support breastfeeding
  - Is appropriate for the baby's age and condition
  - Is appropriate for how long a mother will need to use a pump
  - Cycles quickly and has a rhythm similar to an infant's suck
  - The flange shape is comfortable and the appropriate size for a mother's breast in order to provide the stimulation necessary for her milk to let down
  - Uses standard size bottles for collecting milk
  - The parts are dishwasher safe and easy to assemble, with few parts
  - Is quiet and easy to use with the type of hand or arm motion required
  - If electric, the power source is adequate—has the necessary outlet type (two or three prongs) and amount of voltage
  - Is easy to transport
  - Is affordable for the length of time required
  - Written instructions are provided and service is readily available
  - Provides someone knowledgeable in breastfeeding to answer questions and resolve problems about its use
  - Has a toll free number to call with questions
  - If pumping at work, options may be limited by the type of pump (if any) available, the amount of time available for pumping, and the facilities for pumping
- The following types of breast pumps should be avoided:
  - Those manufactured by companies that sell ABM
  - Those without autocycling suction which may damage breast tissue

Hand-Held Breast Pumps

- There are three types of hand-held pumps:
  - Manual (see Figure 19.10)
  - Battery (see Figure 19.11)
  - Combination of battery and electric
- Pumps that use natural movements will be the most comfortable for mothers to use

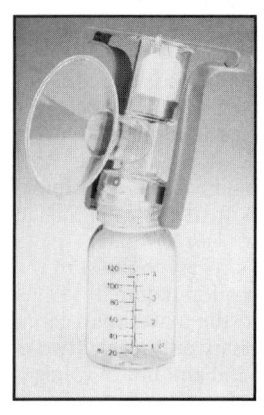

Figure 19.10 Hand-held breast pump
Courtesy of Hollister/Ameda-Egnell, Cary, IL.

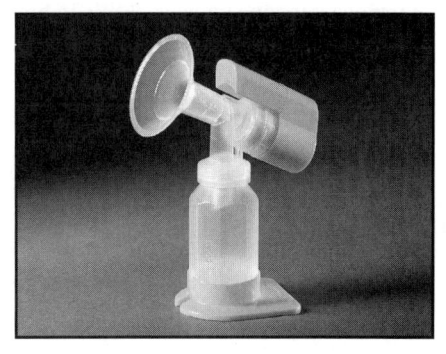

Figure 19.11 Battery-operated breast pump
Courtesy of Medela, Inc., McHenry, IL.

Electric Breast Pumps

- Provide the most efficient pumping (see Figure 19.12)
- Work well for the regular absence of nursing
- Offer the option of pumping both breasts at the same time (see Figure 19.13)
  - Save time
  - Increase breast stimulation
  - Obtain higher milk yields

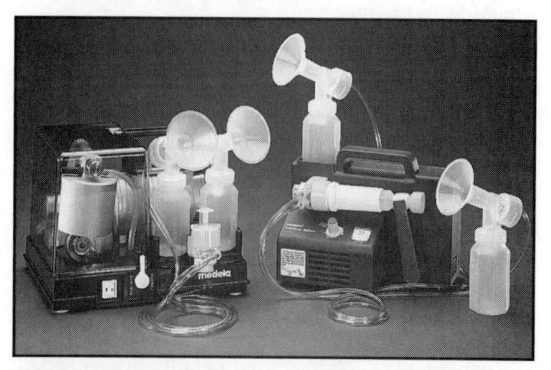

Figure 19.12 Electric breast pump
Courtesy of Medela, Inc., McHenry, IL.

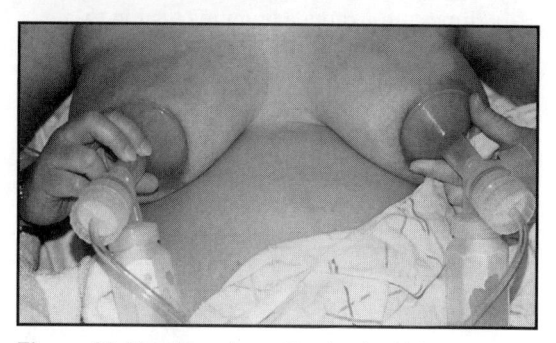

Figure 19.13 A mother using the double pumping feature of an electric breast pump
Printed by permission of Kay Hoover.

Conditioning a Letdown for Pumping
- Arrange to use the pump where there is privacy
- Sit in a comfortable chair
- Have a picture of the baby
- Make a tape recording of the baby's sounds to listen to while pumping
- See Chapter 6 for other techniques to establish a letdown

Pumping Technique
- Wash hands
- Get comfortable
- Massage the breast
- Express a few drops of milk by hand
- Moisten the pump flange for a better seal
- Secure the flange on the breast
- Center the nipple so that breast tissue touches the sides of the flange
- Begin pumping with the suction on the lowest setting
- Provide only the amount of suction needed to maintain milk flow throughout a session
- Increase the suction strength gradually as needed
- When single pumping
  - Alternate between both breasts several times throughout a pumping session to capitalize on the multiple letdowns that occur simultaneously
  - Pump for five to seven minutes on the first breast and repeat that time on the second breast
  - Return to the first breast for three to five minutes and repeat that time on the second breast
  - Finish on the first breast for two to three minutes and repeat that time on the second breast
- When double pumping, 12 to 15 minutes total pumping time may be sufficient

Pumping for a Hospitalized Baby
- Pump at least eight times every 24 hours, regardless of the amount of milk obtained

- Pump during the night when prolactin levels are the highest to produce larger quantities of milk
- A mother needs to maintain her own health and energy by getting a four- to five-hour stretch of sleep
- As the time nears for the baby to come home, begin to pump more regularly at night
- Pump during the night whenever the mother wakes naturally
- Drink extra fluids just before bedtime to facilitate waking naturally for night pumping

Care and Use of Expressed Milk
- There are several types of storage containers
  - Glass
    - Best choice for storage
    - Does not absorb the milk's antibodies or its other proteins
    - Cleans more easily
    - Protects against contamination of the milk during storage
  - Hard plastic (polypropylene)
    - Next best choice for storage
    - Interior surface can scratch and make cleaning difficult
  - Soft plastic (polyethylene) baby bottle liners
    - Frequently used, but not recommended
    - Dramatically reduce certain antibodies in milk
    - Difficult to seal
    - May puncture easily
    - May alter the smell and taste of the milk
  - Breast shells
    - Milk collected in the opposite breast during a feed must be refrigerated immediately after the feed.
    - Milk that drips into the shell between feeds should not be saved, as it has been against the mother's skin for a lengthy time

- Preparation for storage
  - Clean all collection containers and pump parts that have made contact with the milk after every use so they are ready for the next session—wash them with soapy water and rinse thoroughly
  - Store the milk in small amounts—usually two to four ounces—in order to avoid any milk being wasted at feeds
  - If freezing the milk, leave space for the expansion of milk in the container
  - Label the container with the date and time the milk was expressed and the amount of milk, and if the milk is going to be given to a caregiver with multiple children, include the names of the mother and baby
- Storage time
  - Room temperature
    - Research varies on safe storage times
    - Some sources state that milk is safe up to eight hours without a significant increase in the bacteria count
    - Some sources consider four hours to be the maximum time
    - Variables are inherent in the collection of the milk, the milk's contamination, and the definition of "room temperature"
  - Refrigerator
    - Milk is safe for three days
    - Avoid temperature extremes—do not store on the door or near the freezer's defrosting unit
  - Freezer
    - The optimal temperature is 0 degrees F or minus 18 to 20 degrees C
    - Do not store milk on the door
    - Milk is safe for three months in a freezer that has a separate door and is part of a refrigerator unit
    - Depending on its temperature, milk can be safe for six months to one year in a deep freezer

- Special guidelines for an infant in the NICU
  - Place the milk in a separate storage container for each pumping session
  - Whenever possible, express the milk just before the baby is to be fed
  - If the milk is not to be used within one hour, refrigerate it immediately
  - If the milk is not to be used within 48 hours, freezing is recommended
- Combining containers of milk
  - You can combine milk when a mother pumps both of her breasts at the same time
  - When combining milk from different pumping sessions, label it with the date and time of the earliest pumping
  - Newly pumped milk may be added to previously pumped milk after it has been cooled, or to frozen milk after it has been chilled for at least two hours
  - Do not add a larger quantity of newly expressed milk to a container of milk than has already been frozen, to prevent the freshly pumped milk from partially defrosting the frozen milk
- Defrosting and warming human milk
  - If a large stock of milk is in the freezer, use the oldest milk first
  - Arrange the milk in the freezer with the oldest containers the most visible
  - If the milk is frozen, it can be thawed in the refrigerator overnight, and it may remain refrigerated up to 24 hours
  - Rapid thawing of frozen milk
    - In a pan of warm water
    - Under a stream of warm tap water
  - No microwaving
    - Microwaving results in hot spots that may pose a danger to the baby's mouth
    - Microwaving causes a marked decrease in the activity of anti-infective properties in milk

ALTERNATE FEEDING METHODS

Human Milk Banks
- Donors of human milk are screened for infectious diseases
- The donor milk is processed and pasteurized
- Donor milk is dispensed by a prescription for medical need
- Donor milk can be shipped anywhere in the United States overnight
- The decline in the number of milk banks in the United States is due to the use of preterm formulas and the prevalence of HIV
- Each milk bank has its own criteria for the collection and storage of milk

Alternate Feeding Methods

Cup Feeding
- Use a small cup or spoon with rounded edges—"sippy" cups should be avoided because the spout does not allow the baby to trough his tongue correctly
- Cup feeding is a baby-led alternative in which a baby can pace his own intake, his respiration is easier, and his swallowing occurs when he is ready
- Babies as young as 30 weeks in gestation can maintain heart rate, respiration, and oxygenation while cup feeding
- Cup feeding does not invade a baby's oral cavity
- Cup feeding promotes appropriate tongue movement that is used during breastfeeding as the baby learns to extend his tongue to and over the alveolar ridge
- Babies lap milk by protruding their tongues into the milk
- Milk is often held in a baby's mouth for some time before swallowing occurs
- Babies as early as 30 to 34 weeks' gestation may obtain small boluses of milk
- As a baby matures, the sipping action begins to develop

- Procedure for cup feeding (see Figures 19.14 and 19.15)
  - Fill the cup about half way with approximately one-half to one-third of an ounce of expressed mother's milk
  - Tuck a cloth under the baby's chin to catch any spills
  - Have the mother hold the baby in her arms or in a semi-sitting position on her lap
  - Bring the cup to the baby's lips and rest the cup's rim on his lower lip with it touching the corners of his mouth

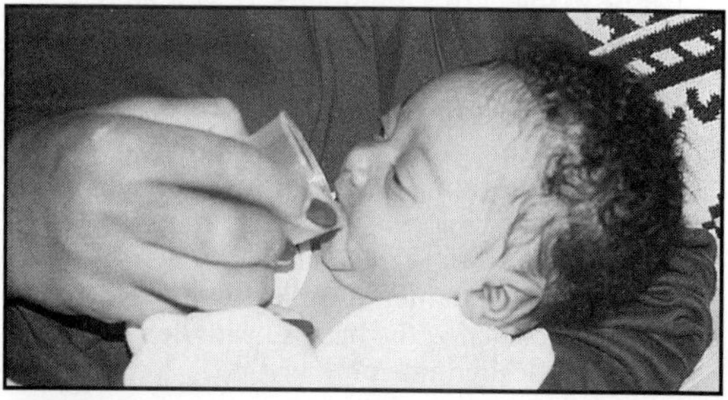

Figure 19.14 A mother cup feeding her baby
Printed by permission of Kay Hoover.

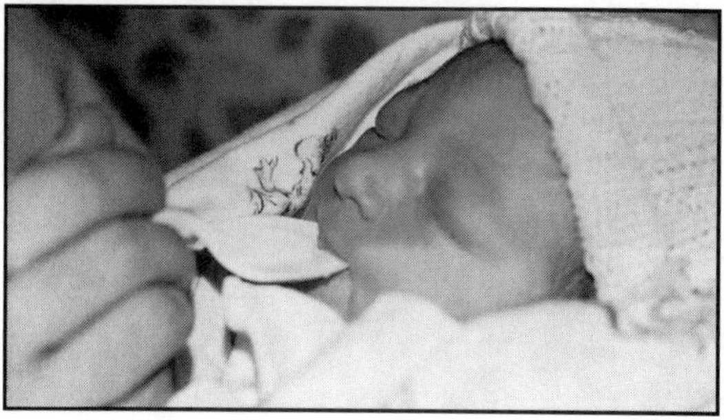

Figure 19.15 A mother spoon feeding her baby
Printed by permission of Kay Hoover.

- Tip the cup so that the milk just barely touches his lips
- Do not pour the milk into the baby's mouth, as this increases the risk of aspiration

Tube-Feeding Device

- Provides supplemental nutrition while a baby suckles at the breast (see Figure 19.16)
- Can be adjusted to deliver more of a supplement when milk production is low and deliver less of a supplement as milk production increases
- An inexpensive, noncommercial supplementer can be made with a Number 5, 6, or 8 French oral gastric tube placed in the end of a syringe or in a bottle (see Figure 19.17 for an example)
- Procedure for tube feeding
  - Caution: Some supplements—powdered formulas and human milk fortifiers—have a potential for clogging, and the infant receives insufficient supplementation
  - Place the container of milk either level with, above, or below the baby's head, depending on the desired rate of flow

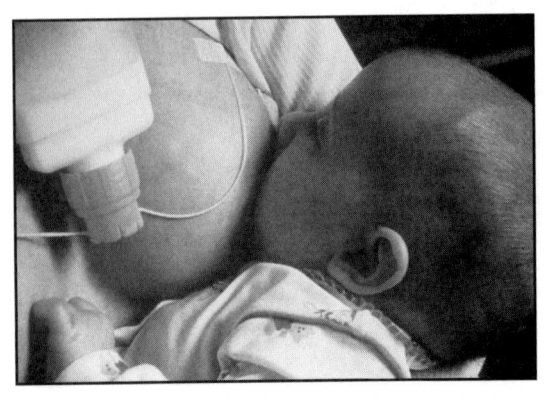

Figure 19.16 A Medela Supplemental Nursing System

Courtesy of Medela, Inc., McHenry, IL.

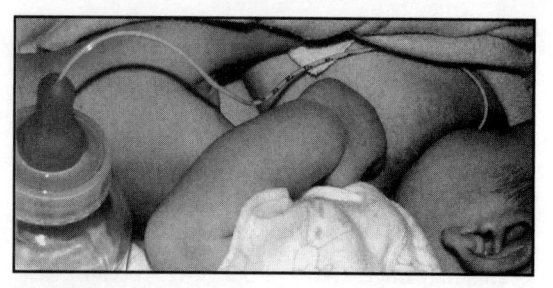

Figure 19.17 A supplementer device made of a baby bottle and tubing

Printed by permission of Kay Hoover.

- Adjust the container's level so that the baby has about one suck per swallow
- Tilt the feeding container so that it is easy to view bubbles rising to the top—this indicates that the baby is sucking and receiving milk effectively
- The tube should extend about one-fourth of an inch beyond the end of the nipple
- The tube can be taped to the mother's breast to keep it in place
- Check the baby's mouth daily to ensure the tube is not irritating the roof of the baby's mouth
- Reduce the supplement at each feed when it is evident that the baby is receiving larger amounts of his mother's milk, as is shown by the following:
  - There is more milk in her breasts
  - Increased amounts of milk are left in the supplementer accompanied by the baby's good weight gain
- Note any changes in the suckling rhythm and supplement flow during feeds, and switch breasts for an optimum stimulation of milk production
- Flush the tubing out with cold water, then wash with hot soapy water, and rinse with clear water after every use

Finger Feeding

- Finger feeding combines a tube-feeding device and finger in a baby's mouth (see Figure 19.18 for an example)
- If finger feeding is used too long, it can become as addictive as an artificial nipple
- Its occasional use may help a baby organize his suck
- A caregiver needs to use a glove, but a baby's parents may finger feed without gloves (because of potential for allergy, latex is not recommended)
- Procedure for finger feeding
  - Prime the tubing with the mother's expressed milk (or ABM if she is unable to express her milk)
  - Crimp the tube to stop the flow until the tube is in position
  - Hold the baby in an upright or semi-upright position at a 45-degree angle to avoid getting milk into his ears
  - Place the container of milk even with, above, or below the baby's head, depending on the desired rate of flow; the container can be raised or lowered to achieve the appropriate flow
  - Position the container so that it will be easy to view the bubbles rising to the top
  - Lay the tubing along the fat pad of your finger and extend it about 1/4 of an inch beyond your finger tip
  - Check the baby's mouth several times daily to ensure that the tubing is not irritating the roof of his mouth
  - Gently tickle the baby's lips so that he will open his mouth for your finger
  - Never push your finger into his mouth—wait until you are invited in by the baby
  - Place the fat pad of your finger with the tube on it into the baby's mouth against his soft palate; your finger nail should be against the baby's tongue

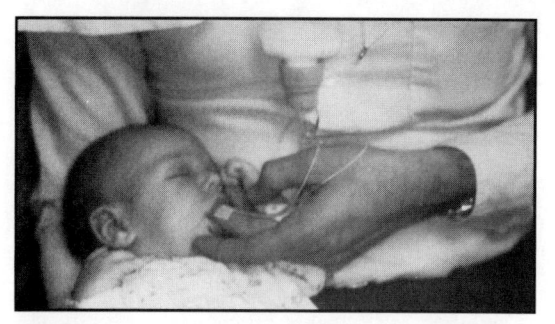

Figure 19.18 A mother finger feeding her baby
Printed by permission of Pat Bull.

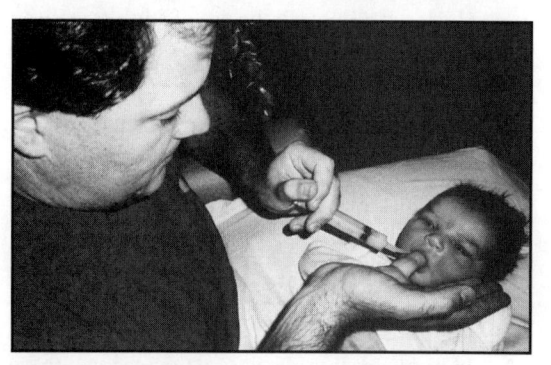

Figure 19.19 A father syringe feeding his baby
Printed by permission of Kay Hoover.

- The goal is for the baby to have one suck per swallow as with breastfeeding
- Note that more than four sucks per swallow may be tiring to a baby

Syringe Feeding

- A periodontal syringe is used by some IBCLCs with finger feeding and at the breast (use of a periodontal syringe is shown in Figure 19.19)

- Fluid is pushed into the baby's mouth in response to sucking
- Syringe feeding places the caregiver in control of the feed
- Extreme caution is advised due to the following potentially harmful consequences:
  - Potential of giving a greater bolus of milk than the baby can handle
  - Is possible to scratch or gouge the baby's tongue, gums, or palate with the syringe

Bottle Feeding

- A mother may select a bottle for feeding for the following reasons:
  - She lacks support in the use of any alternative feeding device
  - She is only comfortable using a bottle
- Bottle feeding compared to breastfeeding:
  - In breastfeeding, the entire oral cavity is filled with breast tissue, versus in bottle feeding where the artificial nipple is not able to fill the baby's oral cavity
  - No artificial nipple conforms to the shape of a baby's mouth the way a human breast does
  - When a baby suckles in breastfeeding, the breast responds with varying milk flows; when he stops suckling, the flow also stops
  - In bottle feeding, a baby's action changes to one of protecting his airway because the bottle provides a continuous drip of fluid—the baby must clamp the teat in order to get a break from the flow
- Choice of artificial nipple
  - Avoid any nipples with a small base—when a baby sucks on this type of nipple he tends to purse his lips (see Figure 19.20 for examples of nipples to avoid)
  - If there is smacking or clicking during a feed, the base of the nipple probably is not large enough

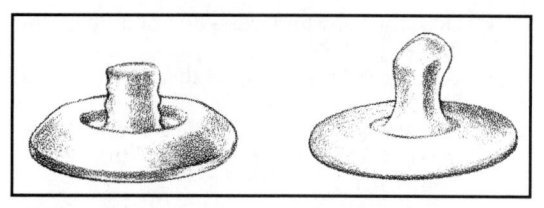

Figure 19.20 A poor choice of a bottle nipple
Illustration by Marcia Smith.

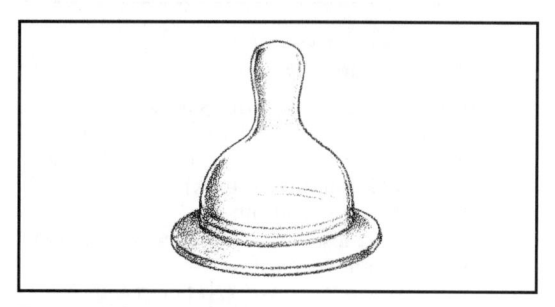

Figure 19.21 An example of a nipple with a larger base
Illustration by Marcia Smith.

- A wide base on a nipple forces a baby to open his mouth wide, as he does with breastfeeding (see Figure 19.21 for an example of a nipple with a wide base)
- Latex nipple
  - These nipples do not last very long
  - They may become gummy after use
  - Boiling latex nipples can release nitrates in them, which may have a cancer-causing effect on the baby
  - An increasing number of people are developing allergies to latex
- Teaching bottle feeding to parents
  - Hold the baby at feeds like in breastfeeding, with the right arm for the first feed and the left arm for the next feed
  - Provide frequent skin-to-skin contact

- Hold the baby for feeds—do not prop up the bottle
- Give the baby a pacifier at the end of the feed for non-nutritive sucking
- Take the baby to bed after he is finished eating so he can spend some special time with his mother

Artificial Baby Milk

Acceptable Medical Reasons for Foods Other Than Human Milk

- Foods other than the mother's milk may be appropriate in certain maternal circumstances (however, in these circumstances the baby may still receive donor human milk):
  - Has Sheehan's syndrome
  - Is receiving long-term drug therapy that uses unacceptable medications
  - Has severe congestive heart failure which is compromising her health
  - Was infected with HIV prior to her baby's birth and has access to a sanitary water supply that would allow for safe preparation of ABM
  - Was infected with HIV after her baby's birth, thus her baby was not exposed to HIV in utero
  - Has tuberculosis prior to receiving appropriate treatment for at least one week
  - Has an active herpes lesion on her breast—the possibility exists that her baby will come into contact with the lesion
  - Is severely ill with a condition such as psychosis, eclampsia, or shock
- Some infant's circumstances indicate a need for food other than human milk:
  - Has galactosemia
  - Has other inborn metabolic errors, such as phenylketonuria (PKU) or maple syrup urine

disease (though these conditions allow for intake of the mother's milk when it is carefully monitored)
- Has a condition—such as hypoglycemia or dehydration—that does not improve by increasing a baby's breastfeeding or intake of human milk
- Had a very low birth weight or was born preterm (less than 32 weeks' gestation) weighing less than 1000 g—may require supplementation for period of time

Choice of Infant Formula
- Powdered formula is the least expensive, but is at risk of being mixed incorrectly
- Concentrated formula is not as expensive as ready-to-feed formulas and is also at risk of being mixed incorrectly
- Ready-to-feed formula is the most expensive and must be discarded if the entire amount is not used within a specified time period
- Instructions vary among companies
- Scoop size varies among manufacturers

Safe Preparation of Artificial Baby Milk
- Read the instructions carefully
- Use the scoop that came with that particular brand of formula
- Check the water supply to make sure it is safe for consumption:
  - Families with well water should have it tested
  - If the safety of the water supply is questionable, purchase bottled water
  - To prevent lead poisoning, obtain water from the cold water tap only and run the cold water for at least one minute—or longer if it has not been used for several hours—before collecting it
  - When traveling, always consider the safety of the water en route

- If you are unsure about the water's bacteria level, use bottled water or boil the tap water for five minutes—boiling the water any longer can cause the lead to concentrate
- Use a clean bottle and sterile utensils for every feed
- Wash the can opener and the top of the can with hot soapy water before opening
- Check the expiration date on each can of formula to ensure that its date has not expired
- Record the lot numbers of the formula cans in the event of a manufacturer's recall

20

Temporary Breastfeeding Situations

Hyperbilirubinemia

Physiologic Jaundice
- One of most commonly treated medical conditions in a healthy newborn
- Up to 50 percent of all full-term infants are jaundiced in the first week of life with no intervention needed and no ill effects
- A healthy newborn's bilirubin level is 1.5 mg/dl or less
- Over the next three to four days, it rises to a peak level of approximately 6.5 mg/dl
- The bilirubin level then returns to a normal level of less than 1.5 mg/dl by around the tenth day of life
- If bilirubin is produced faster than the liver can process it or if the red blood cells break down more quickly than the body can handle them, it results in temporary buildup of bilirubin and a decreased rate of bilirubin conjugation
- Unconjugated bilirubin is then left to circulate freely in the bloodstream
- If bilirubin is bound (attached to albumin), it is not harmful to the baby as long as it remains within the bloodstream

- If bilirubin is unbound, it can migrate to other parts of the body—including the brain, skin, muscle tissue, and mucous membranes
- Bruising or blood incompatibilities can cause a rapid rise in bilirubin levels
- In conditions such as hepatitis, galactosemia, biliary atresia, or sepsis, there is an abnormality of excretion or reabsorption of bilirubin

Pathologic Jaundice
- In pathologic jaundice, bilirubin is elevated due to a disease process
- It can result from conditions such as infections in the blood or liver, diseases of the liver, obstructions in the gastrointestinal system, and interference with binding of bilirubin in the bloodstream
- Must treat the disease as well as the jaundice

Breastfeeding-Associated Jaundice
- Generally results from one of the following iatrogenic causes:
  - Rigid hospital schedules
  - Routine mother-infant separations
  - Unnecessary supplementation of breastfeeding
  - Pacifier use
  - Lack of education among staff
  - Labor medications resulting in sleepy babies who nurse poorly
- Obstetrical care based on the *Ten Steps to Successful Breastfeeding* (See Chapter 1) will eliminate the interference that leads to jaundice
  - Increase the number and quality of feeds
  - Check the baby's attachment and positioning
  - Room in with the baby
  - Provide frequent skin-to-skin contact between mother and baby
  - Observe feeds for swallowing

- If the baby's suck is weak and ineffective, the mother may perform breast compression (alternate massage) during feeds
- If breast compression does not increase the baby's swallowing, a tube-feeding device may be used at the breast
- Before resorting to phototherapy, increase the feeds to promote more stooling and thus lower bilirubin levels

Late-Onset Jaundice—Breastmilk Jaundice

- Believed to be caused by a factor present in the mother's milk
- Occurs in less than one percent of infants
- Develops extremely slowly
- May become apparent between the fourth and seventh days of life when mature milk has begun to replace colostrum
- Bilirubin reaches its maximum concentration by the second or third week
- May persist through the sixth week of life
- The baby will be lively and will not appear to be sick even when his bilirubin levels peak at 15 to 20 mg/dl
- Is a self-limiting and benign condition
- Breastfeeding does not need to be discontinued in most cases
- There are no reports of kernicterus caused by late onset jaundice

Concerns about High Bilirubin

- High levels of bilirubin can cause kernicterus
- Generally, a healthy full-term infant will not develop kernicterus when his bilirubin level is below 20 mg/dl
- Jaundice becomes clinically significant when
  - It develops within the first 24 hours of life
  - Bilirubin levels become exaggerated
  - It is prolonged beyond two weeks in term infants and beyond three weeks in preterm infants

Detection of Jaundice

- Jaundice is visible when the bilirubin level reaches 5 to 7 mg/dl
- Level of the baby's shoulders: 5 to 7 mg/dl
- Level of the umbilicus: 7 to 10 mg/dl
- Below the umbilicus: 10 to 12 mg/dl
- Below the knees: Greater than 15 mg/dl
- When jaundice is suspected or detected, a blood test must be performed to check the bilirubin level
- If the infant is ill or premature, the safe level of bilirubin is lower, and the jaundice must be treated quickly and monitored closely

Treatment of Jaundice

- Active treatment is rarely required as long as bilirubin levels remain within a safe range
- For less severe jaundice, regular visual observations and periodic testing of bilirubin may be sufficient
- Increase feeds to stimulate the gastrocolic reflex and to increase gut motility, which reduces the intestinal reabsorption of bilirubin through increased stooling
- Water supplementation does not reduce serum bilirubin levels
- Place the baby in a crib near a sunny window—bilirubin breaks down when exposed to sunlight or its equivalent
- Discontinue any maternal or infant medications that contribute to the buildup of bilirubin
- When bilirubin approaches a level that requires more active treatment, place the baby under a special fluorescent light—phototherapy ("bili light") or in a fiberoptic blanket
- Bilirubin levels that require active treatment are as follows:
  - Bilirubin level at 15mg/dl or above at 25 to 48 hours of life

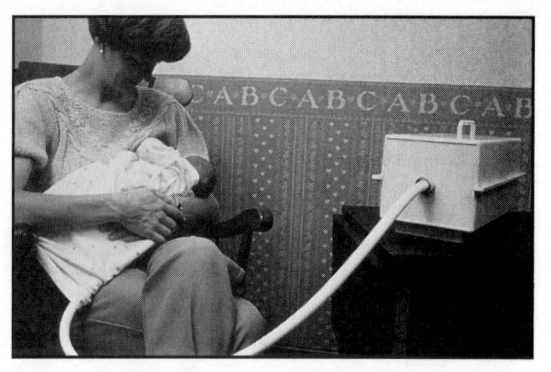

Figure 20.1 Home phototherapy using a bili blanket
Courtesy of Medela, Inc., McHenry, IL.

- Bilirubin level of 18 mg/dl or above at 49 to 72 hours of life
- Bilirubin level of 20 or above at 72 or more hours of life

Phototherapy
- Traditional phototherapy
  - Baby is placed in an isolette to keep him warm
  - The baby's eyes are covered for protection from light
  - The baby is continuously left under the bili light except during brief feeding periods
  - More frequent short feeds and additional fluids are usually recommended
  - Increases the mother-infant separation
- Home phototherapy
  - Uses a fiberoptic blanket
  - Is appropriate for full-term newborns
  - Enables more mother-infant interaction
  - The baby is clothed for better temperature regulation
  - Eye patches are not needed
  - Breastfeeding rates are higher

- Costs less than traditional phototherapy
- Increases parental satisfaction
- Side effects of phototherapy
  - Increased insensible water loss that could lead to dehydration
  - Loose stools
  - Vitamin B_2 deficiency
  - Temperature instability
  - Skin breakdown or rashes
  - Potential eye damage due to lights
  - Apnea
  - Sluggish responses
  - Noticeably weak sucking reflex

Jaundice in a Premature Infant

- A premature infant's brain is especially sensitive to bilirubin
- Digestive system takes longer to detoxify and to eliminate bilirubin
- Bilirubin levels permissible in premature infants are inversely related to the degree of prematurity
- Discontinuing breastfeeding does not help treat this jaundice type and unnecessarily disrupts the establishment of milk production in the early days

Issues for Parents to Explore

- Cause of the jaundice
- Tests that have been done or need to be done
- Test results and what the results mean
- How long it is estimated the jaundice will last
- Criteria for home phototherapy
- If the baby is under a bili light or under observation, when he can be breastfed
- If phototherapy is performed in a hospital, when the parents can have social contact with their baby
- If breastfeeding has been interrupted, how long it will be, and what the bilirubin level must be before breastfeeding can be resumed.
- See Table 20.1 for help with breastfeeding

Delayed Onset of Breastfeeding

Expressing Milk to Maintain Lactation

- Express milk for a total of eight times every 24 hours
- Expressing milk during the night for an extended period of time is not necessary
- Express at night for a short time or closer to the baby's return to the breast
- Use a high-quality, hospital-grade, electric double pump for the best yield
- Milk production will decrease with time, but usually increases again after the baby begins nursing
- Hospitals may provide sterile bottles and instructions for handling milk for a hospitalized baby
- Put small amounts of milk in each bottle—only slightly more than the infant is currently taking
- If the baby has not begun receiving the mother's milk, store no more than one ounce per container until the mother learns how much he takes at a feed
- Do not use soft plastic bottle liner bags to store the milk
- See Chapter 19, Breastfeeding Techniques and Devices, for more information

Transition from Milk Expression to Breastfeeding

- Request a private, quiet place in which to nurse the baby, with a comfortable chair and ample pillows for support
- When a mother learns that her baby can soon nurse, she can begin expressing milk more frequently throughout the day and night
- If the mother is nursing frequently and her baby is not satisfied, she may need to supplement with her expressed milk or ABM until her milk production increases
- Can take several days or even months to reach a goal of exclusive breastfeeding

TABLE 20.1 COUNSELING SUMMARY—JAUNDICED BABY

MOTHER'S CONCERN	SUGGESTIONS FOR MOTHER
Parents are bewildered by procedures and other aspects of baby care.	• Discuss questions with the baby's physician and other care providers. • Read the available literature.
Separation of mother and baby.	• Arrange for bedside treatment of the baby, either using sunlight, a portable bili blanket, or lights. • Arrange for regular intervals of interaction for eye and skin contact.
Treatment is interfering with breastfeeding.	• Arrange for fiberoptic blanket phototherapy. • Arrange for regular contact with the baby and for frequent feeds. • Use relaxation techniques to ensure letdown. • Arrange for uninterrupted feeds.

Baby is sluggish in his responses, with a weak sucking reflex.	• Begin more frequent feeds. • Use breast compression while nursing to encourage suckling. • Use a tube feeding device. • Use cup feeds if the baby's latch is poor.
Physician is considering interruption in breastfeeding.	• Ask for a delay in treatment while the baby is being breastfed frequently to increase his intake of fluids. • Ask for frequent checks of the bilirubin level.
Breastfeeding must be interrupted.	• Begin expressing milk as soon as possible to keep building and maintaining milk production.
Prevention of jaundice.	• Avoid exposure to chemicals during pregnancy. • Avoid jaundice-producing drugs during labor and delivery. • Nurse within one hour after birth and frequently thereafter. • Expose the baby's skin to sufficient sunlight daily.

TABLE 20.2 COUNSELING SUMMARY—DELAYED ONSET OF BREASTFEEDING

- Begin pumping soon after the baby's birth and continue regularly until the baby can nurse.
- Tape a picture of the baby to the breast pump.
- Play a recording of the baby's sounds.
- Express milk directly after visiting the baby.
- Hand express or pump when away from home.
- Place the milk in a clean container and keep it chilled during transport.
- Express milk more frequently to increase production.
- Continue expressing milk until the transition to breastfeeding is complete.
- Offer the baby a supplement if the mother's milk production is low.

- Guidelines for conditioning a baby to breastfeed are as follows:
    - Express milk onto a breast pad, and place it near the baby
    - Place a picture of the mother in the baby's view
    - Insert the gavage tube through a bottle nipple
    - Provide frequent skin contact
    - Conduct practice sessions at the breast
    - Shape and hold the breast for the baby using the Dancer hand position
    - Express milk into the baby's mouth
    - Use a tube-feeding device for feeds
- Refer to Table 20.2

Relactation

- Is defined as the re-establishing of milk production
- A mother who has a greatly reduced milk supply or who has stopped breastfeeding may want to relactate

Issues to Explore with the Mother

- Why the mother initially did not begin or continue with breastfeeding
- How much time has passed since her baby was at the breast
- How the baby has been fed during the time away from the breast
- Mother's breastfeeding management before her decision to wean
- Reason for wanting to relactate
- How the mother will react if her milk production does not meet her baby's full needs
- Support she has in this endeavor
- How those in her immediate household feel
- If she is meeting opposition, how she will deal with lack of support

Determinants of a Mother's Success

- Degree of postpartum breast involution
- Initiating lactation during the first three weeks postpartum, although it is possible to establish lactation beyond that time
- Woman's determination
- Realistic goals
- Amount of breast stimulation that she receives
- Baby's willingness to suckle at breast

Optimizing Her Efforts

- Examine the possible milk-reducing influences in her life such as oral contraceptives, nicotine, and herbal teas like peppermint and sage
- Feed the baby in a relaxed atmosphere without any pressure
- Attempt a feed when the baby is drowsy or in a light sleep state
- Encourage the mother to work toward a correct latch rather than settle for a painful, inappropriate latch

TABLE 20.3 COUNSELING SUMMARY ON RELACTATION AND ADOPTION

MOTHER'S CONCERN	SUGGESTIONS FOR MOTHER
Inadequate letdown.	Use relaxation techniques.
Building milk production.	Begin nursing as early as possible. Use regular supplements and decrease their amount as milk production increases. Use alternate breast massage during feeds. Use frequent feeds. Express milk between feeds. Get sufficient rest. Eat a nutritious diet. Keep a diary of breastfeeds, formula feeds, and weight gain.
Baby reluctant to nurse.	Use soothing techniques for the baby and increased skin-to-skin contact. Apply the mother's milk or a sweet substance to her nipple. Slowly drop the mother's milk inside of the baby's mouth before placing the baby on the breast. Use a nursing supplementer.

Preparation for breastfeeding.	Massage the mother's back and breasts. Stimulate the nipples manually. Stimulate milk production by using an electric breast pump. Avoid using soap and other drying agents on the breasts.
Low milk supply.	Supplement the baby with formula; do not dilute it. View breastfeeding primarily as a means of nurturing the baby's emotional health. Have the baby checked frequently for weight gain. Monitor the baby's weight while replacing formula with breastfeeding.
Nipple preference in baby.	Use a nursing supplementer, cup, spoon, or dropper.
Mother frustrated with part-time breastfeeding.	Simplify bottle preparation techniques or use a nursing supplementer. Learn to appreciate breastfeeding for the nurturing relationship with the baby.

- Perform rebirthing, also referred to as remedial co-bathing
  - Baby and mother spend gentle, calming time together in a warm bath
  - Baby is placed on the mother's abdomen in a bath of warm water
  - After a period of time the mother reclines and places the baby on her abdomen
  - Baby is allowed, without assistance, to crawl up to the breast, to root, and to latch on
  - See Table 20.3
  - See Chapter 13, Infant Attachment and Suckling" and Chapter 16, Problems with Milk Production and Transfer, for more suggestions on increasing milk production and encouraging a baby to nurse

Nursing an Adopted Baby

Factors in Success

- Provides emotional satisfaction for both mother and infant
- The mother needs realistic motives for breastfeeding
- Doubtful that an adopted baby can be nourished entirely on the mother's milk alone
- Women who lactated previously are three times as likely to have milky secretions
- Babies younger than three months are more likely to suckle when placed at the mother's breast
- If inability to give birth resulted from a hormonal imbalance, the same imbalance could affect the chances of inducing lactation
- Success depends greatly on the woman's desire to nurse and the motherly feelings she develops that stimulate letdown reflex

Process of Inducing Lactation

- Perform breast massage and back rubs five to eight times daily over a period of three to six months to increase blood circulation to and within the breast
  - Pump the breasts with a hospital-grade, electric breast pump
  - Use a double setup to stimulate milk production
- Pump several times a day for 10-minute sessions
- Ask the adoption agency to have the baby fed with an alternative method to minimize nipple preference
- Ask for breastfeeding sessions if the infant's placement does not occur soon after birth
- Milk production will increase more rapidly after the baby begins suckling at breast
- Massage and express milk before and after feeds to increase output
- Allow the baby to sleep in bed with the mother so he can suckle sleepily for comfort throughout the night
- Use a tube-feeding device to supplement with donor human milk or ABM to ensure optimal nourishment
- When replacing a supplement with the mother's own milk at the breast, the decrease should not exceed 25 ml per feed
- Monitor the baby's growth and output for four to seven days before another decrease in supplement occurs
- Refer to Table 20.3

Baby Loses Interest in Breastfeeding

Possible Causes of a Baby's Disinterest

- The baby is easily distracted because of his stage of development
- The mother unknowingly rebuffed her baby with

a reaction to being bitten
- The mother is menstruating and the taste of her milk and the scent of secretions on her skin seem less familiar to her baby

Management of Feeds

- Use relaxation techniques and massage before feeds
- Increase skin contact with the baby before feeds
- If the baby's gums are sore, rub them with ice or a finger before feeds
- Nurse in a quiet, dark room without distractions
- Attempt to nurse when the baby is almost asleep
- Increase evening and nighttime feeds
- Use breast compression while the baby is at the breast to increase milk flow
- Hold the baby in an upright position to facilitate easier breathing during feeds
- Express milk onto the nipple or the baby's lips to encourage him to feed
- If the baby prefers one breast, transfer him to the other breast by gently sliding him over rather than turning him around
- Feed the baby in the presence of other breast-feeding babies
- Put the baby to breast when he begins sucking on his thumb or another object
- Nurse before offering any dietary supplements
- Reduce the amount of supplements that are being given to the baby
- Offer liquids by cup or another method that avoids the use of artificial nipples

Other Actions Mothers Can Take

- Skin-to-skin contact between the mother and baby will help to re-establish trust
- Undress and take the baby to bed or into the bath with her
- Promote a feeling of well-being by getting plenty of rest, adding extra protein and fresh vegetables

to her diet, and drinking sufficient fluids
- Discontinue the use of pacifiers
- Hand express or pump the breasts between feeds to maintain milk production
- Check the baby for any illness or teething pain and contact the physician if necessary
- Cleanse the breasts with clear water before feeds to remove deodorant, lotions, or other substances
- Discontinue using any new brands of deodorant or lotion

Baby Who Prefers One Breast

Causes of Breast Preference
- The baby dislikes something about the breast's appearance or feel (mole, hair, or other differences, or the smell of the skin due to deodorant or perfume)
- The baby dislikes the taste of milk in one breast (rare)
- Birth involved trauma to one side of his face, chin, neck, or shoulder, which is causing pain
- A cold or ear infection causes discomfort when the baby is held on the affected side
- The mother has a malignant growth in her breast tissue

Encouraging the Baby to Feed at Both Breasts
- Begin the feed on the preferred breast first
- Express a little milk from the other breast to start the baby suckling on it
- Try feeding at times when the baby is drowsy and less aware of which breast he is suckling
- Entice the baby with expressed milk on the nipple
- Use the clutch hold, which may fool the baby into thinking he is on the preferred breast, especially if he has pain or sensitivity in his ear

21

High-Risk Infants

Prolonged Hospitalization of the High-Risk Infant

Supporting the Mother
- Mothers of high-risk infants who have support are more likely to breastfeed
- Focus on the mother rather than on the baby
- Encourage her to talk about the following:
  - Her birth
  - Her baby
  - Her ability or inability to cope
  - How she is sleeping
  - Her appetite
  - Whether she is taking her pain medication
- See Table 21.1

Infants in the Neonatal Intensive Care Unit (NICU)
- Human milk is vital to the progress of a high-risk infant, who is at risk for developing a variety of infections
- Interactions between parents and baby are important to the baby's progress
  - Babies that are held and cared for by their mothers during hospitalization have better weight gains and quicker recoveries
  - Point out the baby's behavioral capabilities

TABLE 21.1 COUNSELING SUMMARY—PROLONGED HOSPITALIZATION

Mother's Concerns	Suggestions for Mother
Mother's emotional needs unrecognized.	Discuss the birth experience and adjustment factors with a supportive person.
Early separation from baby.	Provide quality interaction through touching, eye contact, and time alone with the baby.
Exhaustion from traveling to and from the hospital and caring for the baby at home.	Arrange for household help.
	Prepare and freeze meals before homecoming.
	Stock grocery supplies before the homecoming.

- Help parents develop realistic expectations
- Eye-to-eye contact between parents and infant is important
- Encourage parents to take part in baby care such as feeding, bathing, and diapering
- Encourage mothers to have private time with their babies whenever the condition permits—arrange for a privacy screen or rooming in when baby is able
- Advocate practices that protect breastfeeding such as the following:
  - Breastfeeding as soon as possible
  - Not requiring successful bottle feeds before the baby is put to breast
  - No artificial nipples
  - Close physical contact

Taking the Baby Home
- Learn if supplements are required and how often they are to be given
- Address any special care procedures or restrictions needed
- Limit visitors
- Address the typical behavior of high-risk infants such as crying, breathing noises, and spitting up
- Discuss the crying behavior of a preterm, high-risk infant
  - Varies according to gestational age
  - Cries may be more high pitched and uneven than those of full-term babies
  - Crying may seem to occur more frequently
  - A greater number of high-risk infants develop colic-like symptoms than do full-term babies

Babies Not Born at Term

Small for Gestational Age (SGA) Infant
- Intrauterine growth was slowed before birth took place
- Is also referred to as intrauterine growth retardation (IUGR)
- Frequently have early feeding problems and may breastfeed poorly
- May require supplementation until the condition stabilizes and the baby begins to gain weight
- After the condition has stabilized, the baby seems to demand very frequent feeds

Premature Infant
- Is an infant born before 37 weeks' gestation
- The usual requirements for discharge:
  - Reach approximately 35 weeks gestational age
  - Demonstrate good sucking reflex
  - Have no respiratory problems
  - Have no signs of disease or complications
  - Good weight gain

Maintaining Lactation Until the Baby Can Nurse

- Mother's milk is important to the baby as it is the same age as her baby and will change to meet her baby's needs as his needs change
- Expressing her milk is something only she can do for her baby—the mother should begin to express milk within six hours of the baby's birth (see Chapter 19, Breastfeeding Techniques and Devices)
- The amount of milk a mother will produce for the rest of breastfeeding is determined in the first two weeks of life
  - Express as frequently as possible in the first few days after birth
  - Express at least eight times every 24 hours
  - Have one expressing session during the late evening or early morning hours
  - Use a hospital-grade, electric pump, and double pump for 12 minutes
- Have colostrum sent to the nursery and spoon fed to her baby if he is able to tolerate oral feeds
- If the baby is unable to tolerate anything oral, drip colostrum on a breast pad and place it in the isolette with the baby to familiarize him with his mother's scent
- Massage the breasts before and during pumping sessions
- Encourage the milk ejection reflex in the following ways:
  - Sensory stimulation with a picture of her baby or the smell of his clothing
  - Auditory and visual relaxation
  - Massage the mother's back while she is pumping
- Use galactogogues such as fenugreek or blessed thistle
- Use prescription medications such as metoclopramide

Preserving the Safety of the Mother's Milk

- Shower daily and wash hands before each pumping session

- After a pumping session, rinse the pump parts that came in contact with the milk in cold water, and then wash them in hot, soapy water
- Boil the pump parts daily
- Store milk from each pumping session separately and label the containers according to the hospital's specifications
- If freezing is required, wrap the containers in newspaper or towels and keep them in a cold-insulated container during transport

Feeding a Preterm Infant Expressed Milk

- Initial feeds often are fed via gavage tubing
- Freshly expressed milk is preferred for feeds when a baby is not yet able to go to breast—its composition is the most suitable for the baby
- Frozen milk loses a small portion of its protective properties, however it is still preferable to ABM in nutrition and protection
- After an infant is able to tolerate oral feeds, he should be fed with a cup, spoon, or dropper in the mother's absence

Putting a Preterm Baby to Breast

- It is possible for a baby to effectively handle feeds at the breast as young as 30 weeks gestation and at weights as small as 1100 g
- It is physiologically easier for a preterm infant to suckle on a human breast than on an artificial nipple
- A preterm baby can suckle well enough at the breast to maintain good weight gain

Kangaroo Care

- Is when a baby is placed skin to skin with his mother in close proximity to her breasts (see Figure 21.1)
- The baby is held skin to skin, upright and prone between the mother's breasts, wearing only a diaper

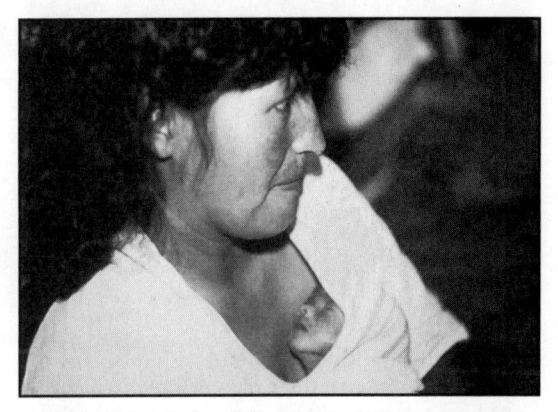

Figure 21.1 A mother and baby in kangaroo care
Printed by permssion of UNICEF.

- The baby and mother are wrapped together to maintain his temperature appropriately
- Advantages to the baby are as follows:
  - Less crying
  - More regular heart rate and respiration
  - Better sleep periods
  - Is better oxygenated
  - Is able to maintain his temperature
  - Has a tendency to gain weight faster
  - Becomes gently familiar with his new feeding environment
- Advantages to parents are as follows:
  - Increases maternal attachment and confidence
  - Increases the breastfeeding outcome
  - The baby can kangaroo during gavage feeds to build his association with sucking and eating
  - Stable infants, even when still on a ventilator, may begin kangaroo care

Feeds at the Breast
- Massage the breasts before and during feeds
- Use a breast pump to initiate milk flow

- Express milk before feeds so that the baby can nurse with a less intense milk flow, which enables the baby to "practice" with low milk flow
- Take care to not overstimulate the baby
- May need to supplement breastfeeds using the following to increase calories:
  - The creamy portion of expressed milk that rises to the top
  - Expressed hindmilk after a breastfeed

Going Home with a Premature Infant

- To ease the transition, room in with the baby in the hospital two or three days before discharge
- At home, continue the hospital routines for the first few days
- Pumping can decrease as the baby breastfeeds more frequently and more efficiently, and it may be necessary until the infant reaches the previously expected due date
- Find out when the baby will be able to discontinue using supplements and special devices
- Use electronic balance scales at home to measure intake—weight gain is a parent's greatest worry
- See Table 21.2

Postmature Infant

- Is a baby born after 42 weeks' gestation
- May be an appropriate size for gestational age in body length
- Often small for its due date because of a progressive increase in placental dysfunction
- May have difficulty maintaining its respiration and blood sugar levels
- May be sluggish during initial attempts at breastfeeding
- May need to be coaxed and prodded in the same ways as a premature infant
- Breastfeeding progresses same as for a full-term infant

Counseling a Mother Whose Baby Has Died

Breastfeeding Concerns
- Relieving fullness of the breasts without stimulating them to the extent that more milk is produced
- Express just enough for comfort
- Use the same comfort measures as for engorgement (see Chapter 14, Breastfeeding Issues in the Early Weeks)
- A continuous application of cabbage leaves to the breasts encourages milk to dry up and offers the mother relief (change cabbage leaves about every two to three hours)
- Mothers who had begun nursing or pumping
  - Will have more difficulty stopping lactation
  - May need to continue pumping and decrease slowly as in a weaning pattern

Counseling Suggestions
- Helpful suggestions for counseling grieving parents
  - DO show your genuine concern and caring
  - DO be available to listen and empathize
  - DO say you are sorry about what happened
  - DO allow the mother to express as much grief as she feels
  - DO encourage parents to be patient with themselves
  - DO allow the mother to talk about her baby
  - DO talk about the special qualities of the baby she lost
  - DO acknowledge the impact of the baby's death
  - DO reassure the parents that they did everything possible for their baby
  - DO refer to the baby by name
  - DO show your sadness and disappointment

TABLE 21.2 COUNSELING SUMMARY—PRETERM INFANT

Mother's Concerns	Suggestions for Mother
Anxiety about taking a small baby home. Anxiety about beginning breastfeeding.	• Continue close medical supervision of the baby. • Keep realistic expectations. • Allow for a transition period.
Baby tires easily at the breast.	• Wake the baby frequently during feeds. • Stimulate the baby to nurse. • Nurse frequently for short time periods as long as the baby is suckling and swallowing.
Weak rooting reflex.	• Provide skin-to-skin contact. • Turn the baby's head toward the breast. • Help the baby open his mouth. • Form the nipple and bring the baby to the breast.
Weak sucking mechanism.	• Use the Dancer hand position to increase intraoral negative pressure.
Intermittent sucking and resting during feeds.	• Plan to allow a lengthy amount of time for each feed.

Nipple preference.	• Express milk until letdown occurs. • Avoid using artificial nipples. • Cup feed when the mother is not present for feeds.
Difficult to interest the baby in her breast.	• Provide frequent skin contact and nuzzling. • Familiarize the baby with the smell of his mother's milk.
Difficult to position the baby at her breast.	• Use pillows to bring the baby to breast level. • Use the clutch hold for positioning and the Dancer hand position under the baby's chin.
Difficult to determine whether the baby is getting enough milk.	• Determine with the NICU staff the number of wet diapers and stools to expect each day. • Determine the follow-up visit schedule with a pediatrician. • Determine the minimum feeding frequency to expect and what to do if the baby does not meet that goal. • Consider renting an electronic scale for daily weighing at home; plan with a pediatrician what weight gain to expect; learn from the nursing staff how to determine accurate weights.

- Things to avoid when you are counseling grieving parents
    - DON'T let your own sense of helplessness keep you from reaching out to the mother
    - DON'T avoid the mother because you are uncomfortable with her situation
    - DON'T say you know how the mother feels
    - DON'T suggest that the mother should be feeling better by a certain time
    - DON'T tell parents what they should feel or do
    - DON'T change the subject when the baby is mentioned
    - DON'T try to find something positive about the baby's death
    - DON'T point out that they can always have other children or suggest that they should be grateful for any other children they already have
    - DON'T suggest that the baby's care by the parents or medical personnel was inadequate
    - DON'T avoid using the baby's name for fear of causing pain for the mother
    - DON'T be overly cheerful or casual

22

When Breastfeeding is Interrupted

Managing Breastfeeding through a Separation

Challenges for the Mother
- The mother may face several challenges
  - Attitudes of family members
  - Child care arrangements
  - Finding time to spend with each family member
  - The baby's willingness to accept nourishment by an alternative feeding method
  - Conflicting emotions and feelings of guilt
  - Being at risk for plugged ducts, engorgement, and mastitis
  - Taxing her energy reserves and needing adequate rest and nutrition
  - The baby may want to remain with his mother or appear to reject her

Feeding Issues
- The management of feeds will require several considerations
  - Better to delay until the baby is old enough to begin solid foods (around six months of age)
  - Consider the separation anxiety that occurs at around nine months of age

- Options for maintaining milk production (milk production will diminish to some extent) are as follows:
  - Remove milk regularly through pumping or hand expression to feed to the baby during the mother's absence
  - Express only enough milk to relieve discomfort, allow milk production to diminish slightly, and feed the baby infant formula during the mother's absence
- Experiment with feeding methods two weeks before the separation
  - Bottles may be convenient, but can cause nipple preference
  - Type of nipple used should encourage the baby to open his mouth wide
  - Use a nipple with a large base (see Chapter 19, Breastfeeding Techniques and Devices)
- Following the separation
  - If milk production declines, hand express or pump to rebuild milk production
  - Entice the baby to nurse by tube-feeding (see Chapter 19) or by dripping milk onto the breast
  - May need to supplement feeds until milk production increases
  - Arrange for help with household chores
- See Table 22.1

Short-Term Separations

When the Mother Is Ill

- The mother produces antibodies in her milk that protect the baby from infection
- In most cases, antibodies against the virus offset a baby's potential harm
- Close contact is more likely a mechanism of disease transmission
- The baby was likely exposed during the mother's most contagious period

TABLE 22.1 COUNSELING SUMMARY—SEPARATION OF MOTHER AND BABY

Mother's Concerns	Suggestions for Mother
Overfullness, leaking.	• Express milk during the absence. • Wear breast pads. • Nurse directly before and after the separation.
Low milk production.	• Express milk regularly during missed feeds. • Drink for thirst. • Nurse frequently when with the baby.
Nourishment for the baby.	• Feed the mother's milk or artificial baby milk.
Nipple preference.	• Use a cup or medicine spoon.
Baby not accepting an alternative.	• Have another person feed the baby with an alternative feeding method before the separation occurs. • Suggest more than one alternative feeding method.
Baby's behavior.	• Recognize a baby's reaction to separation from his mother.
Ability to express milk.	• Practice milk expression before the separation.
Timing the of separation.	• Delay the separation until milk production is established (around two months).
Difficulty obtaining milk.	• Establish a routine to condition a letdown. • Improve the mother's milk expression technique (that is, practice hand expression or acquire a more efficient breast pump).
Avoiding missed feeds.	• Arrange for the mother and baby to be together for feeds by having the baby brought to the mother or the mother going to the baby.

- Breastfeeding can continue while the mother receives most medications
- Decrease the baby's exposure by washing hands or, in extreme cases, by wearing a mask

Hospitalization of the Mother

- In most cases, a mother with an illness or injury can breastfeed
  - If she is not consuming medication harmful to her baby
  - May need another adult to help her care for her baby
- In some situations, weaning may be a better alternative

Hospitalization of the Baby

- A mother who wants to remain with her baby can inquire about rooming-in policies for mothers of sick babies
- Ask to visit the baby regularly and to nurse him if permitted
- In a high-risk center, ask for the baby to be transferred to a facility closer to home after his condition stabilizes
- Babies who must undergo surgery will benefit from their mother's presence immediately before and after the procedure
- Babies can nurse up to three hours before surgery
- Ask how soon the mother can see and nurse the baby following surgery, and whether she can be with him in the recovery room

During and After Hospitalization of the Mother or Baby

- Ask if the mother and baby can stay together continually and about cost and arrangements
- Arrange for them to be together at feeding times
- Ask to use a hospital breast pump while she is there

- The mother will benefit from frequent contact and support
- If breastfeeding is interrupted, milk production may need to be increased
- If the mother and baby are separated for an extended period, the mother may need to relactate (see Chapter 20, Temporary Feeding Situations)
- The mother may need help re-establishing a breastfeeding routine
- The mother may need to discuss her feelings
- See Table 22.2

Supporting the Working Mother

Considerations in Returning to Work
- The mother needs to explore options available to her:
  - How long she will be able to stay on maternity leave
  - Whether working hours can be altered, reduced, or eliminated
  - Options available such as job sharing, on-site child care, working from home, flex hours, or part-time hours
  - Alternatives available that will keep the mother and child together
  - Support she will receive from her supervisor and co-workers
  - Location and time allotment available for lactation breaks

Breastfeeding Management
- Initiate good breastfeeding practices while in the hospital
- Use support systems for information and encouragement
- Begin planning for the separation two to three weeks before returning to work
  - Begin expressing milk and using a breast pump

TABLE 22.2 PREPARATION FOR HOSPITALIZATION

Points to Consider	Suggestions for Mother
Explore your options.	• Learn if hospitalization is necessary. • Request a second opinion. • Learn if hospitalization can be delayed until the baby is older and milk production is established. • Learn whether early discharge is possible if home nursing care is arranged. Contact the local Visiting Nurses Association for home care.
Be assertive regarding your wishes.	• Discuss all concerns and wishes with your physician to avoid separation or to work toward minimizing missed feeds. • Examine hospital policies concerning rooming in and the use of a hospital breast pump.
Become well informed.	• Learn about hospital procedures and the factors surrounding hospitalization. • Review informed consent as discussed in Chapter 3. • Inquire with the local Chamber of Commerce about support groups available.

	• Contact resource groups. • Contact the United States Department of Health and Human Services for literature about the hospitalization of children, including a review of books available commercially.
Keep clear, well-organized records.	• Record expenses for income tax deductions—child care, travel, and breast pump rental—as these may be paid by insurance. • Write down all details of your care plan, and provide copies for yourself, your physician, and the hospital.
Prepare for transportation to and from the hospital.	• Arrange for your partner, a friend, or other relative to take time off from work to drive you to and from the hospital if this is acceptable to your care provider.

- Begin storing milk
- Plan an alternative feeding method
- Have a person close to the baby feed him the mother's expressed milk
- If a bottle nipple is used, warm the nipple
- The mother may need to leave the immediate area
- Do not try a new feeding method when the baby is too hungry
- Perform several trial runs with the baby's care provider
- Ease into a feeding routine that mimics the work schedule
- Plan for quiet nursing time with the baby after returning home from work

Feeding Options during Work Hours

- Breastfeed on breaks with child care onsite or nearby
- Reverse the child's nursing cycle
- Begin collecting milk before returning to work
- Feed ABM during the separation and breastfeed when home with the baby
- Wean completely to ABM
- Regularly remove milk if separated from the baby
- Have an expressing routine
  - Match lactation breaks to the baby's feeding needs
  - Respond to fullness in the breasts
  - If the baby is young, express milk every three hours
  - Must have access to a breast pump at work
  - A double breast pump will require about 10 minutes
  - A single pump or hand expression requires about 20 minutes
  - As the baby grows, the time between pumpings will decrease
- Enhancing the letdown reflex
  - Express milk in a comfortable area
  - Massage the breasts using moist heat

- Use an audiotape, picture, or clothing to remind herself of the baby
- Collecting milk
  - Store in quantities that the baby will take at one feed
  - Can be stored safely at room temperature for up to eight hours
  - Do not allow cooled milk to warm on the way home
  - See Chapter 19 for information on the collection and storage of milk

Mother's Comfort and Adjustment

- A smooth transition for returning to work will increase the mother's comfort and adjustment to the new routines
  - Start out working part time either days weekly or hours daily
  - Return to work on Thursday or Friday for a short first week back to work
  - Pack a bag for the baby and herself the night before work
  - Plan to have extra time before leaving home to snuggle and feed the baby
- Milk production may fluctuate with emotional ups and downs
- If expressing is delayed, the breasts can become quite full
- May experience leaking during the adjustment
  - Keep a change of clothes at work
  - Wear prints rather than solid colors
  - Have a jacket or sweater handy
  - Wear breast pads to absorb leaked milk
- Select a care provider who understands the needs of a breastfeeding baby
- Provide a written list of instructions regarding the following:
  - Care of the milk
  - Baby's special preferences
  - Alternative feeding method

- The hunger signs to watch for so the baby is not overly hungry
- How to hold the baby in the same position as when breastfeeding
- How to allow him to draw the milk or bottle nipple into his mouth
- Avoid feeding him too close to his mother's arrival time

23

Mothers and Babies with Long-Term Special Needs

Breastfeeding Multiples

Breastfeeding Management
- The following suggestions will help the mother manage her breastfeeds:
  - Have plenty of pillows available to help the mother position more than one baby at her breasts during a feed
  - Have the help of another person in the early days with the positioning of the babies
  - Keep a log for each baby's diapers and feeds
- Mastitis may be more common due to fatigue and the mother's abundant milk supply
- A missed feed of one or all babies can result in engorged breasts more quickly than in the case of a mother with one baby
- When the mother misses a feed, she must express milk to avoid engorgement and plugged ducts
- Feeding options
  - Nurse both babies simultaneously and reverse breasts for each baby at the next feed
  - Confine each baby to one breast only and always reserve the same one for the same baby

- Confine each baby to one breast and alternate breasts each day
- If more than two babies
  - Nurse all babies throughout the day so they all receive the mother's milk and have time at the breast
  - Rotate babies at each feed so that all of them spend equal time on each breast
- See Figure 23.1 for positioning options

Parenting Issues with Breastfeeding Multiples

- Breastfeeding encourages the mother to regard each baby's needs individually
- Breastfeeding brings a calming element to an otherwise hectic life
- The mother will need to be more accessible to her babies for feeds

Tandem Nursing

Breastfeeding during Pregnancy

- No proven danger exists for the mother or developing fetus except in a woman who has experienced or is at risk for premature labor
- Nipple tenderness is common in early pregnancy
- The mother may experience discomfort when her child touches her breasts
- A feeling of nausea can occur when the older child nurses
- When colostrum production begins, a child may discontinue nursing
- A decrease in milk yield may cause the child to lose interest in breastfeeding

Breastfeeding Siblings

- The question of adequate milk production is not an issue, as the increased suckling will continue to increase a mother's milk production

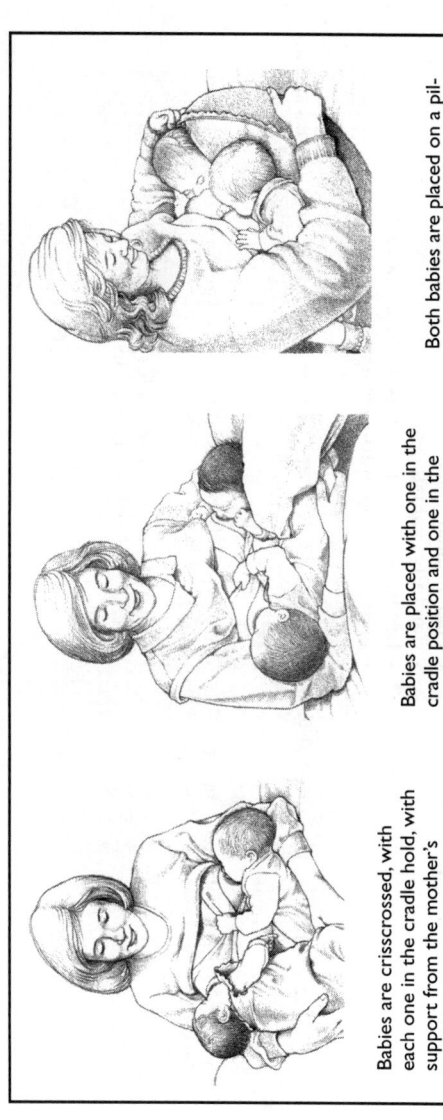

Figure 23.1 Positions for nursing twins
Illustration by Marcia Smith.

Babies are crisscrossed, with each one in the cradle hold, with support from the mother's hands under their buttocks and pillows placed under the mothers' elbows.

Babies are placed with one in the cradle position and one in the clutch position, with pillows supporting the mother's arms. A pillow on her lap may also help.

Both babies are placed on a pillow in the clutch position. A footstool can add to the mother's comfort.

TABLE 23.1   COUNSELING SUMMARY—MULTIPLE BIRTHS

MOTHER'S CONCERNS	SUGGESTIONS FOR THE MOTHER
Lack of time for all tasks.	• Plan a nursing schedule. • Carefully evaluate priorities. • Use time-saving methods for household chores. • Prepare simple nutritious meals. • Enlist help from others.
Bonding with more than one baby.	• Breastfeed separately at least one time every day and spend time alone with each baby every day during the first few weeks. • Regard the babies as individuals and meet their separate needs.
Bonding with a baby who has a delayed homecoming.	• Obtain help with the babies who are already settled in and spend more time with the new arrival.

Nursing two babies at the same time.	- Let each baby nurse exclusively on one breast, or
- Put babies on alternate breasts at each feed, or
- Let each baby nurse on one breast for the entire day and alternate breasts daily.
Spending too much time nursing babies separately.	- Whenever one baby is hungry, nurse both.
Nursing three or more babies.	- Nurse two at a time and get help from another person to feed the other baby with an alternative feeding method.
- Alternate babies so that a different one is fed with alternate means at each feed.
- Nurse the first two babies simultaneously and the other baby on both breasts afterward.
Greater susceptibility to mastitis.	- Avoid long periods away from the babies.
- Remove milk from the breasts when feeds are missed.

TABLE 23.2 COUNSELING SUMMARY—TANDEM NURSING

Mother's Concerns	Suggestions for Mothers
Nursing during pregnancy.	• Give special attention to diet to ensure it has adequate nutrients. • Discontinue breastfeeding if contractions occur frequently.
Mother resents nursing the older child.	• Wean the older child gradually. • Nurse the baby when the older child is otherwise occupied. • Substitute other activities for breastfeeding the older child.
Ensuring the baby gets enough milk.	• Let the baby nurse first, or • Reserve a particular breast for each child and alternate daily.
If the baby is overwhelmed by an abundant milk supply.	• Let the older child nurse first for a short time to reduce flow, then put the baby to breast.

- The emotional needs of the older child and the mother's comfort and physical well-being are important issues
- See Table 23.2

Special Maternal Health Conditions

Diabetes
- A diabetic mother can breastfeed safely regardless of type of diabetes

- Diet-controlled diabetic women have no breast-feeding restrictions
- Oral hypoglycemic use is switched to insulin therapy during pregnancy to ensure the safety of the fetus
  - Insulin is not excreted in human milk
  - Insulin needs will drop dramatically after the delivery of the placenta
  - The mother's blood glucose must be tested frequently in the first days postpartum to determine her requirements
  - Insulin levels will fluctuate erratically until lactation is established
  - Levels will fluctuate again when weaning is initiated
- Breastfeeding issues
  - Breastfeeding early and regularly postpartum is important for assisting Stage II lactogenesis
  - Lactogenesis is delayed in diabetic mothers versus nondiabetic mothers by two to three days
  - Remission of diabetes may be experienced during lactation because of an altered hormone balance
- Generally requires an increase in calories, carbohydrates, and protein
- Mothers with diabetes are prone to yeast infections that can affect both the vaginal area and the nipples
- If mastitis occurs, the mother must monitor her blood sugar closely and make the necessary adjustments in her treatment regimen
- During any interruption in breastfeeding, adjustments will need to be made in the mother's caloric intake and insulin dosage to compensate for the decrease in her utilization of sugar for lactation—this is especially important during weaning
- See Table 23.3

TABLE 23.3 COUNSELING SUMMARY—DIABETES

MOTHER'S CONCERNS	SUGGESTIONS FOR MOTHER
Effect of breastfeeding on diabetes.	• Monitor the condition carefully and adjust the caloric intake accordingly. • Consume enough carbohydrates to avoid acetone being released in the mother's milk.
Monilial infection of nipples.	• Keep the nipples dry between feeds to prevent occurrence. • Closely monitor nipple condition and request a topical fungicide from the physician.
Breast infection.	• Regularly remove milk from the breasts to avoid an infection which may upset the insulin balance.
Weaning.	• Make any changes in insulin and food *gradually*.

Hypothyroidism
- When properly managed, a mother who is receiving thyroid supplementation can breastfeed without a risk to her baby's health
- The thyroid that the baby receives through his mother's milk is equal to that of other breastfeeding mothers
- The following mothers need thyroid testing:
  - Mothers with low milk production and a history of thyroid problems
  - Mothers with low milk production, which has no identifiable cause

Cystic Fibrosis
- A mother with cystic fibrosis can breastfeed with the following cautions:
  - Requires monitoring the baby for bacterial exposure
  - The mother's nutritional status also requires monitoring
  - Is suggested that the mother's milk is analyzed periodically—this is especially important during an exacerbation of symptoms
- More studies are needed regarding the safety of a mother with cystic fibrosis breastfeeding her baby

Maternal Phenylketonuria

No data suggests that breastfeeding would be contraindicated

Tuberculosis
- Breastfeeding can be permitted if tuberculosis is discovered before birth and treatment is initiated immediately
  - Maternal therapy is continued
  - Infant prophylaxis is initiated
- If tuberculosis is diagnosed in the mother after the infant is born
  - All contact between the mother and infant must be suspended
  - Appropriate therapy must be initiated and continued for at least two weeks
  - During the interruption in breastfeeding, the mother should express and discard her milk to establish her milk production

Hepatitis C
- The risk of transmission to the infant through breastfeeding appears to be quite low
- Breastfeeding is acceptable

Herpes

- Breastfeeding is acceptable if no herpetic lesions are in the exposed area
- Avoid possible transmission by covering the lesions
- Epstein-Barr
  - Little is known about how it is transmitted
  - It poses no threat to a breastfeeding infant
- Varicella zoster—shingles and chickenpox
  - If the mother is infected at the time of delivery, she must be isolated from her infant until her lesions heal completely
  - Her milk can still be given to her infant
- Herpes simplex
  - Herpes simplex I (cold sore) usually appears on the mouth and nose areas
  - Herpes simplex II (genitalis) is usually transmitted through sexual contact
  - Neonates who contract this disease usually do so through direct contact with infected tissues
  - Mortality rates are extremely high for infants who are exposed during vaginal birth
  - If an active lesion appears within three weeks of delivery, a cesarean is usually performed
- Cytomegalovirus (CMV)
  - Minimal risk of transmission through the mother's milk
  - Benefits of human milk outweigh the risks of not breastfeeding
  - Passive antibodies enable term infants to breastfeed regardless of whether the mother is shedding the virus in her milk
  - CMV in human milk can be destroyed through pasteurization at 62 degrees C for eight minutes

Human Immunodeficiency Virus (HIV)

- See the AAP guidelines in Figure 23.2
- See the WHO guidelines in Figure 23.3

> The World Health Organization has developed recommendations for breastfeeding in the developing world (AAP, 1995). The following recommendations are made by the American Academy of Pediatrics for the United States, where infectious diseases and malnutrition are not major causes of infant mortality and where safe alternatives to breastfeeding are available.
>
> 1. Women and their health care providers need to be aware of the potential risk of transmission of HIV infection to infants during pregnancy and in the peripartum period, as well as through human milk.
> 2. The AAP recommends documented, routine HIV education, and routine testing with consent of all women seeking prenatal care so that each woman will know her HIV status and the methods available both to prevent the acquisition and transmission of HIV and to determine whether it is appropriate to breastfeed.
> 3. At the time of delivery, provision of education about HIV and testing with consent of all women whose HIV status during this pregnancy is unknown are recommended. Knowledge of the woman's HIV status assists in counseling on breastfeeding and helps each woman understand the benefits to herself and her infant of knowing her sero status and the behaviors that would decrease the likelihood of acquisition and transmission of HIV.
> 4. Women who are known to be HIV-infected must be counseled not to breastfeed or provide their milk for the nutrition of their own or other infants.
> 5. In general, women who are known to be HIV-seronegative should be encouraged to breastfeed.

Figure 23.2 Statement by the American Academy of Pediatrics on HIV and breastfeeding *(continues)*

> However, women who are HIV-seronegative but at particularly high risk of seroconversion (injection drug users and sexual partners of known HIV-positive persons or active drug users) should be provided education about HIV with an individualized recommendation concerning the appropriateness of breastfeeding. In addition, during the perinatal period, information should be provided on the potential risk of transmitting HIV through human milk and about methods to reduce the risk of acquiring HIV infection.
> 6. Each woman whose HIV status is unknown should be informed of the potential for HIV-infected women to transmit HIV during the peripartum period and through human milk and the potential benefits to her and her infant of knowing her HIV status and how HIV is acquired and transmitted. The health care provider needs to make an individualized recommendation to assist the woman in deciding whether to breastfeed.
> 7. Neonatal intensive care units should develop policies that are consistent with the above recommendations for the use of expressed human milk for the nutrition of neonates. Current OSHA standards do not require gloves for the routine handling of expressed human milk. However, gloves should be worn by health care workers in situations where exposure to human milk might be frequent or prolonged, for example, in milk banking.
> 8. Human milk banks should follow the guidelines developed by the United States public health service, which includes screening all donors for HIV infection and assessing risk factors that predispose to infection, as well as pasteurization of all milk specimens.

Figure 23.2 Statement by the American Academy of Pediatrics on HIV and breastfeeding

HIV statement by the World Health Organization

Risks of breastfeeding and replacement feeding

1. The benefits of breastfeeding are greatest in the first six months of life (optimal nutrition, reduced morbidity and mortality due to infections other than HIV, and delayed return of fertility).
2. Exclusive breastfeeding during the first four to six months of life carries greater benefits than mixed feeding with respect to morbidity and mortality from infectious diseases other than HIV.
3. Although breastfeeding no longer provides all nutritional requirements after six months, breastfeeding continues to offer protection against serious infections and to provide significant nutrition to the infant (half or more of nutritional requirements in the second six months of life, and up to one third in the second year).
4. Replacement feeding carries an increased risk of morbidity and mortality associated with malnutrition and associated with infectious disease other than HIV. This is especially high in the first six months of life and decreases thereafter. The risk and feasibility of replacement feedings are affected by the local environment and the individual woman's situation.
5. Breastfeeding is associated with a significant additional risk of HIV transmission from mother to child as compared to non-breastfeeding. This risk depends on clinical factors and may vary according to pattern and duration of breastfeeding. In untreated women who continue breastfeeding after the first year, the absolute risk of transmission through breastfeeding is 10–20 percent.

Figure 23.3 Statement by the World Health Organization on HIV and Breastfeeding

(continues)

(continued)
6. The risk of MTCT of HIV through breastfeeding appears to be greatest during the first months of infant life but persists as long as breastfeeding continues. Half of the breastfeeding-related infections may occur after six months with continued breastfeeding into the second year of life.
7. There is evidence from one study that exclusive breastfeeding in the first three months of life may carry a lower risk of HIV transmission than mixed feeding.

Recommendations:
- When replacement feeding is acceptable, feasible, affordable, sustainable, and safe, avoidance of all breastfeeding by HIV-infected mothers is recommended.
- Otherwise, exclusive breastfeeding is recommended during the first months of life.
- To minimize HIV transmission risk, breastfeeding should be discontinued as soon as feasible, taking into account local circumstances, the individual woman's situation, and the risks of replacement feeding (including infections other than HIV and malnutrition).
- When HIV-infected mothers choose not to breastfeed from birth or stop breastfeeding later, they should be provided with specific guidance and support for at least the first two years of the child's life to ensure adequate replacement feeding. Programs should strive to improve conditions that will make replacement feeding safer for HIV-infected mothers and families.

Cessation of breastfeeding
1. There are concerns about the possible increased risk of HIV transmission with mixed feeding during the transition period between exclusive breastfeeding and complete cessation of breastfeeding. Indirect evidence on the risk of HIV

transmission through mixed feeding suggests that keeping the period of transition as short as possible may reduce the risk.
2. Shortening this transition period, however, may have negative nutritional consequences for the infant, psychological consequences for the infant and the mother, and expose the mother to the risk of breast pathology, which may increase the risk of HIV transmission if cessation of breastfeeding is not abrupt.
3. The best duration for this transition is not known and may vary according to the age of the infant and/or the environment.

Recommendation:
HIV-infected mothers who breastfeed should be provided with specific guidance and support when they cease breastfeeding to avoid harmful nutritional and psychological consequences and to maintain breast health.

Infant feeding counseling
1. Infant feeding counseling has been shown to be more effective than simple advice for promoting exclusive breastfeeding in a general setting. Good counseling may also assist HIV-infected women to select and adhere to safer infant feeding options, such as exclusive breastfeeding or complete avoidance of breastfeeding, which may be uncommon in their environment. Effective counseling may reduce some of the breast health problems, which may increase the risk of transmission.
2. Many women find that receiving information on a range of infant feeding options is not sufficient to enable them to choose, causing them to seek specific guidance. Skilled counseling can provide this guidance to help HIV-infected women make

(continues)

(continued)

a choice appropriate for their situation to which they are more likely to adhere. The options discussed during counseling need to be selected according to local feasibility and acceptability.
3. The level of understanding of infant feeding in the context of MTCT in the general population is very limited, thus complicating efforts to counsel women effectively.
4. The number of people trained in infant feeding counseling is few relative to the need and expected demand for this information and support.

Recommendations:
- All HIV-infected mothers should receive counseling, which includes provision of general information about the risks and benefits of various infant feeding options, and specific guidance in selecting the option most likely to be suitable for their situation. Whatever a mother decides, she should be supported in her choice.
- Assessments should be conducted locally to identify the range of feeding options that are acceptable, feasible, affordable, sustainable, and safe in a particular context.
- Information and education on mother-to-child transmission of HIV should be urgently directed to the general public, affected communities, and families.
- Adequate numbers of people who can counsel HIV-infected women on infant feeding should be trained, deployed, supervised and supported. Such support should include updated training as new information and recommendations emerge.

Breast health
1. There is some evidence that breast conditions including mastitis, breast abscess, and nipple fissure may increase the risk of HIV transmission

through breastfeeding, but the extent of this association is not well quantified.

Recommendation:
HIV-infected women who breastfeed should be assisted to ensure that they use a good breastfeeding technique to prevent these conditions, which should be treated promptly if they occur.

Maternal health
1. In one trial, the risk of dying in the first two years after delivery was greater among HIV-infected women who were randomized to breastfeeding than among those who were randomized to formula feeding. This result has yet to be confirmed by other research.
2. Women who do not breastfeed or stop breastfeeding early are at greater risk of becoming pregnant.

Recommendation:
HIV-infected women should have access to information and follow-up clinical care and support, including family planning services and nutritional support. Family planning services are particularly important for HIV-infected women who are not breastfeeding.

Special Infant Health Conditions

Phenylketonuria
- Infants must immediately be put on a special diet
  - Restricts the level of phenylalanine intake
  - Provides sufficient amounts of phenylalanine to allow the infant to grow appropriately
  - Strictly monitors the intake of the amounts of phenylalanine
- The level of phenylalanine in human milk is approximately 40 mg/dl
- The level of phenylalanine in cow's milk and

ABM is unpredictable, ranging from 73 to 159 mg/dl
- An infant's diet is adjusted for phenylalanine based on weekly blood tests
  - Must maintain a level below 10 mg/dl
  - Determines the amount of phenylalanine-free formula needed
- To meet his requirements of phenylalanine, an infant may be able to consume up to 20 ounces of human milk daily, supplemented with a phenylalanine-free formula
- A physician may interrupt breastfeeding to stabilize the phenylalanine levels
- A physician may recommend that a mother continue breastfeeding without interruption, using one of the following two procedures:
  - The infant receives phenylalanine-free formula at every feed and maintains a consistent daily intake of the prescribed volume of human milk and phenylalanine-free formula
  - Substitute phenylalanine-free formula for one or two breastfeeds per day, with the mother expressing her milk at missed feeds
- Between three and twelve months of age, the baby's diet should be challenged with a phenylalanine load to reconfirm diagnosis
  - The baby is given a natural protein load that is calculated to provide a specific amount of phenylalanine for three days
  - It is usually in the form of cow's milk or an evaporated milk formula
  - If the mother does not wish to interrupt breastfeeding during that time, the phenylalanine content of her milk will need to be measured to minimize error
- Managing feeds
  - Potential difficulties exist in maintaining milk production
  - Worrying about the baby may affect the let-down reflex

- The mother may be prone to plugged ducts or mastitis due to restricted feeds
- Periodic weight checks are required to track the amount of mother's milk that the baby has consumed
- To ensure efficient utilization of amino acids, give a phenylalanine-free formula to the baby within 15 minutes of a supplemental food containing protein, such as human milk
- If the levels of phenylalanine are high during the initial prescription phase, the baby could be breastfed once or twice a day after pumping
- See Table 23.4
- Dietary changes
  - Guidelines for introducing solid foods are the same as for any other breastfeeding infant
  - High-phenylalanine foods such as eggs, meat, cheese, and milk are NOT recommended
  - Weaning a PKU infant from the breast is more structured than the weaning of other breastfeeding babies
  - Monitor the phenylalanine intake closely to maintain balance

Galactosemia

- The infant is unable to metabolize lactose
- Requires an immediate and total weaning from all milk, including human milk, and other foods that contain lactose

Cleft Lip and Cleft Palate Infant

- Immunologic properties of human milk can be particularly valuable
- Children with a cleft palate are apt to have fluid in their middle ear and are prone to ear infections
- Breastfeeding offers improved speech development and aids in visual development
- Cleft may be of the lip, palate or both (see Figure 23.4)

TABLE 23.4 COUNSELING SUMMARY—PKU BABY

Mother's Concerns	Suggestions for Mother
Maintaining proper phenylalanine intake for baby.	• Offer the recommended amounts of phenylalanine-free formula and limit breastfeeding as prescribed by the physician.
Nursing restricted.	• Maintain milk production through regular pumping or manual expression. • Have the baby nurse on the just-expressed breast. • Use an electronic scale to determine the amount of the mother's milk consumed.
Managing feeds.	• Use only one breast per feed. • Offer phenylalanine-free formula and the mother's milk at the same feed, either by using a tube-feeding device or offering first one and then the other.
Weaning.	• Carefully plan weaning and substitute nourishment according to the baby's present weight and projected weight for the date that weaning will be completed. • Closely monitor the phenylalanine intake by replacing a dropped feed with the correct amount of phenylalanine-free or low phenylalanine formula and solid foods.

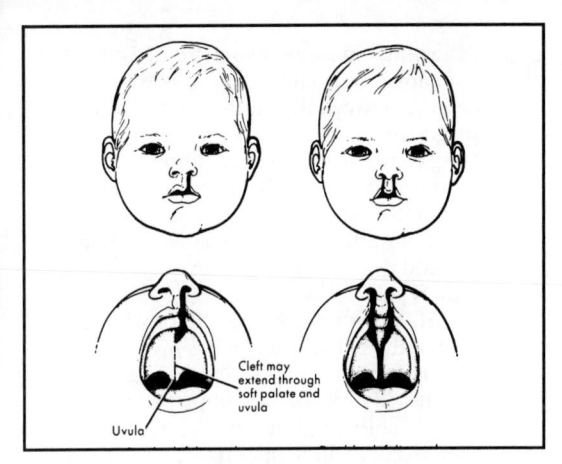

Figure 23.4 Cleft lip and palate, single cleft lip and palate (unilateral) and double cleft lip and palate (bilateral)
Source: The Mosby Medical Encyclopedia. New York; the C.V. Mosby Company 1985; p. 170. Printed with permission.

- Cleft lip
  - An isolated cleft lip presents no physiologic impediment to breastfeeding
  - The infant can nurse at the breast as well as his noncleft peers
  - The infant can mold the open cleft around the breast perhaps more easily than a small rubber nipple
- Cleft palate
  - Creates a hole between the infant's mouth and nose
  - The infant is unable to create a vacuum and hold the breast in his mouth
  - To compensate, a mother can cup her breast as she brings the baby toward her to latch on
  - The mother will need to continue holding the breast in the baby's mouth throughout the feed
  - Often a child finds the beginning of a feed easiest, when the breast is firmer

- Extracting hindmilk is sometimes difficult
- If a baby is reluctant to nurse, skin-to-skin contact between the mother and baby is suggested
- Long-term use of a breast pump for expressing hindmilk is likely to be necessary
- The mother may pump exclusively and provide her milk with an alternative feeding method
* Surgical repair
  - An infant with a cleft lip, with or without a cleft of the palate, usually has lip repair surgery at about three months of age
  - Repair will probably not improve the infant's nursing ability significantly because the breastfeeding difficulties lie with the palate, and not the lip
  - Lip repair will provide an important psychological lift to the mother
  - The infant may be fit with an obturator—a feeding plate placed over part of the cleft palate—which theoretically assists in feeding (see Figure 23.5)
* Counseling issues (see Table 23.5)

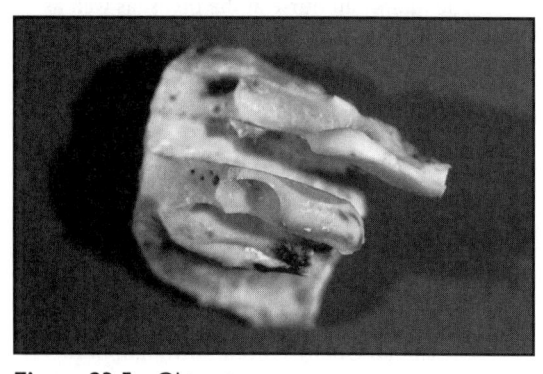

Figure 23.5 Obturator

Reprinted by permission of Sarah Coulter Danner.

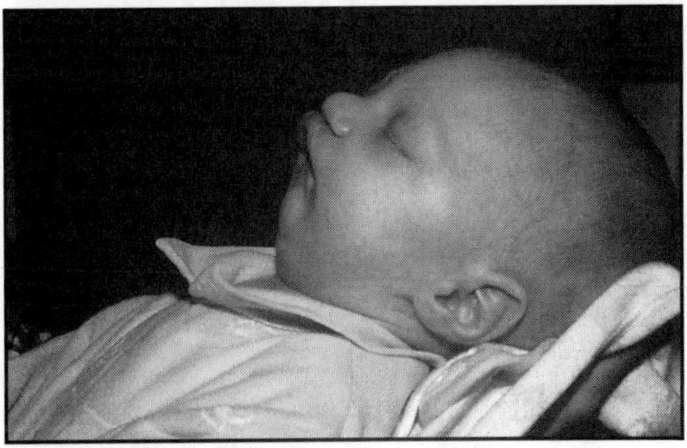

Figure 23.6 Baby with Pierre Robin syndrome
Printed by permission of Linda Kutner.

Pierre Robin Syndrome

- The infant has a receding lower jaw, displacement at the back of the tongue, a cleft palate, and an absence of the gag reflex
- The infant can have difficulty maintaining an airway, particularly during the newborn period
- Pierre Robin syndrome occurs in many different degrees—an infant with a very slight case may be able to breastfeed
- If an infant cannot breastfeed initially, the mother can express and provide milk to him
- See Figure 23.6

Infants with Down Syndrome

- The baby will gain weight and grow in length more slowly than an average infant
- The baby will benefit greatly from human milk's immunologic factors and its easy digestibility
- The baby may have a tendency toward obesity
- Hypotonia will cause the baby's head, arms, and legs to be loose and floppy

TABLE 23.5 COUNSELING SUMMARY—CLEFT LIP AND CLEFT PALATE

MOTHER'S CONCERNS	SUGGESTIONS FOR MOTHER
Nursing with a cleft palate.	• Lip will usually mold around the breast. • If necessary, cover the cleft with a finger to ensure good suction.
Ensuring adequate nourishment.	• Massage the breasts before nursing to fill the lactiferous sinuses. • Hold the breast in the baby's mouth. • With a unilateral cleft, the breast enters on the side of the defect and the baby's cheek on the side of the defect should touch the breast. • With a bilateral cleft, the breast enters at the midline and the baby's body straddles the mother. • Use a feeding plate—obturator—to partially cover the cleft.
Maintaining milk production.	• Closely monitor the baby's weight gain, wet diapers, and frequency of feeds. • Express milk after feeds and feed the milk to the baby in a tube-feeding device or medicine dropper. • Pump or hand express after feeds to adequately remove milk from the breast and to stimulate milk production. • Use breast shells between feeds to stimulate milk production. • Avoid using nipple shields.

Choking and milk leaking out nose during a feed.	• Feed the baby in an upright position. • Push the baby's chin to his chest to stop choking, then resume the feed. • Acceptance of these conditions and having patience during feeds can overcome problems.
Baby reluctant to nurse.	• Use short frequent feeds. • Nurse while the baby is still sleepy. • Use a tube-feeding device at the breast. • After feeds, express milk and feed it in a bottle with a premie nipple.
Interrupting breastfeeding for surgical repair.	• Express to remove milk from the breast and to maintain milk production. • Feed the expressed milk to the baby with an alternative feeding method that avoids nipple preference.
Disappointment due to the baby never being fully breastfed.	• Realize that breastfeeding is worthwhile as a nurturing technique, as well as a feeding method.
Pierre Robin syndrome.	• Breastfeeding is not usually possible; expressed milk is recommended.

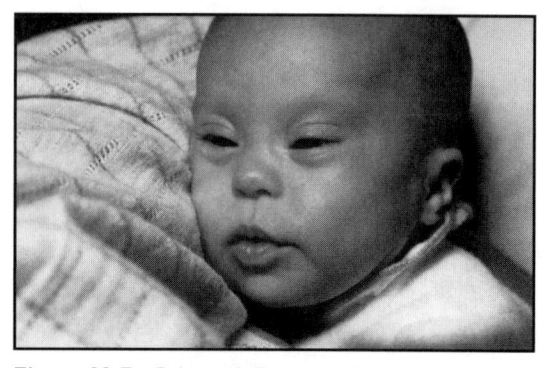

Figure 23.7 Baby with Down syndrome
Printed by permission of Sarah Coulter Danner.

- The baby may have difficulty removing milk from the breast sufficiently and should be fed the thick hindmilk
- The baby may have difficulty rooting and sucking because of weak reflexes
- The infants' flaccid, flat tongue initially may be unable to cup around the nipple to form a trough
- The baby may nurse sluggishly and become easily fatigued at the breast (see Chapter 12, Getting Breastfeeding Started, for a discussion of rousing techniques)
- Minimize the effort required by these babies as follows:
  - Support their bodies well during feeds
  - Massage the breast and express milk to initiate a letdown before putting the baby to breast
  - Watch for signs of fatigue
- See Figure 23.7

Hydrocephalus

- Breastfeeding is possible by making adjustments in positioning
- The infant's head needs to be positioned slightly higher than the breast

- The infant needs to be fed frequently to avoid gastroesophageal reflux (GER)

Spina Bifida

- The baby can be brought to the breast as soon as it is allowable
- The baby's body will need a great deal of support from pillows
- The mother will need someone to carefully lift the baby and bring him to her for feeds
- The mother's position will need to be slightly altered to avoid putting pressure on the baby's spinal column
- Feedings need to be brief until the baby has recovered from surgical repairs

Infants with Brain Damage

- Will be unable to maintain concentration and have extremely poor attention spans
- Reflexes that are instinctive at birth will soon be forgotten and will require reteaching
- Learned abilities will be forgotten and will require constant and continual reinforcement
- Mothers will constantly need to coax their babies to nurse
- May have difficulty swallowing that results in gagging and choking, which can be prevented as follows:
  - Nursing with the baby in an upright position
  - Stroking downward under the baby's chin to aid swallowing
- May lose interest in nursing before they adequately remove milk from the breast, which can be avoided by the following:
  - Nursing for brief five-minute periods
  - Nursing more frequently
- See Table 23.6 for help with breastfeeding

TABLE 23.6 COUNSELING SUMMARY—NEUROLOGICALLY IMPAIRED INFANT

MOTHER'S CONCERNS	SUGGESTIONS FOR MOTHER
Baby has difficulty grasping the breast.	• Position the baby close to the mother's breast and adequately support his body. • Position the baby's lower lip outward from his gum. • Press the baby's tongue down to create a groove for the nipple. • Use the Dancer hand position to support the breast and the baby's chin.
Baby has difficulty sucking.	• Feed milk by a cup, dropper, or spoon.
Maintaining milk production.	• Pump or express to remove milk from the breasts after feeds.
Baby gags or chokes during feeds.	• Position the baby's head so his throat is slightly above the nipple. • Stroke downward under the chin to aid swallowing.
Baby loses interest after several minutes of nursing.	• Pre-express milk to initiate a letdown. • Express milk onto the nipple or into the corner of the baby's mouth. • Nurse more frequently for five-minute periods at a time. • Use a tube-feeding device to maintain milk flow.
Mother overwhelmed with caring for the baby.	• Talk with other parents of handicapped babies.

Professional Considerations

Standards of Practice for the Lactation Consultant

Adhere to the Profession's Standards of Practice
- Work in concert with the primary caregiver of the infant and mother
- Individualize your approach
- Prioritize your practices to meet the physical and emotional needs of your clients

Standards for Clinical Practice
- Assess the mother and child individually
- Evaluate the physical appearance and findings of the mother and child
- Document your findings and take a formal history
- Develop a plan of care and follow up based on the mother's needs and goals
- Implement a plan of care as follows:
  - Explain the risks and benefits of any suggested interventions
  - Demonstrate all suggested techniques
  - Provide written instructions for reinforcement
  - Conform to all safety, hygiene, infection control, and universal precautions

- Inform the primary caregiver(s) of interactions and plans in writing
- Refer to other care providers and support groups when needed
- Document the steps in implementing your plan of care (see Chapter 10, Hospital Practices that Support Breastfeeding)
- Evaluate and document the outcome of your plan of care which has been implemented, and modify it if it is not working

Standards for Breastfeeding Education and Counseling

- Educate mothers and families to make informed decisions
- Provide anticipatory guidance to promote optimal breastfeeding and to minimize difficulties
- Provide support and education to help a mother breastfeed through problems
- Educate caregivers to optimize their breastfeeding care for mothers and babies

Standards for Professional Responsibilities

- Function within the broader standards of the health care industry
- Serve as an advocate for the mother and child at all times
- Be aware of any changes in standards and/or clinical research
- Be clinically competent
- Be accountable for your professional actions
  - Respect the privacy of the mother-child relationship
  - Be aware of changing practices and professional or ethical issues
  - Recognize limitations in your knowledge or skills
  - Obtain your clients' written consent before providing care

- Communicate all relevant information to the primary caregiver(s)
- Collaborate with and refer to other health care professionals
- Participate in appropriate professional organizations
- Lend support to colleagues

Standards for Legal Considerations

- Practice within the laws of the geopolitical region in which you live
- Respect the breastfeeding dyad's rights to privacy and confidentiality
- Retain all client records for the period of time that is acceptable for your geopolitical area
- Obtain liability insurance before practicing as an IBCLC
- Know the legal issues involving the lactation consultant-client relationship
  - Know that expectations and duties are contractual in nature
  - Render the appropriate care unless authorized to withdraw
  - A relationship is established for all contacts—in person and by telephone—and by the act of making an appointment
  - Are obligated to give care or refer to another practitioner
  - Advise a mother if a problem is beyond your competency and refer her to a competent practitioner
  - Know that a telephone conversation creates a relationship if you indicate acceptance or give comments in the nature of treatment
- The relationship lasts until the need for your services no longer exists or until you or the mother withdraw
- Instances that do not create a client relationship
  - Physician requests that you see a patient or review a patient's record (unless you are aware

the physician relies on you for lactation advice)
- You have an affiliation with a hospital (unless you are contacted by the mother via a hospital hot line)
- Informed consent
  - Obtain informed consent before providing care to mothers (see Figure 24.1)
  - Discuss specific areas with mothers (see Chapter 5, Client Consultation)
  - Inform the mother of her chance of success and any inherent risks
  - Standard consent forms ordinarily lack sufficient information
  - Consent should cover the care of both the mother and infant
  - Have the consent form signed by both the IBCLC and the mother
- Retain all details about the health of the mother and infant, correspondence, and appointment calendars
- Avoiding liability
  - Become familiar with your state's laws regulating the practice of medicine and protocols in your practice setting
  - Obtain malpractice insurance and keep it in force continuously
  - Build positive relationships with the mothers in your care
  - Do not guarantee results or create unrealistic expectations
  - Empower mothers to make their own decisions
  - Recognize when you should not accept a case
    - You get an uncomfortable or negative feeling
    - A case may be beyond your level of competence
    - You may not have time to handle it
  - Document everything you do, what you chose not to do, and the reasons why

> I acknowledge that (your name) has explained to me that (I am/I may be/my baby is/my baby may be) affected by (condition) and has made the following treatment recommendation:
>
> I acknowledge that the following information has been provided to me: (information provided)
>
> Purpose of the care/treatment: (purpose)
>
> Alternative forms of care/treatment: (alternative care/treatment)
>
> Risks of alternative care/treatment: (risks)
>
> Risks of not undergoing care/treatment: (risks)
>
> I further acknowledge that I have had full opportunity to discuss this information with (your name) and hereby consent to the following lactation consultant care or treatment (specify care or treatment)
>
> _____ _____
> Date   Patient/client or person
>   authorized to consent for
>   patient/client
>
> _____ _____
> Date   (Your name and credentials)

Figure 24.1 Consent form for breastfeeding care
Printed with permission of Breastfeeding Support Consultants.

- Avoid making negative notations in a mother's record
- Organize your work space to make it convenient for documenting
- Incorporate your private practice to limit personal liability

Adhere to the Ethics of the Profession

- Be careful not to undermine a physician's position:
  - Try to work within the parameters of a physician's advice
  - If you disagree, discuss the discrepancy with the physician
  - If a mother asks you for referral to another physician, suggest at least three names
- Inform clients of all fees at the beginning of a consultation
- Make sure all rental equipment is clean and in good condition

Appendix A

Professional Resources

Academy of Breastfeeding Medicine
ABM Executive Office
P.O. Box 81323
San Diego, CA 92138
Phone: 1-877-836-9947
Fax: 1-619-295-0056
International phone: 1-619-295-0058
E-mail: ABM@bfmed.org
Web address: www.bfmed.org

American Academy of Pediatrics (AAP)
141 Northwest Point Boulevard
Elk Grove Village, IL 60007-1098
Phone: 1-800-433-9016 or 1-847-434-4000
Fax: 1-847-434-8000
E-mail: kidsdocs@aap.org
Web address: www.aap.org

American College of Nurse-Midwives (ACNM)
818 Connecticut Avenue NW
Suite 900
Washington, D.C. 20006
Phone: 1-202-728-9860
Fax: 1-202-728-9897
E-mail: info@acnm.org
Web address: www.midwife.org

American College of Obstetricians and Gynecologists (ACOG)
P.O. Box 96920
Washington, D.C. 20090-6920
Phone: 1-202-863-2518
Fax: 1-202-484-1595
E-mail: resources@acog.org
Web address: www.acog.org

American Dietetic Association (ADA)
216 W. Jackson Boulevard
Suite 800
Chicago, IL 60606-6995
Phone: 1-800-877-1600 or 1-312-899-0040
Fax: 1-312-899-1979
E-mail: cdr@eatright.org
Web address: www.eatright.org

American Medical Association (AMA)
515 North State Street
Chicago, IL 60610
Phone: 1-312-464-5000
Fax: 1-312-464-4184
Web address: www.ama-assn.org

American Public Health Association (APHA)
Clearinghouse on Infant Feeding and Maternal Nutrition
1015 15th Street NW
Washington, D.C. 20005
Phone: 1-202-789-5600
Fax: 1-202-789-5661

Association of Women's Health, Obstetric and Neonatal Nurses (AWHONN)
2000 L Street NW
Suite 740
Washington, D.C. 20036
Phone: 1-202-261-2414 and 1-800-673-8499 (US) and 1-800-245-0231
Fax: 1-202-728-0575
e-mail: chrish@awhonn.org
Web address: www.awhonn.org

Australian Breastfeeding Association
See Nursing Mothers Association of Australia

Baby Friendly USA
8 Jan Sebastian Way
Sandwich, MA 02563
Phone: 1-508-888-8092
Fax: 1-508-888-8050
E-mail: info@babyfriendlyusa.org
Web address: www.mypage.onemain.com/bfusa

Department of Health and Human Services
Administration for Children and Families
200 Independence Avenue SW
Washington, D.C. 20201
Phone: 202-619-0257 or 877-696-6775
E-mail: hhsmail@os.dhhs.gov
Web address: www.dhhs.gov

Healthy Mothers, Healthy Babies
121 North Washington Street
Suite 300
Alexandria, VA 22314
Phone: 1-703-836-6110
Fax: 1-703-836-3470
Web address: www.hmhb.org

Human Milk Banking Association of North America, Inc.
(HMBANA)
Mothers' Milk Bank
P-S-L Medical Center
1719 East 19th St.
Denver, CO 80218
Phone: 1-919-250-8599 or 1-303-869-1888
Web address: www.hmbana.org

Infant Feeding Action Coalition
INFACT Canada
6 Trinity Square
Toronto, Ontario
Canada M5G 1B1
Phone: 416-595-9819
Fax: 416-591-9355
E-mail: info@infactcanada.ca
Web address: www.infactcanada.ca

Institute for Reproductive Health
Georgetown University Medical Center
3PHC Room 3004
3800 Reservoir Road NW

Washington, D.C. 20007
Phone: 1-202-687-1392
Fax: 1-202-687-6846
E-mail: irhinfo@gunet.georgetown.edu

International Baby Food Action Network (IBFAN)
(See INFACT for Canadian address/phone—INFACT is the
North American coordinator for IBFAN)
(Also see National Alliance for Breastfeeding
Advocacy–NABA for the U.S. address/phone)
Web address: www.ibfan.org

International Board of Lactation Consultant Examiners
(IBLCE)
7309 Arlington Boulevard
Suite 300
Falls Church, VA 22042-3215
Phone: 1-703-560-7330
Fax: 1-703-560-7332
E-mail: iblce@erols.com
Web address: www.iblce.org

International Childbirth Education Association (ICEA)
P.O. Box 20048
Minneapolis, MN 55420
Phone: 1-952-854-8660 or 800-624-4934
Fax: 1-952-854-8772
E-mail: info@icea.org
Web address: www.icea.org

International Lactation Consultant Association (ILCA)
1500 Sunday Drive
Suite 102
Raleigh, NC 27607
Phone: 1-919-787-5181
Fax: 1-919-787-4916
E-mail: ilca@erols.com
Web address: www.ilca.org

La Leche League International, Inc.
P.O. Box 4079
1400 N. Meacham Road
Schaumburg, IL 60173-4048
Phone: 1-800-525-3243 or 1-847-519-7730
Fax: 1-847-519-0035
E-mail: lllhq@llli.org
Web address: www.lalecheleague.org

Lamaze International
2025 M St.
Suite 800
Washington, D.C. 20036-3309
Phone: 1-202-367-1128 or 1-800-368-4404
Fax: 1-202-367-2128
E-mail: Lamaze@dc.sba.com
Web address: www.Lamaze-childbirth.com

March of Dimes
1275 Mamaroneck Avenue
White Plains, NY 10605
Phone: 1-914-428-7100 or 888-663-4637
Fax: 1-914-428-8203
Web address: www.modimes.org

National Alliance for Breastfeeding Advocacy (NABA)
254 Conant Road
Weston, MA 02193-1756
Phone: 1-617-893-3553
Fax: 1-617-893-8608
E-mail: marshalact@aol.com
Web address:
http://hometown.aol.com/marshalact/naba/home

National Association of WIC Directors (NAWD)
2001 S. Street NW
Suite 580
Washington, D.C. 20009
Phone: 1-202-232-5492
Fax: 1-202-387-5281
E-mail: nawdnutri@aol.com
Web address: www.wicdirectors.org

National Perinatal Association
3500 E. Fletcher Avenue
Suite 205
Tampa, FL 33613-4712
Phone: 1-813-971-1008 or 888-971-3295
Fax: 1-813-971-9306
E-mail: npa@nationalperinatal.org
Web address: www.nationalperinatal.org

Nursing Mothers Association of Australia
(Name will change to Australian Breastfeeding Association on 8/1/01)
P.O. Box 4000

Glen Iris, Vic 3146
Australia
Phone: 61 3 9885 0855
Fax: 61 3 9885 0866
E-mail: nursingm@nmaa.asn.au
Web address: www.nmaa.asn.au

UNICEF
Nutrition Cluster H-8F
3 United Nations Plaza
New York, NY 10017
Phone: 1-212-326-7000
Fax: 1-212-887-7465
E-mail: netmaster@unicef.org

World Alliance for Breastfeeding Action (WABA)
P.O. Box 1200, 10850
Penang, Malaysia
Phone: 604-6584-816
Fax: 604-6572-655
E-mail: secr@waba.po.my
Web address: www.waba.org.br

World Health Organization (WHO)
Avenue Appia 20
1211 Geneva 27, Switzerland
Phone: 00 41 22 791 21 11
Fax: 00 41 22 791 31 11
E-mail: info@who.ch
Web address: www.who.int

Resources for Lactation Consultants

Resources are available from many of the organizations previously listed. In addition, the following businesses and organizations offer a variety of resources:

BEST START
4809 E. Busch Blvd.
Suite 104
Tampa, FL 33617
Phone: 1- 800-277-4975 or 1-813-971-2119
Fax: 1-813-971-2280
E-mail: beststart@beststartinc.org

Birth and Life Bookstore (a division of Cascade Health Care Products)
141 Commercial Street NE
Salem, OR 97301-3402
Phone: 1-800-443-9942 or 1-503-371-4445
Fax: 1-503-371-5395
E-mail: onecascade@worldnet.att.net
Web address: www.1cascade.com

Breastfeeding Support Consultants, Inc.
Center for Lactation Education
228 Park Lane
Chalfont, PA 18914-3135
Phone: 1-215-822-1281
Fax: 1-215-997-7879
E-mail: info@bsccenter.org
Web address: www.bsccenter.org

Childbirth Graphics (a division of WRS Group, Inc.)
P.O. Box 21207
Waco, TX 76702-1207
Phone: 1-800-299-3366, ext. 287
Fax: 1-254-751-0221
E-mail: sales@wrsgroup.com
Web address: www.childbirthgraphics.com

Geddes Productions
P. O. Box 41761
Los Angeles, CA 90041-0761
Phone: 1-818-951-2809
Fax: 1-818-951-9960
E-mail: orders@geddespro.com
Web address: www.geddespro.com

Hollister Incorporated (Ameda-Egnell)
2000 Hollister Drive
Libertyville, IL 60048-3781
Phone: 1-847-680-1000 or 1-800-323-4060
Fax: 1-847-680-1017
Web address: www.hollister.com

Lactnet
E-mail: Listserv@listserv.net
In the body of the letter (file) put the following all on one line:
Subscribe Lactnet (Your Name)

Lactnews
E-mail: barbara@lactnews.com
Web address: www.jump.net/~bwc/lactnews

Medela, Inc.
P.O. Box 660
McHenry, IL 60051-0660
Phone: 1-800-435-8316 or 1-815-363-1166
Fax: 1-800-995-7867 or 1-815-363-1246
E-mail: customer.service@medela.com
Web address: www.medela.com

Pharmasoft Publishing
21 Tascocita Circle
Amarillo, TX 79124-1317
Phone: 1-800-378-1317
E-mail: books@ibreastfeeding.com
Web address: http://neonatal.ttuhsc.edu/lact/

Seabury and Smith (for liability insurance as an Allied Health Therapist)
332 S. Michigan Avenue
Suite 1400
Chicago, IL 60604
Phone: 1-800-621-3008
Fax: 1-312-427-7938

UCLA Lactation Alumni Association
Carol Follingstad
(To purchase superbill)
2021 Grismer #17
Burbank, CA 91504
Phone: 1-818-841-4182
Fax: 1-818-848-2882
E-mail: cfolling@fmsn.com

WHO Publications
49 Sheridan Avenue
Albany, NY 12210
Phone: 1-518-436-9686
Fax: 1-518-436-7433
E-mail: qcorp@compuserve.com

Drug Hotlines

Brigham and Women's Hospital
Boston, MA
Phone: 1-617-732-5500 ext. 33696

The Lactation Center at the University of Rochester
Rochester, NY
Phone: 1-716-275-0088

Rocky Mountain Poison and Drug Center
(must become a subscriber)
Phone: 1-303-893-3784
Fax: 1-303-739-1119

Appendix B

Breastfeeding Promotion

TABLE B.1 THE INTERNATIONAL CODE OF MARKETING OF HUMAN MILK SUBSTITUTES

CODE PROVISION	IMPLICATIONS TO CONSIDER
Under the scope of the Code, items marketed or otherwise represented to be suitable as human milk substitutes can include foods and beverages such as: • Infant formula. • Other milk products. • Cereals. • Vegetable, fruit, and other puréed preparations. • Juices and baby teas. • Follow-on milks. • Bottled water.	Whether or not a product is considered to be within this definition will depend on how it is promoted for infants. Any products that are marketed or represented as suitable substitutes to human milk will fall into this category. Because babies should only receive human milk for about the first six months, any other food or drink promoted for use during this time will be a human milk substitute.

(continues)

TABLE B.1 THE INTERNATIONAL CODE OF MARKETING OF HUMAN MILK SUBSTITUTES (continued)

Code Provision	Implications to Consider
Regarding advertising and information, the Code recommends that: - Advertising of human milk substitutes, bottles, and teats to the public not be permitted. - Educational materials explain the benefits of breastfeeding, the health hazards associated with bottle feeding, the costs of using infant formula, and the difficulty of reversing the decision not to breastfeed. - Product labels clearly state the superiority of breastfeeding, the need for the advice of a health care worker, and a warning about health hazards; and they show no pictures of babies, or other pictures or text idealizing the use of infant formula.	Health workers such as lactation consultants and breastfeeding counselors need to press their legislators for measures that will implement the Code in full. This would protect mothers from advertising in parent magazines and on television. It would also prevent direct company contact with mothers through hot lines, Internet sites, mailings, home-delivered supplies of formula, and baby clubs.

Regarding samples and supplies, the Code recommends that:

- No free samples be given to pregnant women, mothers, or their families.
- No free or low-cost supplies of human milk substitutes be given to maternity wards, hospitals, or any other part of the health care system.

Under the Code, free or low-cost supplies can be distributed only outside of the health care system and must be continued for as long as the infant needs them. In the United States, this is usually equal to one year. Elsewhere, it is equal to at least six months. The health care system encompasses health care workers, including lactation consultants and breastfeeding counselors.

Regarding health care facilities and health care workers, the Code recommends that:

- There be no product displays, posters, or distribution of promotional materials.
- No gifts or samples be given to health care workers.
- Product information for health professionals be limited to what is factual and scientific.

This provision also covers bottles that are provided and shown in advertisements by breast pump companies that are clearly feeding bottles, even when no teats are shown. Pens and pads of paper with the name of a formula company are examples of gifts.

1. All pregnant women and new mothers will be informed of the nutritional and health benefits, and basic management of breastfeeding.
2. Staff will presume the mother is breastfeeding unless the mother informs the staff otherwise.
3. Mothers will be helped to initiate breastfeeding within an hour of birth unless maternal or neonatal complications intervene.
4. All nursing mothers will be given instructions on the hand expression of milk. If they should be separated from their infants, nursing mothers will be given specific instructions on breastfeeding and how to maintain lactation (pumping). Mothers who have not begun breastfeeding within eight to twelve hours of birth will begin milk expression.
5. Breastfeeding newborns will be given no food or drink other than human milk unless medically indicated and a specific order is written by the physician. A list of medical indications for using human milk substitutes is provided.
6. Breastfeeding babies will be given pacifiers only at the direction of the mother. The risks and benefits of using artificial nipples (on pacifiers, bottles, and so forth) will be explained to the mother.
7. Infants who need supplementation will be tube fed at the breast or cup fed unless medically contraindicated.
8. Rooming in will be encouraged; babies are to be kept with their mothers 24 hours a day. Mothers will be taught how to co-sleep with their infants safely.
9. Mothers will be taught to watch for infant feeding cues, and will breastfeed their babies on demand rather than on a predetermined schedule. Mothers will be encouraged to breastfeed their babies a minimum of eight times in a 24-hour time period.
10. Mothers will be given information about breastfeeding support groups and lactation consultants prior to discharge from the hospital.
11. Each health care professional who cares for mothers and infants at this facility is expected to maintain the skills and knowledge necessary for implementation of this policy.

Figure B.1 A baby-friendly hospital breastfeeding policy

1. Develop or implement a current breastfeeding protocol for use in your practice that is communicated to all staff. Provide copies to those who cover for you.
2. Arrange for all staff to attend inservices that teach the skills necessary to implement the protocol.
3. Inform all pregnant women about the benefits and management of breastfeeding. Give written, noncommercial, prenatal information on breastfeeding. Refer the parents to breastfeeding classes, and encourage fathers to attend.
4. Help mothers to initiate and maintain breastfeeding during your hospital rounds. Perform the newborn's exam in the mother's room, showing her how well-designed her baby is for breastfeeding.
5. If the mother and baby are separated due to illness, prematurity, and so on, confirm that an electric breast pump is available for expressing milk, and that milk is expressed at least eight times in a 24-hour time period. A prescription may be written for human milk, if necessary, to cover the cost of renting an electric breast pump.
6. Avoid the use of sterile water, glucose water, or formula for breastfeeding newborn infants, unless medically indicated. Adequate amounts of milk are present at delivery in the form of colostrum.
7. Encourage mothers to room in with their babies 24 hours a day in the hospital. This protects the baby from disease in the nursery, provides opportunities for unrestricted contact and feeding, and encourages mothers to become aware of their baby's needs and rhythms.
8. Advise mothers to feed their infants on cue, eight to twelve times during a 24-hour time period. Teach behavioral feeding cues to avoid underfeeding or overhunger, which results in infant behavioral disorganization.
9. Avoid the use of artificial nipples and pacifiers in newborn breastfeeding infants. This approach decreases the incidence of nipple preference and its sequelae.
10. Have available on staff a nurse practitioner or lactation consultant whose responsibility can include prenatal teaching, hospital rounds, call-in times, and visits for breastfeeding questions or problems. Or have the staff refer such situations to a lactation consultant in the community. Refer mothers to breastfeeding support groups for mother-to-mother support.

Printed by permission of Marsha Walker.

Figure B.2 Ten steps to a baby-friendly pediatric practice

1. Create and implement a breastfeeding promotion and support policy for use in your practice that is communicated to all staff. Provide copies to those who cover for you.
2. Arrange for all staff to attend inservices that teach the skills necessary to implement the protocol.
3. Inform all pregnant women about the benefits and management of breastfeeding. Give written, noncommercial information on breastfeeding. Recommend that both parents attend prenatal breastfeeding classes. Refer the parents to childbirth education classes.
4. Help mothers initiate breastfeeding within 1/2 hour of birth. Place and leave the infant on the mother's chest to promote the prefeeding sequences of behavior that lead to the proper latch, suck, and organization of breastfeedings.
5. If the mother and baby are separated due to illness, prematurity, and so on, confirm that an electric breast pump is available for expressing milk; that milk is expressed at least eight times in a 24-hour time period; and that no nipple soreness, engorgement, or breast problems arise from the use of the pump.
6. Avoid the use of sterile water, glucose water, or formula for breastfeeding newborn infants, unless medically indicated. Adequate amounts of milk are present at delivery in the form of colostrum.
7. Encourage mothers to room in with their babies 24 hours a day in the hospital. This protects the baby from disease in the nursery, provides opportunities for unrestricted contact and feeding, and encourages mothers to become aware of their baby's needs and rhythms.
8. Advise mothers to feed their infants on cue, eight to twelve times during each 24-hour time period. Teach behavioral feeding cues to avoid underfeeding or overhunger, which results in infant behavioral disorganization.
9. Avoid the use of artificial nipples and pacifiers in newborn breastfeeding infants. This approach decreases the incidence of nipple preference and its sequelae.
10. Have available on staff a nurse practitioner or lactation consultant whose responsibilities can include prenatal teaching, hospital rounds, call-in times, and visits for breastfeeding questions or problems. Or refer such situations to a lactation consultant in the community. Refer mothers to breastfeeding support groups for mother-to-mother support.

Printed by permission of Marsha Walker.

Figure B.3 Ten steps to a baby-friendly obstetric practice

1. Create a written breastfeeding policy that is research-based and provide copies of the policy to all home health staff. Include the WHO/UNICEF Code for Marketing Breastmilk Substitutes in the policy.
2. Train all health care staff in maternal-child services using the WHO/UNICEF 18-Hour Course. Update the staff as new or revised research-based information becomes available. New staff should be given the 18-hour Course, which will begin during orientation, and it should be completed within one year.
3. Inform all pregnant women about the benefits and management of breastfeeding; weave breastfeeding information into every visit. Provide written information that complies with the WHO Code. Refer all pregnant women to the prenatal breastfeeding classes within the community.
4. Inform all pregnant women of the importance of initiating breastfeeding within the first hour of life.
5. If postpartum mothers are separated from their babies, be sure they have the proper equipment for milk expression and provide instruction as needed. Teach hand expression to all breastfeeding mothers. Assess breastfeeding during each home visit.
6. Give the child (ages newborn to about six months) no food or drink other than human milk unless medically indicated. Instruct mothers—prenatal and postpartum—about the risks of artificial baby milks. A list of acceptable medical reasons for human milk substitutes is included in the breastfeeding policy.
7. Encourage a "rooming in" home environment. Explain the importance of close mother-infant contact 24 hours a day by the use of a sling, bathing together, sleeping together, and so on.
8. Teach mothers the importance of their babies' cues. Explain the importance of baby-led feeds versus mother-led feeds, which can place limitations and times on feeds. Advise mothers that eight to twelve or more feeds occurring within 24 hours is normal and expected.
9. Do not give artificial teats or pacifiers to breastfeeding infants. Discourage their use, and instead direct the mother to breastfeed for suckling satisfaction. Explain the negative consequences of such devices.
10. Foster the establishment of breastfeeding support groups within the community, and refer mothers to them at any time.

Printed by permission of Debbie Shinskie.

Figure B.4 Ten steps to a baby-friendly home health agency

1. Have a written breastfeeding policy, and train health care staff caring for breastfeeding infants in skills necessary to implement the policy.
2. When a sick infant is admitted, ascertain the mother's wishes about the infant's feed, and assist mothers in establishing and managing lactation as necessary.
3. Provide parents with written and verbal information about the benefits of breastfeeding and human milk.
4. Facilitate unrestricted breastfeeding and frequent human milk expression by mothers who wish to provide milk for their children, regardless of age.
5. Give breastfed children other food or drink only when age appropriate or medically indicated.
6. When medically indicated, use only those alternative feeding methods that are most conducive to successful breastfeeding, and restrict the use of any oral device associated with breastfeeding problems.
7. Provide facilities that allow parents and infants to remain together 24 hours a day, that encourage appropriate skin-to-skin contact, and that avoid modeling the use of artificial feeds.
8. Administer medications and schedule all procedures so they cause the least possible disturbance of the breastfeeding relationship.
9. Maintain a human milk bank that meets the appropriate standards.
10. At the time of the infant's discharge from the hospital or clinic, provide parents with information about breastfeeding support groups in the community.
11. Maintain the appropriate monitoring and data collection procedures that will permit quality assurance and ongoing research.

Printed by permission of Maureen Minchin from *Breastfeeding Matters*, Alma Publications, Victoria, Australia, 1999.

Figure B.5 Eleven steps to optimal breastfeeding in the pediatric unit

Index

Note: **Boldface** numbers indicate illustrations; italic *t* indicates a table.

ABM (*See* artificial baby milk)
abscessed breasts, 257*t*, 258
acrocyanosis (blueness) in newborn, 163
acquired immunodeficiency syndrome (AIDS) (*See* human immunodeficiency virus)
active listening, 21, 24*t*
active or fussy babies, 182
activity/emotional states of infants, 180
adopted babies, induced lactation and relactation, 354–359, 356–357*t*
adult learning and breastfeeding consultation, 17–19
afterpains, 61
age-range for breastfeeding (WHO), 4
AIDS (*See* human immunodeficiency virus)
alcohol use, 76, 117
allergen foods in maternal diet, 76
allergies, 112, 266, 267*t*
  colic, 189–193, 194–195*t*
alpha2-macroglobulin in milk, 110*t*
alpha-lactoglobulin, 106*t*
alternate feeding methods, 334–342
  bottle feeding as, 340–342

  cup feeding as, 334–336, **335**
  finger feeding as, 338–339, **339**
  spoon feeding as, 334–336, **335**
  syringe feeding as, 339–340, **339**
  tube feeding devices as, 336–337, **336**, **337**
alternate massage, 243
aluminum in milk, 103, 123
alveoli, **46**, 49–51, 53, 57, 58, 59, 67
amenorrhea, 292, 293
American Academy of Pediatrics (1997) breastfeeding recommendations, 8–9
amino acids in milk, 83*t*, 100
amipicillin, 119*t*
amoxacillin, 119*t*
amphetamines, 117, 235
analgesics, 119*t*, 141, 278*t*
anatomy and physiology of breast, 46–71, **46**
  abscessed breasts and, 257*t*, 258
  alveoli in, **46**, 49–51, 53, 57, 58, 59, 67
  areola in, 47, 53, 59, 65
  autocrine control of milk production in, 58–59

435

baby's breast congestion at birth and, 52
blood supply to breast in, 48–49, 53–54
bloody discharge from breast in, 70
breast cancer and, 51, 70
cardiac surgery vs., 51
care of the breast for, 131–132, 147
colostrum in, 50, 52, 53, 54, 57
connective tissue of breast in, 48
Cooper's ligaments of breast in, 48
ductal atresia vs., 51
ducts in breast in, 46, 47, 50–53, 49, 59, 67, 95, 221, 247, 249, 256*t*
ejection of milk (*See* let-down reflex)
engorgement of breast in, 49, 57, 220, 221, 223, 247–249, **248**, 383
epithelial and myoepithelial cells of breast in, 50
estrogen and, 53, 54, 57, 58
examination of breasts and, 61, 65–71, **71**
fatty tissue of breast in, 48
feedback inhibitor of lactation (FIL) in, 58
fibrocystic breasts and lumps in, 67
foremilk in, 60
galactocele cysts in, 67
galactopoesis and, 54
glandular tissue of breast in, 49
hindmilk in, 60
hormonal imbalances vs., 54–57
hypothyroidism and, 56–57
infections in breast and, 67
innervation of breast in, **46**, 47
insufficient milk supply and, 51–52, 55, 150–151*t*
intercostal nerves of breast in, **46**, 47
intraductal papilloma in breast and, 67, 70
inverted nipples in, 65–67, **69**
lactiferous sinus in, **46**, 50, 59, 95, 166, 217, 279*t*, 281*t*
lactogenesis and, three stages of, 53–54
latch and, 129
let-down reflex in, 59–61, 62–63
lobe/lobule of breast in, **46**, 49, 50–51
lumps in breast and, 67
lymphatic system of breast in, 48–49
mastitis and, 253, 257*t*, 249
menstrual cycles and breast changes in, 52
milk-producing tissue of breast in, 49–50
milk-transporting tissue of breast in, 50–51
Montgomery gland in, **46**, 47, 53
nipple in, **46**, 47, 50, 53, 65–67, **68**, 129
oxytocin and, 49, 55, 59
placental retention in, 54, 56
plugged ducts in, 249, 256*t*
pregnancy and breast development in, 52, 53
prenatal breast care for, 129–132
problems (pathology) of breast vs. breastfeeding in, 51–52
progesterone and, 53, 54, 57, 58

prolactin and, 49, 54–59
prolactin inhibitory factor (PIF) in, 58, 59
prolactinomas in, 56
puberty and breast development in, 52
self-examination of breasts in, 70, **71**
Sheehan's syndrome in, 56
size of breast vs. ability to breastfeed in, 51–52
stimulation of nipples in, 65, 66
subcutaneous fat of breast in, **46**
suckling action on breast in, 47–48, 59
supplemental feeding and, 52
supportive and sustaining tissue of breast in, 47
surgery to breast vs. breastfeeding, 51, 65, 150, 235, 278*t*, 281*t*
switching breasts during breastfeeding in, 60
synthesis of milk in, 57–59
transitional milk in, 57
variations in breast structure and function in, 61, 65–71
volume of milk produced/consumed in, 58
weaning and changes in breast in, 54, 270–271
whey and, 58
witch's milk and, 52
anemia, 100
anesthesia, 141, 144, 150
angel dust, maternal use, presence in milk, 117
ankyloglossia (*See* frenulum)
antacids, 119*t*
anthelminthics, 119*t*
antibacterial factors in milk, 106–108*t*
antibiotics, 119*t*
antibodies (antigens) in milk, 94, 103–105
anticancer drugs, 118*t*
anticipatory guidance, 27
anticonvulsants, 118*t*
antifungals, 119*t*
antihistamines, 119*t*
antihypertensives, 119*t*
anti-infective agents in milk, 104–105
antileporetics, 119*t*
antimalarial drugs, 119*t*
antimetabolites, 118*t*
antiparasitic factors in milk, 111*t*
antipyretics, 119*t*
antituberculars, 119*t*
antiviral factors in milk, 109–110*t*, 374
arachidonic acid (AA) in milk, 98
arching during feeding, 167
areola, 47, 53, 59, 65, 211–212, **214**–215, 271
artificial baby milk (ABM) (See also cow's milk), 121–125, 136, 149, 158, 342–344, 351, 380
bifidobacterium bifidum bacteria in infant gut vs., 123
caloric requirements of infants and, 183
choice of, 343
choosing and preparing, 125
cognitive development delays and, 123
community impact of, 124–125
contaminants in, 121
cow's milk as, 123
dangers in preparation of, 123–124
deficiencies in, 121
economic burden of, 124

expiration dates for, 125
gastroesophageal reflux
(GER) and, 170
International Code of
Marketing for, 427–429*t*
necrotizing enterocolitis
(NEC) and sepsis in,
105, 122
phenylketonuria (PKU) in
infants and, 399–401, 402*t*
preparation safety for,
343–344
risks of, 121, 122*t*
soy milk as, 123
artificial nipples and pacifiers
(See also nipple shields), 1, 2,
9, 145, 149, 160, 212, 216,
220, 280*t*, 284, 323, 340–342,
341, 361
aspirin, 119*t*
attachment—latch and sucking,
148–149, 151, 152, **199**,
210–229, 213, 279*t*, 280*t*, 283
areola position in, 211–212,
214–215
assisting baby in, 224
bottle feeding and suckling
motion in, 212, **213**, 216
cleft lip/palate vs., 227
consequences of poor latch
in, 221
crying infants and, 225
difficulty in, 221, 224–229,
225–228*t*
engorgement, 220,
221, 223
evaluator techniques for,
324–325
factors affecting, 211
feeding adjustments to
improve, 219, 220*t*,
222–223*t*
feeding cues, 225
finger examination of oral
cavity for, 324, **324**

frenulum or tongue-tie
vs., 227
hyper- and hypotonic
infants vs., 228
hypoglycemic infants
and, 227
improper position for latch-
on, 217, **217**
inverted nipples and,
220, 226
latch-on assessment for,
148–149, 151, 152, **199**,
216–221, 279*t*, 280*t*
levels of intervention for,
224, 229
lip position for, 216
nipple position in, 211–212,
214–215, 216–217
nutritive vs. non-nutritive
sucking in, 211
pacifiers or artificial
nipples, 220
palate abnormalities, 226
pattern of sucking in, 211
physiology of, 211–212, **213**,
214–215
positioning for, 220–221,
222–223*t*, 226, 228
principles of good latch in,
216–217
problems getting
baby latched on in,
218–221, 220*t*
rhythm or coordination of
suck, swallow, breathe in,
211–212, **214–215**,
217–218, 224, 281*t*
signs of good latch in, 216
signs of good milk transfer
in, 217–218
signs of poor latch in,
218–219
suck reorganization and, 325
suck training interventions
in, 229, 325

sucking and suckling in, 210–216
sucking effects on baby in, 210
sucking effects on mother in, 210
swallowing and, 216
tongue position in, 211, **214–215**, 216
tongue sucking in infant in, 228
what to do when poor latch occurs in, 218
withdrawal or avoidance behavior (infant) in, 218
attending, 21, 24*t*
autocrine control of milk production, 58–59

"baby blues," 286
baby-friendly medical practice policies, 152, 430–433*t*
baby-friendly hospital breastfeeding policy, 152, 430
eleven steps to optimal breastfeeding in the pediatric unit, 443
ten steps to a baby-friendly home health agency, 433
ten steps to a baby-friendly obstetric practice, 432
ten steps to a baby-friendly pediatric practice, 431
backaches, maternal, 289
bacterial infections, 104
bathing newborns, 143
battery-operated breast pumps, **328**
Bauer's response during feeding, 168
behavior patterns in infants, 181–182
benefits to breastfed infants, 1–5
benefits to mothers, 5
bereaved mothers, 369, 372

bifidobacterium bifidum bacteria in infant gut, 94, 99, 103, 104, 106*t*, 123
bile salts in milk, 103
bili blanket (*See* phototherapy for jaundice)
bili lights (*See* phototherapy for jaundice)
bilirubin (See also jaundice), 164, 165, 183, 345–348
biting, 260–261
bloated abdomen in infant, 179
blood supply to breast, 48–49, 53–54
bloody discharge from breast, 70
body language as communication tool, 19
bonding (See also kangaroo care; skin-to-skin contact), 127, 142–143
fathers and infants, 290–291
hospitalized infants, 362–363
bottle feeding (See also artificial baby milk), 212, **213**, 216, 340–342, 374
bottle nipple (*See* artificial nipples and pacifiers)
bowel function, infant, 170–171, 176–177*t*, 178–179, 230, 273, 276 (See also stooling)
bowel function, maternal, postpartum, 289
brain (*See* cognitive development)
brain damaged infants, 409, 410*t*
bras, nursing, 133
breast anatomy (*See* anatomy and physiology of breast)
breast cancer and breastfeeding, 51, 70, 122
breast care, 131–132, 147
breast congestion of baby at birth, 52

breast implants, silicone in milk, 120
breast massage, 314–315, **316**
breast pumps, 67, 242, 243, 283, 327–329
breast rejection, 70
breast self-examination, 70
breast shells, 66–67, 129, 234, 319–320, **320**, 331
BREASTfeed Observation form, 35–36
breastfeeding assessment (*See* feeding assessment)
breastfeeding beyond first month (See also early weeks of breastfeeding), 259–271
   allergies in infants vs., 266, 267t
   biting of breast during, 260–261
   complementary foods during, 262–263
   decrease in milk production during, 264
   growth and weight gain in infants in, 259–260
   iron supplements in, 264
   older children and toddlers, 261–262, 384, 388, 388t
   public breastfeeding and, 260
   solid food introduction during, 263–264, 265
   supplementary foods during, 262–263
   teething and, 260–261
   vitamin and mineral supplements during, 264
   weaning and, 267–271
breastfeeding record/diary for first week, 172–175t
breastfeeding techniques (*See* positioning for breastfeeding)

breastfeeding-associated jaundice, 346–347
breastmilk jaundice, 347
breathing, rhythm or coordination of suck, swallow, breathe, 211–212, **214**–215, 217–218, 222t
bronchitis, 122
bronchodilators, 119t
buccal pads, 166
burping after feeding, 169

cabbage leaves as treatment for engorgement/mastitis, 251, 253
caffeine, 76, 116–117
calcium in milk, 98, 101
calcium requirements, maternal, 72, 73t, 84t
caloric content of milk, 96, 97
caloric requirements for breastfeeding mothers, 77, 91–92, 127
caloric requirements of infants, 182–183
cancers (See also breast cancer and breastfeeding), 5, 51, 122, 235
Candida, 99, 244, 247, 323
caput succedaneum, 164
carbohydrates in human milk, 98–99, 107t
cardiac surgery and breastfeeding, 51
casein, 99, 107t, 108t
cephalhematoma, 165, 225
cesarean deliveries, 127, 197, 144, 278t, 289
changes in composition of milk, 96–97
changes in family (*See* family dynamics)
charting with breastfeeding (*See* documentation)
chickenpox (*See* varicella zoster)

chloramphenicol, 118*t*
chloride in milk, 93, 112, 123
C-hold to support breast, 198, 316, **316**
cholecystokinin (CCK) release during feeding, 231
chondroitin sulfate in milk, 110*t*
ciclopirox, 246
ciprofloxacin, 118*t*
circumcision, 136, 225, 280*t*
clarification skills for IBCLC, 22
classes for breastfeeding, 127–129, **130**, **131**
clavicle fractures, 167, 225
cleft lip/palate, 151, 167, 227, 401, 403–404, **403**, 406–407*t*
"client relationship" defined, 413–414
clothing for breastfeeding, 132–133
clotrimazole, 246
cloxacillin, 119*t*
cluster feeds, 149
clutch (football) hold, 200, **201**, 226
CMV (*See* cytomegalovirus)
cocaine, maternal use, presence in milk, 117, 120
cognitive development and breastfeeding, 113, 121, 123
colic, 189–193, 194–195*t*, 196, 221
color of milk, 95
colostrum, 50, 52, 53, 54, 57, 93–94, 97, 99, 103, 143, 129, 132, 227, 247
comfort of mother and infant, 20
common nipple, **68**
communication by infant, 179–181
crying infants, 187–189, 207–209
community impact of ABM, 124–125

community resources for breastfeeding, 147
complement factors in milk, 107*t*
complementary feeding, 1–5, 262–263
conditioning the baby to breastfeed, delayed onset of breastfeeding, 354
connective tissue of breast, 48
consent, 29, 413–415
constipation in infant, 178
consultations with client, 27–45
consumer rights and responsibilities, 16
containers for storing expressed milk, 331–333
contraceptives, 118*t*, 293–295
Cooper's ligaments of breast, 48
copper in milk, 103
corticosteroids, 119*t*
cosleeping, 185–186, 283
co-trimaoxazole, 118*t*
counseling processes, 20–26
cow's milk (*See also* artificial baby milk), 101
  allergies and, 112
  colic, 190–193, 194–195*t*
  health risks of use, 123
  phenylketonuria (PKU) in infants, 399–401
Coxsackie B virus antibodies in milk, 94
cracked nipples, 244, 245*t*
cradle hold, 199, **200**
crisis intervention, 27
Crohn's disease, 103, 122
cross-cradle hold, 226
crying infants, 187–189, 207–209, 225
cultural differences, special counseling, 308–312, 311*t*
cup feeding, 334–336, **335**
cystic fibrosis in mother, 391
cytomegalovirus (CMV), 392

441

Dancer hand position to support breast, 198, 317, **317**
dapsone, 118*t*, 119*t*
decrease in milk production, 264
dehydration in newborns (See also hydration status), 273–274
delayed onset of breastfeeding, 351, 354*t*
    conditioning the baby to breastfeed after, 354
    expressing milk to maintain lactation in, 351
    transition from expressed milk to breastfeeding after, 351
Depo-Provera, 295
depression (*See* postpartum depression)
descriptors of breastfeeding in, for documentation, **43–45**
devices
    breast shells, 319–320, **320**
    inverted syringe for flat or inverted nipples, 318–319, **319**
    lubricant for breasts, 317–318
    nipple shields, 320–323, **321**
    pacifiers and artificial nipples, 323
diabetes, 103, 119*t*, 122, 388–389, 390*t*
diaper rash in newborn, 164
diarrhea in infant, 178
diary, breastfeeding record/diary for first week, 172–175*t*
dieldrin, 121
diets, 77 (See also maternal health and lactation)
difficulty in suckling, in infants, 221, 224–229, 225–228*t*
digestive function in infants, 168–171, 210, 230, 273, 276
    bloated abdomen in, 179
    bowel or stool behavior in, 170–171, 176–177*t*, 178–179, 230, 273, 276
    burping after feeding and, 169
    colic in, 189–193, 194–195*t*
    constipation in, 178
    diarrhea in, 178
    elimination in, 170–171, 230, 273, 276
    gastroesophageal reflux (GER) and, 169–170
    Hirschsprung's disease and, 179
    infrequent stools in, 178–179
    meconium and, 171
    projectile vomiting during or after feeding and, 169
    pyloric stenosis and vomiting in, 169
    spitting up during or after feeding in, 168–169
    voiding in, 170–171, 230, 273, 276
digoxin, 119*t*
discharge from hospital, 34, 147, 152
    early discharge (less than 48 hours), 272
discharge from vagina, postpartum, 288–289
diseases contraindicating breastfeeding, 342
diuretics, 118*t*
docosahexaenoic acid (DHA) in milk, 98
documentation, 32, 415
    BREASTfeed Observation form, 35–36
    descriptors of breastfeeding, 43–45
    IBFAT, 40–42
    information gathering and history taking, 30

LATCH assessment, 37
mother-baby assessment,
38–39
dominant hand hold position,
200, **201**, 202
donor milk, human milk
banks, 334
doulas, 140
Down syndrome infants, 405,
408, **408**
drug/medication use, 75,
114–116, 118–119*t*, 225,
278*t*, 342
drugs of abuse, 117, 120
ductal atresia and.
breastfeeding, 51
ducts of breast, **46**, 47, 50–53,
49, 59, 67, 95, 221, 247,
249, 256*t*
duration of feeds, 97, 231,
280*t*, 283

ear infections (otis media) and
breastfeeding, 105
early weeks of breastfeeding (See
also breastfeeding beyond first
month; initial breastfeeding
help and support), 230–258
abscessed breasts in,
257*t*, 258
alternating positions for
sore nipples during, 243
cholecystokinin (CCK)
release during feeding
in, 231
cracked nipples during,
244, 245*t*
decreases in feeding frequency during, 233
duration of feeds in, 231,
280*t*, 283
engorgement of breasts during, 247–249, **248**
establishing milk production during, 230–233

foremilk feeding in, 231
frequency of feeds during,
231–232
galactorrhea and hyperprolactinemia in, 235
hindmilk feeding
during, 231
increases in feeding frequency during, 232–233
interruption of breastfeeding for sore nipples during, 243
leakage from breasts during,
234–235
mastitis during, 249,
253, 257*t*
nipple soreness during, 231,
235–243, 236–242*t*
one vs. two breasts in feeding during, 230–231
plugged ducts and,
249, 256*t*
sleepy babies and, 231
sufficient milk intake during, signs of, 230
yeast infections (thrush)
during, 244–247
easy or placid babies, 181–182
eclampsia, 342
E coli (*See Escherichia coli* antibodies in milk)
economic burden of ABM, 124
ejection of milk (*See* let-down
reflex)
electric breast pumps, 329, **329**
elimination in the newborn,
170–171, 230, 273, 276
emergency or untimely
weaning, 270
emotional support for
parents, 20
empathetic listening, 21, 24*t*
empowering women to breastfeed, 15–19
ending feeding session, 209, **209**

energy or caloric requirements of infants, 274
engorgement, 49, 57, 220, 221, 223, 247–249, **248**, 383
    massaging the breast in, 315, **316**
    occurrence of, 248
    prevention of, 249
    treatment of, 249, 250–251*t*, 252*t*, 254–255*t*
environmental contaminants, maternal exposure, 120–121
enzymes in milk, 99–100, 103, 104
epidermal growth factors in milk, 103
epidural anesthesia, 141, 150, 278*t*, 289
episiotomies, 141, 289
epithelial/myoepithelial cells of breast, 49, 50
Epstein–Barr virus, 392
ergometrine, 118*t*
erythromycin, 119*t*
Escherichia coli antibodies in milk, 94, 99
estrogen, 53, 54, 57, 58, 118*t*, 293
ethics for IBCLC, 416
evaluating counseling contact, questions for, 25–26
evaluator techniques, 324–325
examination of breasts, 61, 65–71, **71**
exclusive breastfeeding, 1–3, 5, 9
exercise and breastfeeding, 92, 289
expressed milk, 351, 366
    feeding expressed milk after, 366
    freezing or refrigerating milk after, 332, 333, 366
    for hospitalized babies, 330
    for human milk banks, 334
    storing expressed milk after, 331–333, 365–366, 381
expressing milk, 8, 9, 148, 149, 157, 223, 234, 243, 282, 325–334, **326**, 377, 380–381, 404
    battery-operated breast pumps for, **328**
    breast pump selection criteria in, 327–329
    electric breast pumps for, 329, **329**
    hand-held breast pumps for, 328, **328**
    let-down reflex for, 330
    maintaining lactation through, 351, 365, 374
    manual expression in, 325–326, **326**
    massaging the breast for, 315, **316**
    technique for, 330
    transition from expressed milk to breastfeeding in, 351
eye treatment at birth, 136, 142

facial asymmetry in newborn, 165
facilitating skills for IBCLC, 21–22, 24*t*
factor-finding proteins in milk, 106*t*
failure to thrive (FTT) (See also growth and weight gain in infants), 276–277
    causes of, 277, 281*t*
    interventions for infant in, 277, 281–282
    issues to address with the mother in, 277
    signs of, 276
    supplementing the baby vs., 282, 284

total required intake of
milk by infant vs., 282,
284, 285*t*
family dynamics, 286–297
fathers and infants, 129, 149,
290–291, 300–301, **339**
fatigue, 278*t*
fats in milk, 94, 96–98, 107*t*,
109*t*, 111*t*
fatty acids in milk, 98, 109*t*, 111*t*,
121, 123
fatty tissue of breast, 48
feedback inhibitor of lactation
(FIL), 58
feeding adjustments to improve
latch, 219, 220*t*, 222–223*t*
feeding assessment (*See* attachment), 31
feeding cues, 1, 2, 8, 127, 143,
145–146, 148, 149, 159,
179–181, 196, 225
fertility and breastfeeding, 292
fetal position in newborn,
161–162, **162**
fibrocystic breasts and lumps,
67, 235
finger as pacifier, 324
finger examination of oral
cavity, 324, **324**
finger feeding, 338–339, **339**
flanged, lips (*See* lip position in
latch)
flat nipple, **68**
fluoride in milk, 102
focusing skills for IBCLC, 22
folic acid/folate, maternal,
87*t*, 106
follow-up care after hospital
discharge, 147
follow-up method of counseling, 25
fontanels, 165
food pyramid, 77, **78**
football hold (*See* clutch hold)
forceps deliveries, 142, 151,
165, 225

foremilk, 60, 94, 98, 221, 231
formula (*See* artificial baby milk)
forty-eight hour plan of care for
breastfeeding in hospital,
148–149
freezing or refrigerating human
milk, 332, 333, 366
frenulum (ankyloglossia), 151,
165–166, **166**, 227, 242, 281*t*
frequency of feeds, 231–232,
280*t*, 283
FTT (*See* failure to thrive)
fucosylated oligosaccharides, 108*t*
fussy babies, 182

galactocele cysts in breast, 67
galactogogues, 283, 365
galactopoesis, 54
galactorrhea, 235
galactosemia, 342, 401
gangliosides in milk, 107*t*
gasteroenteritis, 122
gastroesophageal reflux (GER),
169–170, 409
general anesthesia, 144
gentian violet, 246
getting breastfeeding started (*See
also* feeding cues; latch; positioning for breastfeeding),
196–209
 allowing baby to set
  pace in, 196
 assisting at, 205–209
 baby-led feeding in, 196
 baby's body position
  (zone 3) in, 198
 baby's mouth position
  (zone 4) in, 198
 cesarean deliveries
  and, 197
 C-hold to support breast in,
  198, 316, **316**
 clutch (football) hold in,
  200, **201**
 cradle hold in, 199, **200**
 cues, 196

Dancer hand position to support breast in, 198, 317, **317**
dominant hand hold position in, 200, **201**, 202
ending feeding session in, 209, **209**
hands-and-knees position for, 203, **204**
latch-on process in, **199**
lying down position for, 202, **202**
mother's body position (zone 1) in, 197
mother's breast position (zone 2) in, 197–198
no restrictions on length of feed in, 196
nutritive vs. non-nutritive sucking in, 205
over-the-shoulder position in, 204, **204**
positioning for feeding in, 197–204
posture feeding position in, 202–203, **203**
skin-to-skin contact in, 207
sleepy infants and, 205–207
special or unconventional nursing postures for, 203–204, **204**
glandular tissue of breast, 49
glucose, 98, 389
glycolipids, 108*t*
glycopeptides, 106*t*
glycoproteins in milk, 107*t*
grasp reflex, 167
grief (*See* bereaved mothers)
growth and weight gain in infants (See also failure to thrive), 98, 128, 147, 182–184, 184*t*, 230, 259–260, 272–285
appropriate growth for age in, 272
breastfed vs. bottle fed, 3–4
caloric requirements of infants for, 182–183
cow's milk vs. human milk in, 101
decreases in feeding frequency and, 233
dehydration in newborns and, 273–274
differences in infant growth in, 274
energy or caloric requirements of infants for, 274
factors influencing milk production and transport and, 276–280*t*
failure to gain/thrive and, 221, 276–277
head circumference in, 260
increases in feeding frequency and, 232–233
increasing milk production for, 283*t*
insufficient milk supply for, 55, 150–151*t*
intrauterine growth retardation (IUGR) and, 364
length in, 260
poor-weight-gaining infants and, 275–276
postmature infants and, 368
preterm infants and, 368
signs that breastfeeding is going well and, 273
slow weight-gaining infants and, 274–275
small for gestation age (SGA) infants and, 364
supplemental feeding and, 282, 284
total required intake of milk by infant for, 282, 284, 285*t*

warning signs of inadequate weight gain in, 276
warning signs that breastfeeding is not going well and, 153–154*t*
weight loss in growing babies and, 221
weight loss in newborns and, 151, 183–184
growth factors in milk, 104, 106*t*
guiding method of counseling, 21–23, 24*t*

haemagglutinin inhibitors in milk, 110*t*
hand expression (*See* manual expression of milk)
hand-held breast pumps, 328, **328**
hands-and-knees nursing position, 203, **204**
head circumference of growing infant, 260
head of newborn, 164–165
health benefits of human milk, 103–113
health consumerism and role of IBCLC, 15
heart disease in infants, 103, 279*t*
heart disease, maternal, 342
hepatitis in mother, 391
heroin, maternal use, presence in milk, 117, 120
herpes in mother, 235, 342, 392
high-risk infants (*See* preterm and high-risk infants)
hindmilk, 60, 98, 231, 280*t*, 283, 404, 408
Hirschsprung's disease, 179
HIV (*See* human immunodeficiency virus)
Hoffman technique, 66
home health agency, baby-friendly, 433*t*

home health care-based lactation consulting, 13
home help and support, 133
hormonal imbalances vs. lactation, 55–57, 281
hospital-based lactation consulting, 11–12
hospital practices to support breastfeeding, 9, 136, 139–160, 272, 278*t*, 330–331, 362–363, 376–379*t*
   baby-friendly practices for, 152, 430*t*
   Eleven Steps to Optimal Breastfeeding in Pediatric Unit for, 434
   in labor and delivery, 140–144, 148
   in neonatal intensive care unit (NICU), 362–363
   in postpartum unit, 144–147
   Ten Steps to Successful Breastfeeding program and, 155–160
hospitalization of baby, 330–331, 362–363, 376–377, 378–379*t*
hospitalization of mother, 376–377, 378–379*t*, 376
human immunodeficiency virus (HIV/AIDS), 334, 342, 392–399
human milk banks, 334
human milk properties, 93–125, 126
   allergy protection from milk, 112
   amino acids in milk, 100
   anti-infective agents in milk, 104–105
   antibacterial factors in milk, 106–108*t*

antibodies (antigens) in milk, 94, 103–105
antiparasitic factors in milk, 111*t*
antiviral agents in milk, 374
antiviral factors in milk, 109–110*t*
artificial baby milk (ABM) vs. human milk, 121–125, 342–344
bifidobacterium bifidum bacteria in infant gut and, 94, 103–104, 106*t*, 106
calcium in milk, 98, 101
caloric content of milk, 96, 97
carbohydrates in milk, 98–99, 107*t*
casein in, 99
changes in composition of milk, 96–97
chloride in milk, 93, 112
color of milk, 95
colostrum in, 93–94, 97, 99, 103
complement factors in milk, 107*t*
cow's milk vs., 101, 112
diseases contraindicating breastfeeding, 342
ear infections (otis media) vs. breastfeeding, 105
enzymes in milk, 104
factor-finding proteins in milk, 106*t*
fats in milk, 94, 95, 96–98, 107*t*, 109*t*, 111*t*
fluoride in milk, 102
foremilk, 94, 98
gangliosides in milk, 107*t*
growth factors in milk, 104, 106*t*
health benefits of human milk, 103–113

hindmilk, 95, 98
immunization vs. breastfeeding, 111
immunoglobulin A (IgA) in milk, 94, 104
immunoglobulin G (IgG) in milk, 94, 106*t*, 109*t*, 111*t*
immunoglobulin M (IgM) in milk, 94, 106*t*, 109*t*
immunoglobulins in milk, 96, 104
immunologic properties of milk, 103
impurities in milk, 113–121
iron in milk, 102
lactase and lipase in milk, 104
lactoferrin in milk, 93, 106*t*, 107*t*, 110
lactose in milk, 98–99
laxative effect of colostrum, 94
lymphocytes and macrophages in milk, 104, 108*t*
lysozyme, 99–100, 104, 107*t*
mature milk, 94–95, 97
mother's diet and milk components, 94
mucins in milk, 104, 107*t*, 110*t*
necrotizing enterocolitis (NEC) and sepsis vs. breastfeeding, 105, 113, 122
nitrogen in milk, 112
oligosaccharides in milk, 105, 106*t*, 108*t*
potassium in milk, 93
preterm/premature delivery and milk components, 112–113
protein in milk, 93, 96, 97, 99–100, 107*t*, 113

secretory immunoglobulin (sIgA) in milk, 94, 106*t*, 109*t*, 111*t*
sodium in milk, 93, 112
supplements to milk, 113
thyroid hormones in milk, 105
trace elements in milk, 103
transitional milk, 94
vegetarian diets and milk composition, 100
viral antibodies in milk, 94
Vitamin B complex in milk, 100
Vitamin C in milk, 102
Vitamin D in milk, 100
Vitamin E in milk, 100
Vitamin K in milk, 100–101
vitamins and minerals in milk, 93, 100–103
volume of milk produced/consumed, 95–96
water content of milk, 102
whey, 99
humor as communication tool, 17–18
hydration status of newborn, 164, 171, 273–274, 343
hydrocephalic infants, 408–409
hyperbilirubinemia (*See* jaundice)
hyperprolactinemia, 235
hyperthyroidism, 235
hypertonia in infant, 162–163, **163**, 228
hypoglycemic infants, 227, 343
hypoglycemic mothers (*See* diabetes)
hypoprolactinemia, 279*t*, 281*t*
hypothalamus and let-down reflex, 59
hypothyroidism, 56–57, 105, 235, 278*t*, 279*t*, 281*t*, 390
hypotonia in infant, 162, **162**, 228, 405, 408

IBCLC (*See* International Board Certified Lactation consultant)
IBFAT, 40–42
ibuprofen, 119*t*
illness in mothers (*See* maternal illnesses)
immunization and breastfeeding, 111
immunoglobulin A (IgA) in milk, 94, 104
immunoglobulin G (IgG) in milk, 94, 106*t*, 109*t*
colic, 190–193, 194–195*t*
immunoglobulin M (IgM) in milk, 94, 106*t*, 109*t*
immunoglobulins in milk, 96, 104
immunologic properties of milk, 103
impurities in milk, 113–121, 119*t*
alcohol as, 117
breast implants and, 120
caffeine as, 116–117
cocaine as, 120
drugs and medications as, 114–116, 118–119*t*
drugs of abuse as, 117, 120
environmental contaminants as, 120–121
heroin as, 120
marijuana as, 117
nicotine, tobacco, and smoking as, 116
passing of, to baby, 113–114, **115**
increasing milk production, 283*t*, 365
induced lactation, 359
infant assessment and behavior, 162–163, 166, 175, 177*t*, 195*t*, 205–209, 211, 225, 230, 273–274, 276, 359–361
infant breastfeeding assessment tool (IBFAT), **40–42**

infections in breast, 67 (See also mastitis)
infectious diseases, 5
influencing mothers, 22–23, 24t, 126
information gathering and history taking, 30
informed consent, 29, 413–415
infrequent stools in infant, 178–179
initial breastfeeding help and support (See also early weeks of breastfeeding; getting breastfeeding started), 146–147, 157, 196
innervation of breast, 46, 47
Innocenti Declaration, 5–8
insufficient milk supply, 51–52, 55, 150–151t
insulin, 389
insurance, 414
intercostal nerves of breast, 46, 47
International Board Certified Lactation Consultant (IBCLC), 10
International Code of Marketing for ABM, 427–429t
interpretational skills for IBCLC, 22
interruption of breastfeeding, 373–382
    bottle feeding during, 374
    following separation and, increasing milk production, 374
    hospitalization of baby and, 376–377, 378–379t
    hospitalization of mother and, 376–377, 378–379t
    illness in mother and, 374, 376, 374
    maintaining lactation until baby can nurse in, 374
    separation anxiety in, 373
    separation of mother and baby in, 373–377, 375t
    short-term separations and, 374, 376
    for sore nipples, 243
    for surgery for baby, 376
    working mothers and, 377
interventions during labor and delivery, 140–141
intraductal papilloma in breast, 67, 70
intravenous (IV) fluid administration during labor, 150, 278t
inverted nipple, 65–67, **69**, 69, 129, 150, 220, 226, 278t, 318–319
    inverted syringe to draw out, 318–319, **319**
inverted-appearing nipple, **69**
inverted syringe, 318–319
iodine requirements, maternal, 85t, 119t
IQ (*See* cognitive development)
iron, 84–85t, 102, 119, 264

jaundice, 136, 151, 164, 221, 279t, 345–350
    bilirubin in, 345–348
    breastfeeding-associated, 346–347
    detection of, 348
    kernicterus and, 347
    late-onset (breastmilk jaundice), 347
    parental concerns about, 350, 352–353t
    pathologic causes of, 346
    phototherapy for, 348–350, **349**
    physiological causes of, 345–346
    in preterm infants, 350
    treatment of, 348–349

kangaroo care, 366–367, **367**
kappa-casein in milk, 107t
Kegel exercises, 289

kernicterus, 347
ketoconazole, 246

labor and delivery, 140–144, 148
    cesarean deliveries and, 127, 197, 144, 278*t*, 289
    clavicle fractures in, 167, 225
    doulas and, 140
    epidural anesthesia and pain medications in, 141, 150, 278*t*, 289
    episiotomies in, 141, 289
    forceps deliveries in, 142, 151, 165, 225
    general anesthesia in, 144
    medical interventions during, 140–141
    pitocin to induce, 142, 150, 278*t*
    separation of mother and baby after, 140, 142–143
    suctioning of baby's breathing passages in, 141, 151, 225
    vacuum deliveries in, 142, 151, 164, 225
    warmers and incubators after, 142
lactase and lipase in milk, 104
lactation consulting (See also special counseling situations), 411–416
    counseling process for, 20–26
    documentation for, 32, 43–45, 415
    education and skills required in, 10–14, 20–26
    hospital staff education/support in breastfeeding in, 139, 155–156
    situations where you must see mother in, 29
    special counseling situations for, 298–313
    standards of practice in, 411–415
lactational amenorrhea method (LAM), 293, **294**
lactiferous sinuses, 46, 50, 59, 95, 166, 217, 279*t*, 281*t*
lactoferrin, 99, 106*t*, 107*t*, 110*t*
lactogenesis, three stages of, 53–54
lactoperoxidase, 107*t*
lactose, 98–99, 191, 401
latch (*See* attachment)
LATCH assessment method, 37, 37
late-onset jaundice (breastmilk jaundice), 347
laxative effect of colostrum, 94
leading method of counseling, 23
leaking from breasts, 61, 129, 234–235, 271, 381
legal considerations for IBCLCs, 413–415
length of growing infant, 260
let-down reflex, 59–63, 97, 114, 210, 221, 234, 283, 330
levels of intervention for suckling difficulty, 224, 229
levonorgestrel, 295
liability, 414–415
linoleic/linolenic acids in milk, 98
lip position in latch-on, 216
lipase in milk, 104
lipids (*See* fats in milk)
listening skills, 21, 24*t*
liver function in newborn (See also jaundice), 345–346
lobe/lobule of breast, 46, 49–51
lochia, 288–289
long-term special needs (See also maternal illness; preterm and high-risk infants), 383–388

for brain damaged infants, 409, 410t
for cleft lip/palate, 401, 403–404, **403**, 406–407t
for Down syndrome infants, 405, 408, **408**
for galactosemia, 401
for hydrocephalic infants, 408–409
for multiple births, 383–384, **385**, 386–387t
for phenylketonuric (PKU) infants, 399–401, 402t
for Pierre Robin syndrome infants, 405, **405**
for spina bifida infants, 409
for tandem nursing, 384, 388, 388t
loss of interest in breastfeeding, infant, 359–361
low-income mothers, special counseling, 301–303, 304t
lumps in breast, 67
lying down position, 202, **202**
lymphatic system of breast, 48–49, 247–249, **248**
lymphocytes and macrophages in milk, 104, 108t
lymphoma, 103
lysozymes, 57, 99–100, 104, 107t

macromolecules in milk, 109t
macrophages in milk, 104, 108t
magnesium requirements, maternal, 86t
magnesium sulfate, 278t
maintaining lactation through expressing, 351, 365, 374
manganese in milk, 103
manual expression of milk, 325–326, **326**
maple syrup urine disease, 342–344

marijuana use, maternal use, presence in milk, 117
massaging the breast, 243, 314–315, **316**
masseter muscles, 212
mastitis, 221, 249, 253, 257t, 383
    abscessed breasts and, 257t, 258
    causes of, 253
    diabetic mothers and, 389
    treatment of, 253, 257t
maternal health and nutrition, 6, 12, 72–92, 279t, 360
    alcohol use and, 76, 117
    allergen foods in diet and, 76
    caffeine use and, 76, 116–117
    calcium requirements for, 72, 73t, 84t
    caloric requirements for breastfeeding mothers in, 77, 91–92, 127
    colic and milk components from, 190–193, 194–195t
    diabetic mothers and, 389
    drug and medication use in, 75, 114–116, 118–119t
    exercise and, 92, 289
    folic acid/folate in, 87t
    food pyramid for, 77, **78**
    improving the diet tips for, 79t
    increasing milk production in, 283t, 365
    iodine requirements in, 85t, 119t
    iron requirements in, 84–85t
    magnesium requirements in, 86t
    menu suggestions for, 74t, 80–81t
    nicotine, tobacco, and smoking in, 75, 116

phosphorus requirements in, 84*t*

protein requirements in, 83*t*

special diets for pregnancy and lactation and, 77

substances to limit or avoid in, 75–76, 114–121

vegetarian diets and, 82, 90

Vitamin A requirements in, 86–87*t*

vitamin and mineral chart for, 83–89*t*

Vitamin B complex requirements in, 87–89*t*, 91

Vitamin C requirements in, 89*t*

Vitamin D requirements in, 87*t*

Vitamin E requirements in, 87*t*

water intake requirements in, 73, 75, 83*t*

weight management in, 77, 91–92, 127

zinc requirements in, 85*t*

maternal illness

cystic fibrosis as, 391

cytomegalovirus (CMV) as, 392

diabetic mothers and, 388–389, 390*t*

Epstein–Barr virus as, 392

hepatitis as, 391

herpes as, 392

human immunodeficiency virus (HIV/AIDS) as, 334, 342, 392–399

hypothyroidism as, 390

phenylketonuria (PKU) as, 391

short-term separation because of, 374, 376

tuberculosis as, 391

varicella zoster as, 392

mature milk, 94–95, 97

meconium, 61, 94, 143, 151, 171, 183

medications, 74, 92, 114, 116, 124, 140, 141, 191, 205, 235, 289, 342

medroxyprogesterone, 295

mefloquine, 119*t*

meningitis, 104

menstrual cycles, 52, 270, 292, 360

lactational amenorrhea method (LAM), 293, 294, 293

metabolic disorders in infants, 279*t*, 342

metoclopramide, 365

metronidazole, 118*t*

miconazole, 246

milk ejection reflex (*See* let-down reflex)

milk production (See also growth and weight gain in infants), 272–285

factors influencing milk production and transport, 276–280*t*

insufficient milk supply, 51–52

milk-producing tissue of breast, 49–50

milk transfer, 31, 66, 166, 211, 217, 274, 320 (See also growth and weight gain in infants)

milk-transporting tissue of breast, 50–51

minocycline and black milk, 95

misconceptions about breastfeeding, 126

monoglycerides in milk, 109*t*, 111*t*

Montgomery gland, 46, 47, 53, 271

453

moro (startle) reflex, 167
morphine, 119*t*
mother–baby assessment method, **38–39**
mother's diet and milk components, 94
mucins in milk, 104, 107*t*, 110*t*
multiple births, 383–384, **385**, 386–387*t*
multiple sclerosis, 103

naftifine hydrochloride, 246
National Center for Health Statistics (NCHS), 3
natural family planning (NFP), 293
necrotizing enterocolitis (NEC) and sepsis vs. breastfeeding, 105, 113, 122
neonatal intensive care unit (NICU), 362–363
nervous system development, 99, 104
neurodevelopmental therapist (NDT), 229, 325
neurologically impaired infants, 279*t*, 281*t*, 409, 410*t*
niacin (See also Vitamin B complex requirements, maternal), 88*t*
nicotine, tobacco, and smoking, 75, 116
NICU (*See* neonatal intensive care unit)
nighttime feeding, 280*t*, 283, 288
nipple creams/ointments, 243
nipple shields, 226, 239, 242, 278*t*, 281*t*, 320–323, **321**
nipples, 46, 47, 50, 53, 65–67, **68**, 129, 211–212, **214–215**, 216, 226
    alternating positions for soreness in, 243
    cracks in, 244, 245*t*
    interruption of breastfeeding for soreness in, 243
    inverted, 65–67, **69**, 69, 129, 150, 220, 226, 278*t*, 318–319
    lubricant for breasts and, 317–318
    pinch test for, 314, **315**
    soreness of, 149, 150, 166, 221, 231, 235–243, 236–242*t*, 278*t*, 283, 317–318
    yeast infections (thrush) in, 244–247
nitrogen in milk, 103, 112
non-nutritive sucking, 148, 149, 168, 205, 211
Norplant, 295
number of breastfeedings per day, 1, 149, 151, 159
nursing bras, 133
nutrition (*See* maternal health and nutrition)
nutritive sucking, 148, 149, 168, 205, 211

obstetric practice, baby-friendly, 432*t*
obturator for cleft lip/palate, 404
older children and toddlers, breastfeeding of, 261–262, 384, 388, 388*t*
oligosaccharides in milk, 106*t*, 108*t*
olive oil, 82, 243
one vs. two breasts in feeding, 230–231
opposition to breastfeeding, 6, 15–19, 298–301
    employer's, 299
    father's, 300–301
    grandmother's, 299–300
    for older children and toddlers, 261–262
    physician's, 137–138, 299

oral cavity of infant, 165–167, 281*t*
    bottle feeding and suckling motion in, 212, **213**
    buccal pads, 166
    cleft lip/palate in, 151, 167, 227, 401, 403–404, **403**, 406–407*t*
    difficulty in suckling and, 221, 224–229, 225–228*t*, 224
    finger examination of, 324, **324**
    frenulum (ankyloglossia) in, 151, 165–166, **166**, 227, 242, 281*t*
    lip position in, 216
    masseter muscles in, 212
    orbicularis oris muscles in, 212
    palate formation in, 166–167, 226
    suckling and milk transfer and, 211–212, **213**, **214–215**
    thrush of mouth and, 167, 244–247
    tongue condition and position in, 165, 211, 216
orbicularis oris muscles, 212
osteoporosis, 72, 123
otis media and breastfeeding, 105
ovarian cancers, 122
over-the-shoulder nursing position, 204, **204**
oxytocin, 49, 55, 59, 143, 210, 234, 314

pacifiers (*See* artificial nipples and pacifiers)
palate formation in infant, 166–167, 226
palliative care, 236
parental role, 15–16, 286–287
passive listening, 21, 24*t*

pediatric practice, baby-friendly, 431*t*
Pediatric Unit, Eleven Steps to Optimal Breastfeeding, 434
peer counselors, IBCLC relationship with, 14
penicillins, 119*t*
perineum, postpartum, 289
perspiration, maternal, postpartum, 289
pesticides, 121
pethidine, 119*t*
phencyclidine hydrochloride, maternal use, presence in milk, 117
phenylalanine, 399–401, 402*t*
phenylketonuria (PKU), 342, 391, 399–401, 402*t*
phosphatidylethanolamine, 107*t*
phosphorus requirements, maternal, 84*t*
phototherapy for jaundice, 348–350, **349**
physical assessment of mother and infant by IBCLC, 30
physical recovery following birth, maternal, 288–289
physician care for mother and baby, 134–138
    physician's advice detrimental to breastfeeding, what to do, 137–138, 299
    questions to ask baby's physician, 136–137
    recommending physicians to clients, 135
    selecting a physician, 134–135
    working with the physician, 137
physician report, 33
physician-group based lactation consulting, 12–13
physiology of breast (*See* anatomy and physiology of breast)

physiology of suckling and milk transfer, 211–212, **213**, **214–215**
Pierre Robin syndrome, 405, **405**
pinch test, 314, **315**
pitocin to induce labor, 142, 150, 278*t*
pituitary disorders, 56, 235
placental retention, 54, 56, 281*t*
placid babies, 181–182, 281*t*
planning for breastfeeding, 132–134
plugged ducts, 221, 249, 256*t*, 383
pneumonia, 122
polio antibodies in milk, 94
poor latch, 153–154*t*, 218–219
poor-weight-gaining infants, 275–276
positioning for breastfeeding, 197–204, 220, 221, 222–223*t*, 226, 228, 283, 314–344, 360
  alternate feeding methods for, 334–342
  baby's body position (zone 3) in, 198
  baby's mouth position (zone 4) in, 198
  breast massage and, 314–315, **316**
  cesarean deliveries and, 197
  C-hold to support breast in, 198, 316, **316**
  clutch (football) hold in, 200, **201**, 226
  cradle hold in, 199, **200**
  cross-cradle hold in, 226
  Dancer hand position to support breast in, 198, 317, **317**
  dominant hand hold in, 200, **201**, 202
  finger as pacifier in, 324
  hands-and-knees position in, 203, **204**
  lying down position in, 202, **202**
  mother's body position (zone 1) in, 197
  mother's breast position (zone 2) in, 197–198
  for multiple babies, 383, **385**
  over-the-shoulder position in, 204, **204**
  pinch test for, 314, **315**
  posture feeding position in, 202–203, **203**
  for sore nipples, alternating positions for, 243
  special or unconventional nursing postures in, 203–204, **204**
postmature infants, 368
postpartum depression ("baby blues"), 286
postpartum psychosis, 287
posture feeding position, 202–203, **203**
posture of newborn, 161–162, **162**
potassium in milk, 93
practice setting for IBCLCs, 11–14
preference for one breast, 361
pregnancy and breast development, 52, 53
  breastfeeding a child during pregnancy, 384, 388, 388*t*
pregnant women education/support for breastfeeding, 140, 156–157
prenatal breastfeeding class, 302
prenatal considerations, 126–138
preparation for breastfeeding, 127–129

preterm and high-risk infants (See also long-term special needs), 150, 362–372
  artificial baby milk (ABM) and, 343
  bereaved mothers and, 369, 372
  cognitive development in, 113
  colic, 189–193, 194–195*t*
  crying patterns in, 187
  feeding expressed milk to, 366
  initiating breastfeeding in, 367–368
  intrauterine growth retardation (IUGR) and, 364
  jaundice in (See also jaundice), 350
  kangaroo care for, 366–367, 367
  maintaining lactation until baby can nurse in, 365
  milk components after preterm delivery and, 112
  necrotizing enterocolitis (NEC) and sepsis vs. breastfeeding in, 113
  neonatal intensive care unit (NICU) and, 362–363
  postmature infants and, 368
  "premature" defined, 364
  in putting preterm infant to breast, 366
  small for gestation age (SGA) infants as, 364
  special counseling needs of, 368, 370–371*t*
  storing expressed milk for, 365–366
  supplements to milk for, 113
  support for mothers of, 362, 363*t*
  in taking baby home, 364, 368
  weight gain in, 368
primipara, 278*t*
private practice lactation consulting, 13–14
problems (pathology) of breast and breastfeeding, 51–52
problems getting baby latched on, 218–221, 220*t*
problem-solving approach, 23, 28–29
progesterone, 53, 54, 57, 58, 293
projectile vomiting, 169
prolactin, 49, 54–55, 57–59, 210, 280*t*
prolactin inhibitory factor (PIF), 58, 59
prolactinomas, 56
promoting breastfeeding, 1–9, 426–434
prostaglandins in milk, 103
protein casseroles, vegetarian, 90
protein in milk, 93, 96, 97, 99–100, 107*t*, 113
protein requirements, maternal, 83*t*
psychiatric drugs, 118*t*
puberty and breast development, 52
public breastfeeding, 260, 298
pyloric stenosis and vomiting, 169
pyrodoxine (See also Vitamin B complex requirements, maternal), 88*t*

questioning skills for IBCLC, 22
quinolone, 118*t*

radioactive pharmaceuticals, 118*t*
rashes, 189

recommending physicians to clients, 135
recommendations for breastfeeding, 1, 8–9
recordkeeping (*See* documentation)
reflective listening, 21, 24*t*
reflexes of infants, 167–168
reflux (*See* gastroesophageal reflux)
relactation, 354–358, 356–357*t*
relaxation techniques for mother, 63
removing baby from breast, 209, **209**
reproductive technology and pregnancy, 55
respiratory infection in infants, 279*t*
rest and relaxation through breastfeeding, 127–128, 184–185, 283
retracted nipple, 69
rhythm or coordination of suck, swallow, breathe, 211–212, **214–215**, 217–218, 224, 281*t*
riboflavin (See also Vitamin B complex requirements, maternal), 88*t*
ribonuclease in milk, 110*t*
rickets, 98
risk factors for breastfeeding problems, 148, 150–151*t*
rooming-in, 145–146, 159
rooting reflex, 142, 168, 198, 218, 408
rotavirus, 104

salbutamol, 119*t*
scheduled feedings, 151, 159, 232
secretory immunoglobulin (sIgA) in milk, 94, 106*t*, 109*t*
secretory leukocyte protease inhibitor in milk, 110*t*

self-examination of breasts, 70, **71**
separation anxiety, 373
separation of mother and baby, 140, 142–143, 151, 157–158, 248, 373–377
sexual adjustments for parents, 291–292
Sheehan's syndrome, 56, 281*t*, 342
shells (*See* breast shells)
shingles (*See* varicella zoster)
sialyllactose, 106*t*, 107*t*
sibling reaction and adjustment to baby, 295–297
SIDS (*See* Sudden Infant Death Syndrome)
signs that breastfeeding is going well, 273
signs of poor latch, 153–154*t*, 218–219
silicone implants, presence in milk, 103, 120
single mothers, special counseling, 303–304, 305*t*
situations where you must see mother, 29
size of breast vs. ability to breastfeed, 51–52, 126
skin condition in newborn, 163–164, 230, 273, 276
skin-to-skin contact (See also bonding; kangaroo care), 142, 143, 144, 148, 207, 360, 366–367, **367**
sleep-wake states of infants, 179–181, 184–187
sleeping arrangements for breastfeeding, 133–134, 278*t*
sleeping patterns in infants, 179–181, 184–187
sleepy infants, 151, 205–207, 231, 279*t*, 281*t*
slow weight-gaining infants, 274–275

small for gestation age (SGA) infants, 364
smoking (*See* nicotine, tobacco, and smoking)
sodium in milk, 93, 112
solid food introduction, 136, 189–193, 194–195*t*, 263–265
sore nipples (*See* nipples)
soy milk, 123, 190–193, 194–195*t*
special counseling situations, 298–313
    bereaved mothers and, 369, 372
    cultural differences and, in immigrant populations, 308–312, 311*t*
    low-income mothers and, 301–303, 304*t*
    opposition to breastfeeding and, 298–301
    preterm infants and, 368, 370–371*t*
    sexual abuse survivors and, 287–288
    single mothers and, 303–304, 305*t*
    support groups for breastfeeding and, 312–313
    teenage mothers and, 305–308, 308*t*
    widowed mothers and, 304
spina bifida, 409
spitting up during or after feeding, 168–169
spoon feeding, 334–336, **335**
Staphylococcus antibodies in milk, 94
startle reflex, 167
stimulation of nipples, 65, 66
stooling, 170–171, 176–177*t*, 178–179, 230, 273, 276

storing expressed milk, 331–333, 365–366, 381
stretch marks, 271
subcutaneous fat of breast, 46
suck reorganization, 325
suck training interventions, 229, 325
sucking (See also attachment), 142, 143, 168, 408
    rhythm or coordination, 211–212, **214–215**, 217–218
suckling action on breast, 47–48, 59
suctioning of baby's breathing passages, 141, 151, 225
Sudden Infant Death Syndrome (SIDS), 122, 185, 186–187
sulphonamides, 118*t*
supplemental feeding, 52, 113, 145, 158, 262–263, 280*t*, 282, 284
    tube feeding devices, 336–337, **336**, **337**
support for nursing mothers, 2, 10, 11, 20
support groups for breastfeeding, 2, 160, 312–313
supportive and sustaining tissue of breast, 47
surgery for baby, 376, 404
surgery to breast and breastfeeding, 51, 65, 150, 235, 278*t*, 281*t*
swaddling, 195*t*, 207–208
swallowing reflex, 60, 61
    rhythm or coordination, 211–212, **214–215**, 217–218
    signs of, 216
switching breasts during breastfeeding, 60
synthesis of milk, 57–59
syringe feeding, 339–340, **339**

syringe, inverted (*See* inverted syringe)

teaching/learning approaches, 17–18, 23, 127–129
teenage mothers, special counseling, 305–308, 308*t*
teething, 260–261
Ten Steps to Successful Breastfeeding, 1, 2, 7, 155–160
tetracyclines, 118*t*, 118
theophyllines, 235
thiamin (See also Vitamin B complex requirements, maternal), 88*t*
thiazide, 118*t*
thrush, 167, 241, 244–247 (See also *Candida*)
thyroid disorders, 56–57, 56
thyroid hormones, 390
thyrotropin-releasing hormones, 235
titanium in milk, 103
toddlers, breastfeeding of, 261–262, 384, 388, 388*t*
tongue condition and position, 165, 211, **214–215**, 216
tongue sucking in infant, 228
tongue tie (*See* frenulum)
toxins in milk (*See* impurities in milk)
tranquilizers, 235
transition from expressed milk to breastfeeding, 351
transitional milk, 57, 94
trypsin, 110*t*
tube feeding, 336–337, **336**, **337**
tuberculosis, 342, 391
twins (*See* multiple births)

ulcerative colitis, 122
UNICEF, 7
untimely weaning (*See* emergency or untimely weaning)
urinary infection in infants, 279*t*

urination, maternal, postpartum, 289
uterus, postpartum, 288

vacuum extraction, 142, 151, 164, 225
variations in breast structure and function, 61, 65–71
Varicella zoster, 392
vasospasm (blanching) in nipple, 242
vegetarian diets, 82, 90, 100
vernix, 143
viral antibodies in milk, 94, 109–110*t*
visitors to newborn and mother, 144
visual development in infants, 98, 121
Vitamin A requirements, maternal, 86–87*t*, 86
Vitamin B complex, 87–89*t*, 91, 100, 106*t*
Vitamin C, 89*t*, 102
Vitamin D, 87*t*, 100, 123
Vitamin E, 87*t*, 100
Vitamin K in milk, 100–101
vitamins and minerals, 93, 100–103
  chart of recommended daily intake (RDI), 83–89*t*
  maternal requirements, 119*t*
  supplements of, 1, 9, 136, 264
voiding, infants, 170–171, 230, 273, 276
voiding, maternal, 289
volume of milk produced/consumed, 58, 95–96, 126
vomiting, 168–169

warmers and incubators, 142
warning signs that breastfeeding is not going well, 153–154*t*
water intake required for infants, 102, 136

water intake required for mothers, 73, 75, 83*t*
weaning, 54, 137, 248, 267–271
weight loss in newborns (See also growth and weight gain in infants), 151, 183–184
weight management in mothers, 77, 91–92, 127, 150, 278*t*
whey, 58, 99
widowed mothers, special counseling, 304, 305*t*
witch's milk, 52
withdrawal or avoidance behavior in nursing infant, 218
Women, Infants, and Children (WIC) lactation consulting, 12
working mothers, 377
    artificial baby milk (ABM) for, 380
    employer's opposition to breastfeeding by, 299
    expressing and storing milk for, 377, 380–381
    feeding options during work hours for, 380–381
    leakage from breasts in, 381
    let-down reflex enhancement in, 380–381
    managing breastfeeding for, 377
    mother's comfort and adjustment issues in, 381–382
    returning to work by, 377
    storing expressed milk by, 381
World Health Organization (WHO) recommendations, 2–4, 7
    HIV, 334, 342

yeast infections and thrush, 164, 167, 241, 244–247

zinc, 85*t*, 103, 106*t*

Notes

Notes

Notes

Notes

Notes

Notes

Notes

Notes

Notes

Notes

Notes